Recent Advances in Dual Disorders (Addiction and Other Mental Disorders)

Recent Advances in Dual Disorders (Addiction and Other Mental Disorders)

Editors

Marta Torrens
Ana Adan

MDPI • Basel • Beijing • Wuhan • Barcelona • Belgrade • Manchester • Tokyo • Cluj • Tianjin

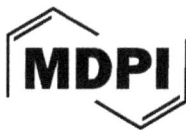

Editors
Marta Torrens
Universitat Autònoma
de Barcelona,
Barcelona, Spain

Ana Adan
University of Barcelona,
Barcelona, Spain

Editorial Office
MDPI
St. Alban-Anlage 66
4052 Basel, Switzerland

This is a reprint of articles from the Special Issue published online in the open access journal *Journal of Clinical Medicine* (ISSN 2077-0383) (available at: https://www.mdpi.com/journal/jcm/special_issues/Dual_Disorders).

For citation purposes, cite each article independently as indicated on the article page online and as indicated below:

LastName, A.A.; LastName, B.B.; LastName, C.C. Article Title. *Journal Name* **Year**, *Volume Number*, Page Range.

ISBN 978-3-0365-7700-5 (Hbk)
ISBN 978-3-0365-7701-2 (PDF)

© 2023 by the authors. Articles in this book are Open Access and distributed under the Creative Commons Attribution (CC BY) license, which allows users to download, copy and build upon published articles, as long as the author and publisher are properly credited, which ensures maximum dissemination and a wider impact of our publications.

The book as a whole is distributed by MDPI under the terms and conditions of the Creative Commons license CC BY-NC-ND.

Contents

About the Editors vii

Marta Torrens and Ana Adan
Recent Advances in Dual Disorders (Addiction and Other Mental Disorders)
Reprinted from: *J. Clin. Med.* **2023**, *12*, 3315, doi:10.3390/jcm12093315 1

Beatriz Puértolas-Gracia, María Gabriela Barbaglia, Mercè Gotsens, Oleguer Parés-Badell, María Teresa Brugal, Marta Torrens, et al.
Lifetime Dual Disorder Screening and Treatment Retention: A Pilot Cohort Study
Reprinted from: *J. Clin. Med.* **2022**, *11*, 3760, doi:10.3390/jcm11133760 5

Viviana E. Horigian, Renae D. Schmidt, Dikla Shmueli-Blumberg, Kathryn Hefner, Judith Feinberg, Radhika Kondapaka, et al.
Suicidality as a Predictor of Overdose among Patients with Substance Use Disorders
Reprinted from: *J. Clin. Med.* **2022**, *11*, 6400, doi:10.3390/jcm11216400 23

Teresa Ferrer-Farré, Fernando Dinamarca, Joan Ignasi Mestre-Pintó, Francina Fonseca and Marta Torrens
Dual Disorders in the Consultation Liaison Addiction Service: Gender Perspective and Quality of Life
Reprinted from: *J. Clin. Med.* **2021**, *10*, 5572, doi:10.3390/jcm10235572 35

Sharleen M. Traynor, Renae D. Schmidt, Lauren K. Gooden, Tim Matheson, Louise Haynes, Allan Rodriguez, et al.
Differential Effects of Patient Navigation across Latent Profiles of Barriers to Care among People Living with HIV and Comorbid Conditions
Reprinted from: *J. Clin. Med.* **2023**, *12*, 114, doi:10.3390/jcm12010114 45

Ana De la Rosa-Cáceres, Marta Narvaez-Camargo, Andrea Blanc-Molina, Nehemías Romero-Pérez, Daniel Dacosta-Sánchez, Bella María González-Ponce, et al.
Bridge Nodes between Personality Traits and Alcohol-Use Disorder Criteria: The Relevance of Externalizing Traits of Risk Taking, Callousness, and Irresponsibility
Reprinted from: *J. Clin. Med.* **2022**, *11*, 3468, doi:10.3390/jcm11123468 63

Cinta Mancheño-Velasco, Daniel Dacosta-Sánchez, Andrea Blanc-Molina, Marta Narvaez-Camargo and Óscar Martín Lozano-Rojas
Changes in the Care Activity in Addiction Centers with Dual Pathology Patients during the COVID-19 Pandemic
Reprinted from: *J. Clin. Med.* **2022**, *11*, 4341, doi:10.3390/jcm11154341 79

Vincenzo Oliva, Michele De Prisco, Maria Teresa Pons-Cabrera, Pablo Guzmán, Gerard Anmella, Diego Hidalgo-Mazzei, et al.
Machine Learning Prediction of Comorbid Substance Use Disorders among People with Bipolar Disorder
Reprinted from: *J. Clin. Med.* **2022**, *11*, 3935, doi:10.3390/jcm11143935 91

Ana Belén Serrano-Serrano, Julia E. Marquez-Arrico, José Francisco Navarro, Antonio Martinez-Nicolas and Ana Adan
Circadian Characteristics in Patients under Treatment for Substance Use Disorders and Severe Mental Illness (Schizophrenia, Major Depression and Bipolar Disorder)
Reprinted from: *J. Clin. Med.* **2021**, *10*, 4388, doi:10.3390/jcm10194388 105

Ana Adan, José Francisco Navarro and on behalf of ADDISCHRONO Group
Protocol for Characterization of Addiction and Dual Disorders: Effectiveness of Coadjuvant Chronotherapy in Patients with Partial Response
Reprinted from: *J. Clin. Med.* **2022**, *11*, 1846, doi:10.3390/jcm11071846 . . . . **121**

Cristina Vintró-Alcaraz, Gemma Mestre-Bach, Roser Granero, Elena Caravaca, Mónica Gómez-Peña, Laura Moragas, et al.
Exploring the Association between Gambling-Related Offenses, Substance Use, Psychiatric Comorbidities, and Treatment Outcome
Reprinted from: *J. Clin. Med.* **2022**, *11*, 4669, doi:10.3390/jcm11164669 . . . . **141**

About the Editors

Marta Torrens

Marta Torrens, MD, PhD, Specialist in Psychiatry, Full Professor of Psychiatry at the University Vic-Central de Catalunya and University Autònoma de Barcelona. Director of the Addiction Research Group at IMIM-Hospital del Mar Research Institut, Barcelona. Elected member of the Scientific Committee of the European Monitoring Centre for Drugs and Drug Addiction and the Informal Scientific Network of UNODC and WHO. She is also is an executive member of the Dual Pathology and Addiction Psychiatry section of the WPA. In research, her main areas of interest are the assessment and treatment of substance addictions, dual disorders, and the gender perspective in addictions. The results of her research have been published in the main specialized journals with an h-index of 48. She has received several international and national awards, including "Honorary Member" of the Spanish Society of Dual Pathology (2013) and the EUFAS European Addiction Research Award 2020.

Ana Adan

Ana Adan is a Full Professor at the Department of Clinical Psychology and Psychobiology at the University of Barcelona (UB). She directs the Substance Use and Dual Disorders research line integrated in the Consolidated Group of Neuropsychology and the Institute of Neurosciences of the UB, and has published more than two hundred scientific papers (h-index of 40). Her research has been supported by 21 projects/networks, and recognized with three extraordinary awards for her PhD supervision. She is a member of the editorial board of various specialized journals and has served on the scientific committee for clinical trials. She developed extensive teaching work in master's and doctoral courses, and currently coordinates the compulsory subject of Psychopharmacology of the degree of Psychology and that of Addictions of the master's degree in General Health Psychology of the UB. She is the director of the online Master's in Drug Addiction of IL3-UB. She received the "Honorary Member" award from the Spanish Society of Dual Pathology in 2021.

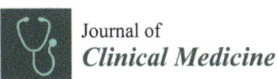

Editorial

Recent Advances in Dual Disorders (Addiction and Other Mental Disorders)

Marta Torrens [1,2,3] and Ana Adan [4,5,*]

1. Addiction Research Group (GRAd), Neuroscience Research Program, Hospital del Mar Medical Research Institute (IMIM), 08003 Barcelona, Spain; mtorrens@psmar.cat
2. School of Medicine, Universitat de Vic-Central de Catalunya, 08500 Vic, Spain
3. Psychiatry Department, School of Medicine, Universitat Autònoma de Barcelona (UAB), 08093 Cerdanyola del Vallès, Spain
4. Department of Clinical Psychology and Psychobiology, School of Psychology, University of Barcelona, Passeig de la Vall d'Hebrón 171, 08035 Barcelona, Spain
5. Institute of Neurosciences, University of Barcelona, 08035 Barcelona, Spain
* Correspondence: aadan@ub.edu; Tel.: +34-933-125-060

In clinical mental health practice, the presence of Dual Disorders (DDs), defined as the comorbidity of at least one Substance Use Disorder (SUD) and another mental disorder in the same person [1,2], is very high and in recent years, the epidemiological data have been steadily increasing. It can be affirmed that the existence of DDs is more the rule than the exception in the care setting. Currently, a multidisciplinary and comprehensive response to the needs of persons with DDs is required. Our previous publication of a first Special Issue on the subject, prepared before the COVID-19 pandemic, compiled a set of topics, from basic to clinical perspectives, with a very positive impact on scientists and professionals in the field [3]. The evidence leaves no doubt about the need for and interest in considering the existence of psychiatric comorbidities in the therapeutic management of patients with SUD. Additionally, it is even more important, if possible, to carry it out comprehensively by expert interdisciplinary teams since dual patients have greater difficulties in both clinical management and stabilization compared to those with only SUD or other mental health disorders (i.e., increases admissions in emergency rooms, hospitalizations, suicide, etc.).

There is currently a long way to go in understanding DDs and with this second Special Issue, we aimed to compile recent advances, considering different levels of approach that provide interesting data, with a view to being transferred as soon as possible to health care. In addition, the impact of the COVID-19 pandemic has already had a negative impact on mental health, especially in the young population. Thus, the detection of both substances and behavioral addictions and many other mental disorders (major depression, anxiety, eating disorders, etc.) has been alerted. All of this takes place in health systems that are already traditionally stressed in the field of mental health, regardless of the country and the model of care, and where there is a need for specialized centers and professionals trained in the management of DDs. This situation will only be overcome with rigorous work from multiple approaches (biological, psychological, social) that allows for inter-disciplinary integration which will result in future advances in knowledge and overcoming the deficits that exist today and new opportunities to improve them.

Puértolas-Gracia et al. [4] showed in a cohort study of 1356 patients with alcohol or cocaine use disorder, which were admitted to treatment in the public addiction outpatient services in Barcelona, that the lifetime prevalence of screening positive for DDs was 74%, with depression being the most frequent (76.4%). These patients were more frequently women, younger, unemployed, reported higher polysubstance use, poorer self-perceived health, and other medical conditions. The results highlighted the prevalence and clinical relevance of DDs and the need to screen to diagnose and treat properly in these services for addiction disease. In the study of Horigian et al. [5], they confirmed the existence of

Citation: Torrens, M.; Adan, A. Recent Advances in Dual Disorders (Addiction and Other Mental Disorders). *J. Clin. Med.* **2023**, *12*, 3315. https://doi.org/10.3390/jcm12093315

Received: 20 March 2023
Accepted: 15 April 2023
Published: 6 May 2023

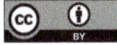

Copyright: © 2023 by the authors. Licensee MDPI, Basel, Switzerland. This article is an open access article distributed under the terms and conditions of the Creative Commons Attribution (CC BY) license (https://creativecommons.org/licenses/by/4.0/).

accidental overdoses and intentional overdoses, and even suicidal attempt, in patients with SUD. In a novel way, they use the Concise Health Risk Tracking Self-Report, a measure that assesses associated symptoms related to suicide as ideation, intent, pessimism, lack of social support, helplessness, and despair. Both studies [4,5] strongly support that entry into treatment for SUD as an invaluable opportunity to assess the presence of other mental disorders or DDs, evaluate suicide risk, and apply adequate treatment and early prevention plans.

However, not only those who request outpatient treatment have a high presence of DDs. Ferrer-Farré et al. [6] studied the existence of DDs among patients with SUD admitted to a general hospital for any pathology and attended by a consultation liaison addiction service, and its association with addiction severity and quality of life. They applied a gender perspective in the study related to the increase in interest in the topic in health in general and in addiction diseases in particular [7]. Again, although the most prevalent DD was depression for both sexes (33.8%), it was higher in women (46.2%) than men (30.9%). Additionally, when DDs were present, women suffered a worse quality of life than men. The study confirms a high prevalence of DDs among patients with SUD admitted to a general hospital for any pathology, and its being associated with a worse quality of life, particularly in women.

Traynor and colleagues [8] developed a trial of patient navigation to reduce barriers to care in people with HIV (human immunodeficiency virus) who reported substance use. Of the 801 participants, 55.3% had a history of substance use treatment in the 6 months prior to treatment, about one-third reported injection drug use in the last 12 months, and 22% had a recorded psychiatric history or DD. Greater severity of alcohol and drug use, less readiness for substance use treatment, and more negative attitudes towards drug treatment were indicators associated with the profiles of patients with increased barriers to care. The results emphasize the need to identify and meet needs at the complex intersection of substance use and HIV services, whose integration can improve patient outcomes.

In recent years, interest in the study of personality traits in DD patients has shown to have differences with respect to those with diagnoses of only SUD or only comorbid mental disorder. It is currently suggested that this could be an endophenotype whose consideration would improve both prevention and treatment programs in mental health [9]. This may be specifically useful in the comorbidity between SUD and personality disorders. The research by De la Rosa-Cáceres et al. [10] focused on the study of the personality facets of the Alternative Model of Personality Disorder of DSM-5 [11] in patients with alcohol use disorder by means of a network analysis. The data show a connection with the facets related to the disinhibition (risk taking, irresponsibility, impulsivity, and rigid perfectionism) and antagonism (callousness, grandiosity, and hostility) domains, which are also associated with premature patient dropout. These facets are relevant to antisocial and borderline personality disorder diagnoses, and their assessment can help to determine whether the personality disorder of patients with SUD is primary or secondary.

Restrictions due to the COVID-19 pandemic had an evident impact on the attention of specialized addiction centers. The study by Mancheo-Velasco et al. [12] evaluated the admissions to treatment of dual patients together with their main sociodemographic and clinical characteristics, considering three key periods in the first wave of the pandemic in Spain: pre-confinement, confinement, and post-confinement. The period of confinement meant there was a large decrease in admissions in general, although in percentage terms, the number of dual patients even increased. There are few differences in the sociodemographic and clinical profile of the patients admitted between time periods, although the increase during the confinement of women, opioid users, and those with mixed anxiety–depressive disorders stand out. Among other indicators, during the confinement, a decrease in the number of toxicological tests and planned therapeutic sessions was observed, even though the patients attended a greater percentage of scheduled sessions.

In recent years, great progress has been made in the development of explanatory models through machine learning in mental health, which could improve both the detection and diagnosis of multiple disorders [13] and be a future tool for precision psychiatry. The research by Oliva et al. [14] is the first to apply machine learning to predict the presence of comorbid SUD in bipolar disorder and using random forest models to identify the type of SUD (any, alcohol, and alcohol with at least another). Although with a low or moderate specificity of the models, due to the consideration of socio-demographic or clinical factors alone, alcohol use disorder with at least one other SUD correctly classifies up to 75% of the sample studied. In addition, this consumption pattern of bipolar patients was positively associated with a hypomanic episode at the onset of bipolar disorder and the presence of hetero-aggressive behavior.

Circadian rhythmicity is an aspect seldom studied in patients with DDs; most of the previous research focuses on sleep problems and/or disorders. The work of Serrano-Serrano et al. [15], studying the circadian rhythm of distal skin temperature and the sleep–wake rhythm, observed that in dual patients with severe mental illness (schizophrenia, bipolar disorder, and major depression) undergoing treatment, after three or more months of abstinence, there is a normalization of sleep, but a more marked impairment of wakefulness persists in dual patients with schizophrenia and bipolar disorder. Consideration of the treatment modality shows a more morning-focused pattern with a better quality of both sleep and wakefulness in residential patients compared to outpatients, regardless of severe mental illness. The data suggest that including in the treatment aspects of regular time habits (activity, intake, exposure to light, etc.) and with a morning-type pattern to promote rhythmic reorganization, this can improve adherence to treatment and the prevention of relapses, especially in outpatients.

The Adan and Navarro [16] protocol proposes a characterization of dual patients, focused on comorbid major depression and schizophrenia, with aspects of genetic polymorphisms, circadian rhythmic functioning, neurocognition, and personality traits with the aim to elucidate the possible markers of vulnerability and prognosis (with a follow-up of one year) useful in clinical practice. In this direction, the same group of researchers has suggested that in dual schizophrenia, the evaluation of the circadian rhythmic expression may be a biomarker [17]. In addition, it is proposed that we carry out a pioneering study with a light exposure intervention in SUD and dual depressed outpatients of both sexes who show difficulties in rhythmic reorganization during treatment.

Finally, the study carried out by Vintró-Alcaraz et al. [18] with gambling disorder outpatients under group cognitive–behavioral treatment is one of the first to explore substance use (tobacco, alcohol, and illegal drugs) in this behavioral addiction. It should be noted that the consumption of substances in these patients exceeds 55%, and that those with the presence of gambling-related illegal acts present a higher likelihood of substance use, specifically tobacco and illegal drugs. These results should encourage future studies on gambling disorders to consider the coexistence of SUD and its implications both in committed gambling related-offenses and in adherence to treatment.

Author Contributions: Conceptualization, M.T. and A.A.; writing—original draft preparation, M.T. and A.A.; writing—review and editing, M.T. and A.A. All authors have read and agreed to the published version of the manuscript.

Funding: This work was supported by the Spanish Ministry of Science and Innovation (MCIN/AE1I/01303910.13039/501100011033; grant: PID2020-117767 GB-I00), the ISCIII-Redes de Investigación Cooperativa Orientadas a Resultados en Salud (RICORS)-Red de Investigación en Atención Primaria de Adicciones (RIAPAd) under grant number RD21/0009/0001, the European Union Next GenerationEU, Mecanismo para la Recuperación y la Resiliencia (MRR), and la Generalitat de Catalunya (2021SGR-801and 2021SGR-00041).

Institutional Review Board Statement: Not applicable.

Informed Consent Statement: Not applicable.

Conflicts of Interest: The authors declare no conflict of interest.

References

1. World Health Organization. *Lexicon of Alcohol and Drug Terms*; World Health Organization: Geneva, Switzerland, 1994.
2. Szerman, N.; Torrens, M.; Maldonado, R.; Pal Singh Balhara, Y.; Salom, C.; Maremmani, I.; Sher, L.; Didia-Attas, J.; Chen, J.; Baler, R.; et al. Addictive and other mental disorders: A call for a standardized definition of dual disorders. *Transl. Psychiatry* **2022**, *12*, 446. [CrossRef] [PubMed]
3. Adan, A.; Torrens, M. Diagnosis and management of addiction and other mental disorders (dual disorders). *J. Clin. Med.* **2021**, *10*, 1307. [CrossRef] [PubMed]
4. Puértolas-Gracia, B.; Barbaglia, M.G.; Gotsens, M.; Parés-Badell, O.; Brugal, M.T.; Torrens, M.; Treviño, L.; Rodríguez-Díaz, C.; Vázquez-Vázquez, J.M.; Pascual, A.; et al. Lifetime dual Disorder screening and treatment retention: A pilot cohort study. *J. Clin. Med.* **2022**, *11*, 3760. [CrossRef] [PubMed]
5. Horigian, V.E.; Schmidt, R.D.; Shmueli-Blumberg, D.; Hefner, K.; Feinberg, J.; Kondapaka, R.; Feaster, D.J.; Duan, R.; Gonzalez, S.; Davis, C.; et al. Suicidality as a predictor of overdose among patients with substance use disorders. *J. Clin. Med.* **2022**, *11*, 6400. [CrossRef] [PubMed]
6. Ferrer-Farré, T.; Dinamarca, F.; Mestre-Pintó, J.I.; Fonseca, F.; Torrens, M. Dual disorders in the consultation liaison addiction service: Gender perspective and quality of life. *J. Clin. Med.* **2021**, *10*, 5572. [CrossRef] [PubMed]
7. Fonseca, F.; Robles-Martínez, M.; Tirado-Muñoz, J.; Alías-Ferri, M.; Mestre-Pintó, J.I.; Coratu, A.M.; Torrens, M. A Gender perspective of addictive disorders. *Curr. Addict. Rep.* **2021**, *8*, 89–99. [CrossRef] [PubMed]
8. Traynor, S.M.; Schmidt, R.D.; Gooden, L.K.; Matheson, T.; Haynes, L.; Rodriguez, A.; Mugavero, M.; Jacobs, P.; Mandler, R.; Del Rio, C.; et al. Differential effects of patient navigation across latent profiles of barriers to care among people living with HIV and comorbid conditions. *J. Clin. Med.* **2023**, *12*, 114. [CrossRef] [PubMed]
9. Río-Martínez, L.; Marquez-Arrico, J.E.; Prat, G.; Adan, A. Temperament and character profile and its clinical correlates in male patients with dual schizophrenia. *J. Clin. Med.* **2020**, *9*, 1876. [CrossRef] [PubMed]
10. De la Rosa-Cáceres, A.; Narvaez-Camargo, M.; Blanc-Molina, A.; Romero-Pérez, N.; Dacosta-Sánchez, D.; González-Ponce, B.M.; Parrado-González, A.; Torres-Rosado, L.; Mancheño-Velasco, C.; Lozano-Rojas, Ó.M. Bridge nodes between personality traits and alcohol-use disorder criteria: The relevance of externalizing traits of risk taking, callousness, and irresponsibility. *J. Clin. Med.* **2022**, *11*, 3468. [CrossRef] [PubMed]
11. Skodol, A.E.; Morey, L.C.; Bender, D.S.; Oldham, J.M. The alternative DSM-5 model for personality disorders: A clinical application. *Am. J. Psychiatry* **2015**, *172*, 7. [CrossRef] [PubMed]
12. Mancheño-Velasco, C.; Dacosta-Sánchez, D.; Blanc-Molina, A.; Narvaez-Camargo, M.; Lozano-Rojas, Ó.M. Changes in the care activity in addiction centers with dual pathology patients during the COVID-19 pandemic. *J. Clin. Med.* **2022**, *11*, 4341. [CrossRef] [PubMed]
13. Shatte, A.B.R.; Hutchinson, D.M.; Teague, S.J. Machine learning in mental health: A scoping review of methods and applications. *Psychol. Med.* **2019**, *49*, 1426–1448. [CrossRef] [PubMed]
14. Oliva, V.; De Prisco, M.; Pons-Cabrera, M.T.; Guzmán, P.; Anmella, G.; Hidalgo-Mazzei, D.; Grande, I.; Fanelli, G.; Fabbri, C.; Serretti, A.; et al. Machine learning prediction of comorbid Substance use disorders among people with bipolar disorder. *J. Clin. Med.* **2022**, *11*, 3935. [CrossRef] [PubMed]
15. Serrano-Serrano, A.B.; Marquez-Arrico, J.E.; Martinez-Nicolas, A.; Navarro, J.F.; Adan, A. Circadian characteristic in patients under treatment for substance use disorders and severe mental illness (schizophrenia, major depression and bipolar disorder). *J. Clin. Med.* **2021**, *10*, 4388. [CrossRef] [PubMed]
16. Adan, A.; Navarro, J.F. on behalf of ADDISCHRONO group. Protocol for characterization of addiction and dual disorders. Effectiveness of coadjuvant chronotherapy in patients with partial response. *J. Clin. Med.* **2022**, *11*, 1846. [CrossRef] [PubMed]
17. Adan, A.; Marquez-Arrico, J.E.; Río-Martínez, L.; Navarro, J.F.; Martinez-Nicolas, A. Circadian rhythmicity in schizophrenia male patients with and without substance use disorder comorbidity. *Eur. Arch. Psychiatry Clin. Neurosci.* **2023**, 1560. [CrossRef] [PubMed]
18. Vintró-Alcaraz, C.; Mestre-Bach, G.; Granero, R.; Caravaca, E.; Gómez-Peña, M.; Moragas, L.; Baenas, I.; del Pino-Gutiérrez, A.; Valero-Solís, S.; Lara-Huallipe, M.; et al. Exploring the association between gambling-related offenses, substance use, psychiatric comorbidities, and treatment outcome. *J. Clin. Med.* **2022**, *11*, 4669. [CrossRef] [PubMed]

Disclaimer/Publisher's Note: The statements, opinions and data contained in all publications are solely those of the individual author(s) and contributor(s) and not of MDPI and/or the editor(s). MDPI and/or the editor(s) disclaim responsibility for any injury to people or property resulting from any ideas, methods, instructions or products referred to in the content.

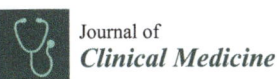

Article

Lifetime Dual Disorder Screening and Treatment Retention: A Pilot Cohort Study

Beatriz Puértolas-Gracia [1,2,3,4,†], María Gabriela Barbaglia [1,2,3,5,6,*,†], Mercè Gotsens [1,†], Oleguer Parés-Badell [1,†], María Teresa Brugal [1,†], Marta Torrens [2,6,7,8], Lara Treviño [1,†], Concepción Rodríguez-Díaz [1,†], José María Vázquez-Vázquez [1,†], Alicia Pascual [1,†], Marcela Coromina-Gimferrer [1,†], Míriam Jiménez-Dueñas [1,†], Israel Oliva [1,†], Erick González [1,†], Nicanor Mestre [1,†] and Montse Bartroli [1,3,5,6,†]

[1] Agència de Salut Pública de Barcelona, 08023 Barcelona, Spain; bpuertolas@imim.es (B.P.-G.); mgotsens@aspb.cat (M.G.); opares@vhebron.net (O.P.-B.); tbrugal@aspb.cat (M.T.B.); ext_ltrevino@aspb.cat (L.T.); ext_crodriguez@aspb.cat (C.R.-D.); ext_jvazquez@aspb.cat (J.M.V.-V.); ext_apascual@aspb.cat (A.P.); ext_mcoromin@aspb.cat (M.C.-G.); miriamjd@gmail.com (M.J.-D.); israelos77@hotmail.com (I.O.); ext_egonzale@aspb.cat (E.G.); ext_nmestre@aspb.cat (N.M.); mbartrol@aspb.cat (M.B.)
[2] Institut Hospital del Mar d'Investigacions Mèdiques (IMIM), 08003 Barcelona, Spain; mtorrens@imim.es
[3] Department of Experimental and Health Sciences, Universitat Pompeu Fabra (UPF), 08002 Barcelona, Spain
[4] CIBER Epidemiology and Public Health (CIBERESP), 28029 Madrid, Spain
[5] Biomedical Research Institute Sant Pau, IIB Sant Pau, Sant Antoni Mª Claret 167, 08025 Barcelona, Spain
[6] Red de Investigación en Atención Primaria en Adicciones (RIAPAd), 28029 Madrid, Spain
[7] Faculty of Medicine, Universitat Autònoma de Barcelona (UAB), 08193 Barcelona, Spain
[8] Faculty of Medicine, Universitat de Vic i Catalunya Central, Vic, 08500 Barcelona, Spain
* Correspondence: mgbarbag@aspb.cat; Tel.: +34-93202-7702
† On behalf of the Dual Diagnosis Study Group.

Abstract: The coexistence of a substance use disorder and another mental disorder in the same individual has been called dual disorder or dual diagnosis. This study aimed to examine the prevalence of lifetime dual disorder in individuals with alcohol or cocaine use disorder and their retention in treatment. We conducted a pilot cohort study of individuals ($n = 1356$) with alcohol or cocaine use disorder admitted to treatment in the public outpatient services of Barcelona (Spain) from January 2015 to August 2017 (followed-up until February 2018). Descriptive statistics, Kaplan–Meier survival curves and a multivariable Cox regression model were estimated. The lifetime prevalence of screening positive for dual disorder was 74%. At 1 year of follow-up, >75% of the cohort remained in treatment. On multivariable analysis, the factors associated with treatment dropout were a positive screening for lifetime dual disorder (HR = 1.26; 95% CI = 1.00–1.60), alcohol use (HR = 1.35; 95% CI = 1.04–1.77), polysubstance use (alcohol or cocaine and cannabis use) (HR = 1.60; 95% CI = 1.03–2.49) and living alone (HR = 1.34; 95% CI = 1.04–1.72). Lifetime dual disorder is a prevalent issue among individuals with alcohol or cocaine use disorders and could influence their dropout from treatment in public outpatient drug dependence care centres, along with alcohol use, polysubstance use and social conditions, such as living alone. We need a large-scale study with prolonged follow-up to confirm these preliminary results.

Keywords: dual disorder; mental disorders; screening; cocaine use disorder; alcohol use disorder; substance-related disorders; treatment retention

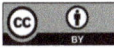

1. Introduction

The coexistence of a substance use disorder (SUD) and another mental disorder in the same individual has been called dual disorder or dual diagnosis (DD) [1]. Several epidemiological studies have shown a high positive association between SUD and other mental health problems [2–4]. According to the National Institute for Health and Care Excellence (NICE) [5], the prevalence of DD is estimated to be between 0.05% and 0.2%

in the general population. In the clinical population, the prevalence of DD ranges from 34% in mental health care service samples to 46% in drug dependent care service samples. This heterogeneity of DD prevalence estimates could be explained by the distinct health care settings, the primary substance of use, the type of comorbid mental disorder and the assessment method used in DD evaluation [6,7]. Regarding DD evaluation, few validated instruments are currently available to assess DD in people with SUD. The Composite International Diagnostic Interview (CIDI) [8] contains a section to screen for DD; however, the Spanish version of this instrument showed low specificity for the diagnosis of mental disorders in the population of substance users [9,10].

SUDs are most frequently associated with affective, anxiety and personality disorders [11]. For example, individuals with alcohol use disorder (AUD) are three times more likely to develop a depressive disorder in their lifetime than those without this [4]. In addition, between 40% and 73% of people with cocaine use disorder (CUD) would meet the diagnostic criteria for another mental disorder, mainly affective or anxiety disorders [12–14]. Individuals with DD have more clinical and social problems than individuals with a single mental disorder. At the clinical level, these individuals show increased psychopathological severity. For example, individuals with dual schizophrenia have more positive symptomatology (i.e., hallucinations, delusions, disorganised speech) [15]. They are also more likely to have infectious diseases (e.g., AIDS, hepatitis or sexually transmitted diseases) [16] and to overdose, with a higher number of hospital emergency department visits and psychiatric hospitalisations than individuals with an SUD alone [15]. In addition, these individuals have an increased risk of premature death, mainly from preventable causes such as suicide [17,18]. At the social level, several studies have suggested that the prevalence of unemployment, homelessness and risk of violent behaviours are higher in individuals with DD [15].

The high complexity of individuals with DD may explain their difficulty in maintaining abstinence or remaining in treatment [19–21]. Studies based on health care professionals' experiences report partial or non-adherence to treatment plans [22,23]. Some studies highlight that individuals with DD are more likely to have more symptoms and medication side effects, polysubstance use, longer substance use, a legal history, less family support, lower socioeconomic status and poor treatment motivation, which have been associated with lower treatment retention.

However, there are few studies on the topic, and some of these provide contradictory results regarding the prevalence of DD and its influence on treatment retention [15,24,25]. Therefore, according to the previous literature review, our study hypotheses are: the prevalence of lifetime DD in a drug dependence care setting would be around 50%; sociodemographic and clinical characteristics and treatment retention would differ between individuals screening positive for lifetime DD and individuals with a SUD alone; and differences in treatment retention among patients screening positive for lifetime DD and patients with a SUD alone would be explained by some sociodemographic, clinical and follow-up characteristics.

The present study aimed to examine: (i) the prevalence of lifetime DD in individuals with AUD or CUD admitted to treatment in four public outpatient drug dependence care centres in Barcelona (Spain); (ii) the sociodemographic and clinical differences between individuals screening positive for lifetime DD and individuals with AUD or CUD alone; (iii) the differences in treatment retention between individuals screening positive for lifetime DD and individuals with AUD or CUD alone; and (iv) the factors associated with treatment retention during the study period from January 2015 to February 2018.

2. Materials and Methods

2.1. Design and Study Population

This was a retrospective/prospective dynamic pilot cohort study comprising all inhabitants of Barcelona (Catalonia, Spain) aged ≥18 years admitted to treatment in 4 public outpatient CAS (Catalan acronym for drug dependence care centres) in Barcelona. The study was based on the first years after the implementation of a DD screening interview in the routine clinical practice of these 4 outpatient drug dependence care centres (from a total of 6) managed by the Public Health Agency of Barcelona. We started the study in January 2017, the cohort was identified and assembled at an earlier point in time based on existing Electronic Health Records (EHR), and was followed prospectively until August 2017 (total follow-up time = 38 months). This was a dynamic cohort because patients could be recruited or leave the cohort at different times. These centres offer the following services: biopsychosocial diagnosis; harm reduction; individual, group and family therapy; psychopharmacological treatment; social and occupational assistance; legal advice; health education; and coordination with other social and health care services. The therapeutic programmes of the CAS include alcohol, heroin, cocaine, cannabis, DD and severe addictive disorders. The teams are multidisciplinary with psychiatry, general medicine, psychology, nursing, social work, and social education professionals [26].

The study population included individuals meeting AUD or CUD criteria of the International Classification of Diseases Tenth Edition (ICD-10) [27] and screened with the Dual Diagnosis Screening Interview (DDSI-IV) [28]. We excluded individuals who started treatment by court order. We used a non-probabilistic sampling. Individuals admitted to treatment for AUD or CUD were included in the study by convenience, i.e., as a pilot study, the lifetime DD screening was administered according to staff capacity in the centres, and mostly to those individuals who showed or reported psychiatric symptoms. The first admission to treatment during the recruitment period (January 2015–August 2017) was considered as an incident case, regardless of whether the individual had been in treatment before the cohort.

2.2. Information Sources

We used the centralised Electronic Health Record (EHR) system of the public Drug Dependence Care Centres of Barcelona, which is managed by the Public Health Agency of Barcelona. Sociodemographic and clinical information of all patients was collected using a standardised survey that is routinely administered during the first treatment visit. We used the Dual Diagnosis Screening Interview (DDSI-IV) [28] to screen for lifetime DD. This brief structured interview of 63 items screens for 11 lifetime mental disorders: depression (7 items), dysthymia (2 items), mania (5 items), panic disorder (3 items), generalised anxiety disorder (3 items), specific phobia (7 items), social phobia (2 items), agoraphobia (2 items), psychosis (24 items), post-traumatic stress disorder (2 items) and attention deficit hyperactivity disorder (6 items), according to the criteria of the Diagnostic and Statistical Manual of Mental Disorders (DSM), 4th version. The DDSI-IV is an adaptation of the screening section of the Composite International Diagnostic Interview (S-CIDI) [8]. It includes some questions to differentiate between primary and substance-induced disorders (e.g., psychosis and attention deficit hyperactivity disorder) and is easy to administer in routine clinical assessments. This screening interview was validated in a Spanish population of substance users from health care settings and research units on drugs of abuse (non-health care settings), showing good psychometric properties, with a sensitivity ranging from 0.80 to 0.93 and a specificity ranging from 0.82 to 0.97 depending on the psychiatric disorder [28,29]. The DDSI-IV was administered by a trained psychologist or psychiatrist during the second or third treatment visit at each centre. Individuals were followed-up annually, and their treatment data recorded (e.g., number of visits, therapeutic programme, services received, status and cause of passive status) in the centralised EHR. We followed the STROBE guidelines for reporting observational studies [30].

2.3. Variables

The dependent variable was treatment retention, defined as total days in treatment from the first face-to-face treatment visit to treatment dropout. To our knowledge, there is no standard definition of treatment retention. We considered the definition of treatment dropout of the National Plan of Drugs of the Spanish Government [31], which follows the

European Guidelines [32], that define dropout as a lack of face-to-face contact between the individual and the treatment centre for 6 months. Each year was reviewed to determine whether the individual was in treatment or not (passive status) and the cause of passive status: dropout, therapeutic discharge, referral, or exitus (Latin language term indicating the death of the patient). The treatment procedures protocol of the Barcelona Public Health Agency defines therapeutic discharge as occurring when the individual in treatment has a favourable outcome, without compulsion or thoughts about future or occasional drug consumption, at least in the last 6 months before the date of discharge; referral when the individual is referred to another health service; and exitus when the patient dies. Individuals in treatment at the end of the study follow-up were censored at the end date (28 February 2018). The primary explanatory variable was the result of the DDSI-IV. Other covariates were sociodemographic (sex, age, educational level, living arrangements, employment status, and legal history), clinical (substance of use, frequency and years of substance use, previous substance use treatment, previous psychiatric treatment, medical or psychiatric history, family history of substance use, self-perceived health and treatment centre) and follow-up (number of visits with a physician or psychiatrist, psychologist, or social worker during the study period) (Appendix A, Table A1).

2.4. Statistical Analysis

We conducted a descriptive analysis of the sample characteristics. We stratified the analyses by the DDSI-IV result, a positive result for one or more mental disorders (dual disorder) or a negative result (AUD or CUD alone, no dual disorder). Sociodemographic and clinical differences between individuals screening positive for DD and individuals with AUD or CUD alone were assessed using Pearson's chi-square test or Fisher's exact test for qualitative/categorical variables, and Student's *t*-test or the Mann–Whitney U test for quantitative variables, using an alpha significance level of 0.05. We estimated Kaplan–Meier survival curves to analyse differences in treatment retention between individuals screening positive for DD and patients with AUD or CUD alone. We studied whether differences were statistically significant using the Wilcoxon and Log-Rank tests.

A multivariable Cox regression model was estimated and was adjusted for potential confounders. Firstly, we estimated a model with the significant variables (*p*-value < 0.2) in the descriptive analysis. We used a manual backward elimination method and theoretical criteria to construct 4 blocks of variables introduced in the model in the following order: explanatory, sociodemographic, clinical and follow-up variables. The final model included explanatory variables (DDSI-IV result and substance of use), sociodemographic variables (sex, age and living arrangements), clinical variables (previous psychiatric treatment) and follow-up variables (visits with a physician/psychiatrist, psychologist or a social worker). Finally, we checked whether the final model met the Cox proportional hazards assumption. We performed all analyses using STATA 14.0 (Lakeway Drive College Station, TX, USA) statistical software.

3. Results

3.1. Sociodemographic and Clinical Characteristics

The study sample consisted of 1356 individuals with AUD or CUD screened for lifetime DD with the DDSI-IV. This study sample represented 48.0% of the total number of individuals who started treatment due to AUD or CUD in the four CAS during the study period. The prevalence of individuals screening positive for lifetime DD was 74.0% ($n = 1000$). Among these, the lifetime comorbid mental disorders were depression (76.4%), dysthymia (27.2%), mania (13.1%), panic disorder (37.5%), generalised anxiety disorder (26.5%), specific phobia (13.4%), social phobia (17.9%), agoraphobia (13.2%), psychosis (30.1%), post-traumatic stress disorder (23.5%) and attention deficit hyperactivity disorder (19.3%). A total of 71.4% ($n = 971$) were individuals with AUD and 77.5% ($n = 386$) were individuals with CUD (data not shown in Table 1).

Table 1. Sociodemographic, clinical and treatment retention characteristics of a cohort of individuals with alcohol or cocaine use disorder (n = 1356) by DDSI-IV result. Outpatient drug dependence care centres in Barcelona, January 2015–February 2018.

		Dual Disorder [1]				No Dual Disorder			
		n (%) [2]	Dropouts [3]	T [4]	n (%) [2]	Dropouts [3]	T [4]	p-Value [5]
All participants [6]		1000 (74.0%)	295 (29.5%)	458,941	356 (26.0%)	101 (28.4%)	151,543	
Sociodemographic								
Sex	Male	697 (70.0%)	216 (31.0%)	312,230	297 (83.0%)	92 (31.0%)	124,244	<0.001 * [9]
	Female	303 (30.0%)	79 (26.1%)	146,711	59 (17.0%)	9 (15.3%)	27,299	
Age [$\bar{x}$, SD] [7]		44.6 (11.1)			46.5 (12.1)			
Age	18–44 years	555 (56.0%)	179 (32.3%)	243,111	176 (49.0%)	58 (33.0%)	76,605	0.049 *
	>45 years	445 (44.0%)	116 (26.1%)	215,830	180 (51.0%)	43 (23.9%)	74,938	
Educational level	Primary education or lower	272 (27.2%)	69 (25.4%)	126,968	87 (24.4%)	26 (30.0%)	32,479	0.141
	Secondary or University education	715 (71.5%)	218 (30.5%)	327,271	268 (75.3%)	74 (27.6%)	118,901	
	Missing values	13 (1.3%)			1 (0.3%)			
Living arrangements	Alone	189 (18.9%)	63 (33.3%)	83,853	58 (16.3%)	20 (34.5%)	26,768	0.140
	With others	702 (70.2%)	200 (28.5%)	325,739	265 (74.4%)	71 (26.8%)	110,836	
	Homeless or institutionalised	89 (8.9%)	23 (26.0%)	37,248	25 (7.0%)	6 (24.0%)	9630	
	Missing values	20 (2.0%)			8 (2.3%)			
Employment status	Employed	380 (38.0%)	119 (31.3%)	169,839	184 (51.7%)	56 (30.4%)	76,531	<0.001 *
	Unemployed	395 (39.5%)	118 (29.9%)	181,709	97 (27.3%)	26 (26.8%)	44,690	
	Retired and others	220 (22.0%)	56 (25.5%)	103,913	75 (21.1%)	19 (25.3%)	30,322	
	Missing values	5 (0.5%)						
Legal history	Yes	262 (26.2%)	78 (29.8%)	123,045	79 (22.2%)	25 (31.7%)	36,456	0.060
	No	729 (73%)	211 (28.9%)	332,220	277 (77.8%)	76 (27.4%)	115,087	
	Missing values	9 (0.8%)						
Clinical								
Treatment initiation	Family or self-initiative	436 (43.6%)	142 (32.6%)	194,750	170 (47.8%)	52 (30.6%)	73,179	0.288
	health care or social services recommendation	560 (56.0%)	153 (27.3%)	261,666	184 (51.7%)	49 (26.6%)	77,574	
	Missing values	4 (0.4%)			2 (0.6%)			
Substance of use	Alcohol only	584 (58.0%)	171 (29.3%)	274,360	245 (69%)	69 (28.2%)	100,997	0.006 *
	Cocaine only	229 (23.0%)	70 (30.6%)	99,287	66 (19.0%)	17 (25.8%)	30,921	
	Alcohol + stimulants	134 (13.0%)	32 (23.9%)	64,471	33 (9.0%)	9 (27.3%)	15,330	
	Alcohol or cocaine + cannabis	53 (6.0%)	22 (41.5%)	20,823	12 (3.0%)	6 (50.0%)	4295	

Table 1. Cont.

		Dual Disorder [1]				No Dual Disorder			p-Value [5]
		n (%) [2]	Dropouts [3]	T [4]	n (%) [2]	Dropouts [3]	T [4]		
Substance use frequency	No consumption or <1 day/week	315 (31.5%)	85 (27.0%)	150,490	98 (27.5%)	28 (28.6%)	43,886		0.528
	Less than daily (weekly)	273 (27.3%)	87 (31.9%)	122,708	104 (29.2%)	31 (29.8%)	46,745		
	Daily	409 (41.0%)	123 (30.1%)	184,001	153 (43.0%)	42 (27.5%)	60,575		
	Missing values	3 (0.2%)			1 (0.3%)				
Substance use in years [ME (IQR)] [8]		21 (12–30)			21 (12–34)				0.165
Previous substance use treatment	Yes	573 (57.3%)	169 (29.5%)	261,005	150 (42.1%)	36 (24.0%)	65,839		<0.001 *
	No	420 (42.0%)	124 (29.5%)	194,726	205 (57.6%)	65 (31.7%)	84,906		
	Missing values	7 (0.7%)			1 (0.3%)				
Previous psychiatric treatment	Yes	451 (45.1%)	114 (25.3%)	217,925	85 (23.9%)	23 (27.1%)	38,390		<0.001 *
	No	446 (44.6%)	147 (33.0%)	192,902	248 (69.7%)	73 (29.4%)	101,804		
	Missing values	103 (10.3%)			23 (6.5%)				
Medical or psychiatric history	None	210 (21%)	65 (31.0%)	93,830	102 (28.7%)	27 (26.5%)	39,198		<0.001 *
	Organic disease history	186 (18.6%)	71 (38.2%)	77,934	131 (36.8%)	42 (32.1%)	56,408		
	Psychiatric disorder history	202 (20.2%)	49 (24.3%)	97,531	31 (8.7%)	8 (25.8%)	14,145		
	Organic and psychiatric history	356 (35.6%)	93 (26.1%)	169,628	76 (21.4%)	19 (25.0%)	33,554		
	Missing values	46 (4.6%)			16 (4.5%)				
Family history of substance use	Yes	445 (44.5%)	141 (31.7%)	200,047	122 (34.3%)	41 (33.6%)	47,591		0.002 *
	No	543 (54.3%)	150 (27.6%)	253,615	231 (64.9%)	60 (26.0%)	102,045		
	Missing values	12 (1.2%)			3 (0.8%)				
Self-perceived health	Very good or good	562 (56.2%)	169 (30.1%)	259,066	252 (70.3%)	76 (30.2%)	103,068		<0.001 *
	Poor, bad or very bad	436 (43.6%)	126 (29.0%)	198,814	103 (28.9%)	25 (24.3%)	47,677		
	Missing values	2 (0.2%)			1 (0.3%)				
Treatment centre	Centre A	361 (36.0%)	124 (34.4%)	163,590	74 (21%)	31 (41.9%)	32,198		<0.001 *
	Centre B	256 (26.0%)	86 (33.6%)	110,029	87 (24%)	34 (39.1%)	31,506		
	Centre C	238 (24.0%)	48 (20.2%)	111,855	132 (37%)	26 (19.7%)	60,639		
	Centre D	145 (14.0%)	37 (25.5%)	73,467	63 (18%)	10 (15.9%)	27,200		

[1] Dual disorder: individual diagnosed with a cocaine or alcohol use disorder with a positive result for one or more mental disorders using the Dual Diagnosis Screening Interview (DDSI-IV); [2] n, number of cases and %, relative frequency; [3] Dropouts: absolute values and relative frequencies (%) of people not attending treatment visits for more than 6 months; [4] t: time of follow-up in person-days; [5] p-value: Pearson's chi-square test or Fisher's exact test; Student's t-test or the Mann–Whitney U test to analyse differences between individuals with and without a dual disorder; [6] All participants: all study participants with a cocaine or alcohol use disorder screened using the Dual Diagnosis Screening Interview (DDSI-IV); [7] $\bar{x}$, Mean and SD, standard deviation; [8] ME, median and IQR, interquartile range; [9] *, indicates that differences between individuals with and without a dual disorder are statistically significant (p-Value < 0.05).

Table 1 details the individuals' sociodemographic and clinical characteristics. Compared with individuals screening negative for lifetime DD, those screening positive at baseline were more frequently women (30.0% vs. 17.0%, *p*-value < 0.001), younger (56.0% vs. 49.0%, *p*-value = 0.049), unemployed (39.5% vs. 27.3%, *p*-value < 0.001) and reported higher polysubstance use (13.0% vs. 9.0% of alcohol and stimulants, respectively, and 6.0% vs. 3.0% of alcohol/cocaine and cannabis, respectively, *p*-value = 0.006). Moreover, a higher proportion had received previous treatment for an SUD (57.3% vs. 42.1%, *p*-value < 0.001), previous treatment for a psychiatric disorder (45.1% vs. 23.9%, *p*-value < 0.001), and more frequently reported a history of organic and psychiatric problems (35.6% vs. 21.4%, *p*-value < 0.001), a family history of substance use (44.5% vs. 34.3%, *p*-value = 0.002) and poorer self-perceived health (43.6% vs. 28.9%, *p*-value < 0.001). The median number of medical or psychiatric treatment visits (8 [IR: 4–13] vs. 6 [IR: 4–10], social care visits (2 [IR: 1–5] vs. 1.5 [IR: 1–3]) and follow-up time (423 vs. 369 days) were relatively higher and were significant in those screening positive for lifetime DD (data not shown in Table 1).

3.2. Characteristics of Treatment Retention

At one year of follow-up (Figure 1), treatment retention was more than 75% in both groups. Moreover, more than 50% of individuals remained in treatment for the entire follow-up period (38 months). Treatment retention decreased similarly in both groups during the study period, and the difference was not statistically significant (Wilcoxon *p*-value = 0.659; Log-Rank test *p*-value = 0.769). The proportion of dropouts in individuals screening positive for lifetime DD was 29.5% and was 28.4% in those screening negative. There were 458,941 person-days of follow-up among individuals screening positive for lifetime DD and 151,543 person-days of follow-up among those screening negative (Table 1).

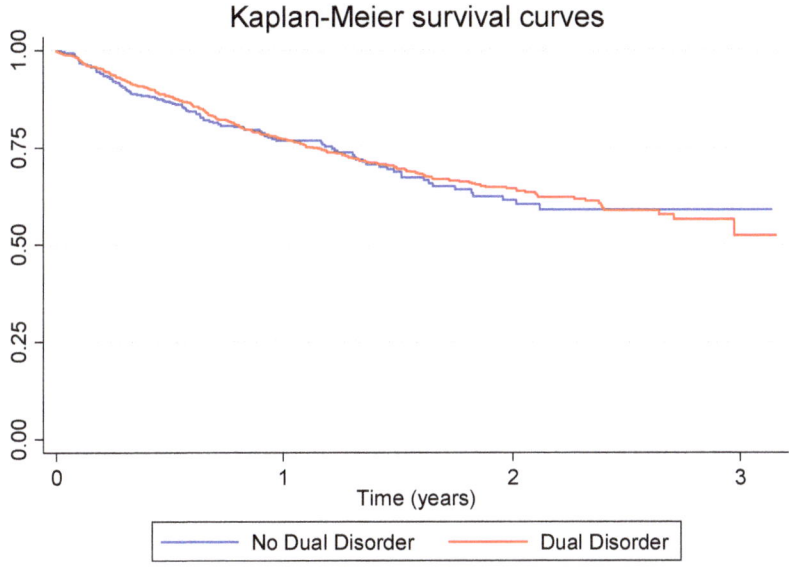

Figure 1. Kaplan–Meier survival curves for treatment retention by DDSI-IV result in a cohort of individuals with alcohol or cocaine use disorder (*n* = 1356). Outpatient drug dependence care centres in Barcelona, January 2015–February 2018.

3.3. Multivariable Explanatory Models of Treatment Dropout

Table 2 shows the different multivariable Cox regression models estimated. After adjustment for different sociodemographic, clinical and follow-up covariates, individuals screening positive for lifetime DD had a 26% increased risk of treatment dropout (HR = 1.26; 95% CI = 1.00–1.60) than those with SUD alone (no DD). According to the substance of use, those who used alcohol only and those who used alcohol or cocaine with cannabis had a 35% (HR= 1.35; 95% CI 1.04–1.77) and a 60% (HR = 1.60; 95% CI = 1.03–2.49) higher risk of treatment dropout, respectively, than those using cocaine only. Individuals who lived alone had a 34% (HR = 1.34; 95% CI = 1.04–1.72) increased risk of treatment dropout than those living with a partner and/or children. The risk of treatment dropout was reduced by 22% with one additional medical visit (HR = 0.78; 95% CI = 0.75–0.80), by 4% with one additional psychologist visit (HR = 0.96; 95% CI = 0.94–0.97) and by 3% with one additional visit with a social worker (HR = 0.97; 95% CI = 0.95–1.00). The Cox proportional hazard assumption (p-Value > 0.05) was observed for all variables included in the final model (model 4), except for the variables of previous psychiatric treatment and number of visits with a physician/psychiatrist and with a psychologist (Appendix A, Table A2).

Table 2. Association of sociodemographic, clinical and follow-up characteristics and treatment dropout in a cohort of individuals with alcohol or cocaine use disorder (n = 1356). Outpatient drug dependence care centres in Barcelona, January 2015–February 2018.

		Model [1] 1		Model [1] 2		Model [1] 3		Model [1] 4	
		HR [2]	95% CI [3]	HR [2]	95% CI [3]	HR [2]	95% CI [3]	HR [2]	95% CI [3]
DDSI-IV [4] result	No dual disorder	1		1		1		1	
	Dual disorder	0.96	0.77–1.21	1.00	0.79–1.25	1.01	0.79–1.28	1.26	1.00–1.60
Substance of use	Cocaine only	1		1		1		1	
	Alcohol only	0.95	0.74–1.22	1.12	0.86–1.46	1.20	0.92–1.57	1.35	1.04–1.77
	Alcohol + stimulants	0.78	0.53–1.12	0.76	0.52–1.10	0.73	0.50–1.08	0.89	0.61–1.30
	Alcohol or cocaine + cannabis	1.57	1.02–2.42	1.60	1.04–2.47	1.62	1.04–2.51	1.60	1.03–2.49
Sociodemographic									
Sex	Female			1		1		1	
	Male			1.34	1.05–1.72	1.27	1.00–1.64	1.11	0.86–1.42
Age	>45 years			1		1		1	
	18–44 years			1.40	1.13–1.75	1.47	1.17–1.85	1.10	0.88–1.39
Living arrangements	With others			1		1		1	
	Alone			1.26	0.98–1.61	1.26	0.98–1.63	1.34	1.04–1.72
	Homeless or institutionalised			0.99	0.67–1.45	0.94	0.64–1.38	0.86	0.58–1.27
	Missing values			1.25	0.71–2.20	0.99	0.55–1.77	1.93	1.09–3.39
Clinical									
Medical or psychiatric history	None					1			
	Organic disease history					1.34	1.00–1.78		
	Psychiatric disorder history					0.68	0.42–1.08		
	Organic and psychiatric history					0.76	0.50–1.17		
	Missing values					1.41	0.75–2.66		
Previous psychiatric treatment	Yes					1		1	
	No					0.83	0.56–1.25	1.03	0.82–1.29
	Missing values					0.85	0.49–1.47	0.97	0.67–1.40
Treatment centre	Centre A					1			
	Centre B					1.09	0.84–1.41		
	Centre C					0.53	0.40–0.71		
	Centre D					0.58	0.41–0.81		

Table 2. Cont.

	Model [1] 1		Model [1] 2		Model [1] 3		Model [1] 4	
	HR [2]	95% CI [3]	HR [2]	95% CI [3]	HR [2]	95% CI [3]	HR [2]	95% CI [3]
Follow-Up								
Physician/Psychiatrist visits							0.78	0.75–0.80
Psychologist visits							0.96	0.94–0.97
Social worker visits							0.97	0.95–1.00

[1] Model: Cox regression model; [2] HR: hazard ratio; [3] 95% CI: confidence interval at 95% normal approximation; [4] DDSI-IV: Dual Diagnosis Screening Interview (DDSI-IV).

4. Discussion

The main findings of this study were: (i) the high prevalence of positive screening for lifetime DD among individuals with AUD or CUD; (ii) the sociodemographic and clinical differences between individuals screening positive for lifetime DD and those with AUD or CUD alone; (iii) the high treatment retention during the study period; and (iv) the risk of treatment dropout was increased by screening positive for lifetime DD, living alone, alcohol use and polysubstance use.

The prevalence of individuals screening positive for lifetime DD (74%) is consistent with some previous studies conducted in clinical samples but using diagnostic tests. About 62% [33] to 85% [34] of individuals undertaking outpatient substance use treatment were diagnosed with DD using the Psychiatric Research Interview for Substance and Mental Disorders (PRISM). Another study, which administered the Mini-International Neuropsychiatric Interview, found that about two out of three individuals with CUD or AUD had a lifetime mental disorder (73.4% and 76.1%, respectively) [14,35].

In Spain, there is a gatekeeping system at the primary care level and general practitioners can medicate individuals with psychiatric symptoms. This might explain our finding that 23.9% and 8.7% of individuals screening negative for a lifetime mental disorder reported they had previous psychiatric treatment or a previous psychiatric history. This reinforces the importance of incorporating screening tools with good psychometric properties and DSM-IV-based criteria into specialised primary addiction care to allow better identification of psychiatric comorbidities among individuals with SUD [36].

Treatment retention in the cohort was more than 75% at one year of follow-up. This percentage is higher than that reported in another study in Barcelona [37]. Almost 50% of individuals treated in outpatient drug dependence care centres dropped out at one year of follow-up. These individuals had been referred from a hospital emergency department. However, in our study, more than 43% of individuals sought treatment on their own initiative or by family recommendation.

After adjustment for different covariates, screening positive for lifetime DD, alcohol use, polysubstance use and living alone showed the potential to explain treatment retention in our study. The risk of treatment dropout was modestly (26%) higher in individuals with a positive result for lifetime DD than in those with AUD or CUD alone. However, we could not accept or reject our study hypothesis because we did not find a significant association on the bivariate analysis and the association on the multivariate analysis was almost not statistically significant. The previous literature also found contradictory results related to retention in the treatment of individuals with DD. For example, Daigre et al. (2019) reported that DD was not an associated factor for treatment retention [25]. However, in their study, they only selected patients with prolonged treatment stays. In contrast, other studies showed that DD is related to poor treatment adherence in individuals with SUD [19–21,23]. Studies conducted in different health care settings (e.g., outpatient clinics, hospitals, therapeutic communities) concluded that the main obstacle to improving health outcomes in these individuals is the difficulty of enhancing their adherence to therapeutic plans. These studies also highlight several related factors, such as symptom severity, medication side effects, years of substance use, polysubstance use or more unfavourable socioeconomic conditions [15,24].

In our study, social living conditions, such as living alone, increased the risk (34%) of treatment dropout. Previous studies also reported a higher risk of treatment dropout when individuals had poor social support or family cohesion, or family conflict. Social and family support has been reported to have a buffering effect on stress related to illness and the treatment process and a motivating effect on treatment follow-up [38]. Likewise, several studies have found an association between social support and recovery in individuals with SUD, showing a reduction in substance use, relapses, stress levels and enhanced general well-being [39,40].

We observed that individuals with alcohol use alone presented a higher risk (35%) of treatment dropout than individuals with cocaine use alone. Likewise, a recent study found that patients with cocaine use and a higher education were more likely to complete treatment than patients with alcohol use [25]. A possible explanation could be the legal status of alcohol use and its advertising and availability in the urban environment [41]. Some studies have observed a positive relationship between the concentration of advertising and sale points of alcoholic beverages and risky alcohol consumption and higher associated morbidity and mortality [42,43].

In our study, individuals with polysubstance use of alcohol or cocaine and cannabis had a higher risk of treatment dropout (60%) than those with cocaine use alone. Previous studies have shown a relationship between polysubstance use and worse treatment outcomes and premature dropout [44,45]. For example, polysubstance use hampers treatment adherence, i.e., remembering to take prescribed medications, attend treatment appointments, etc. [46]. Likewise, a previous study reported a relationship between polysubstance use and a lower percentage of therapeutic discharges in DD patients [47].

This study has several limitations. First, the participants were recruited from four public drug dependence care centres (CAS) in Barcelona, and therefore the study results cannot be extrapolated to other contexts with a significant private supply of drug dependence care. However, these centres are distributed across the city and account for approximately 55% of all SUD treatment admissions. Therefore, we believe that different patient profiles are represented in our study. Second, we used a lifetime DD screening instrument (DDSI-IV) to determine the presence of comorbid mental disorders. Consequently, we may have overestimated the prevalence of DD. However, this instrument has shown ease of administration in routine evaluations, was validated in a population of substance users and, when compared with the Psychiatric Research Interview for Substance and Mental Disorders (PRISM), as the gold standard, showed high sensitivity and specificity ($\geq 80\%$) [28]. Third, we screened for lifetime DD, which might hamper the detection of more significant differences in treatment retention. However, because this was a cohort pilot study, recruitment could only be conducted by convenience, and the DDSI-IV was mostly administered to individuals who showed or reported current psychiatric symptoms when starting treatment. However, the present study has allowed us to identify how to improve clinical interview procedures to introduce DD screening systematically as a part of routine clinical practice (i.e., the DD screening is administered by therapists in training supervised by their referent in the centre). Following this preliminary study, the DDSI-IV has been adapted to the DSM-5 criteria, considering current comorbid mental disorders. However, screening for personality disorders has not been introduced in this version either. Fourth, we were unable to differentiate between primary and substance-induced diagnoses for some of the disorders screened. Therefore, an additional routine assessment was recently introduced during the first treatment visits for individuals screening positive in the DDSI-IV.

The main strengths of this study are the cohort study design, with prospective follow-up of participants, the large sample of a clinical population, the inclusion of several public drug dependence care centres and the use of a centralised EHR system with sociodemographic, clinical and follow-up information. Moreover, the study includes many potential confounders of treatment retention, identified through a comprehensive literature review.

5. Conclusions

Our study shows that DD is a prevalent issue among individuals with alcohol or cocaine use disorders and could influence their dropout from treatment in public outpatient drug dependence care centres, along with alcohol use, polysubstance use and social conditions, such as living alone. We have designed a new large-scale study, which introduces all the above changes and an extended follow-up to confirm these preliminary results. We believe that introducing DD evaluation in the routine biopsychosocial assessments of individuals with a SUD when starting treatment could help the design of more tailored treatment strategies and improve the prognosis of those individuals.

Author Contributions: Conceptualisation, M.T.B.; formal analysis, B.P.-G.; investigation, L.T., C.R.-D., J.M.V.-V., A.P., M.C.-G., M.J.-D., I.O., E.G., N.M. and The Dual Diagnosis Study Group; writing—original draft preparation, B.P.-G.; writing—review and editing, B.P.-G., M.G.B., M.B., M.T.B., M.G., O.P.-B. and M.T.; visualisation, B.P.-G.; supervision, M.G.B., M.B., M.T.B. and M.T.; project administration, M.T.B., M.B. and M.G.B.; funding acquisition, M.T.B. and M.T. All authors have read and agreed to the published version of the manuscript.

Funding: This research was funded by: Instituto de Salud Carlos III, PI16/01075; Instituto de Salud Carlos III—European Regional Development Fund -Red de Trastornos Adictivos (RTA), UE-FEDER 2016 RD16/0017/0010; Instituto de Salud Carlos III, Redes de Investigación Cooperativa Orientadas a Resultados en Salud (RICORS), Red de Investigación en Atención Primaria (RIAPAd), RD21/0009/0001 and the European Union NextGenerationEU, Mecanismo para la Recuperación y la Resiliencia (MRR).

Institutional Review Board Statement: The study was conducted in accordance with the Declaration of Helsinki and approved by The Parc de Salut Mar Clinical Research Ethics Committee (Barcelona, Spain) (2019/6422/I).

Informed Consent Statement: Written informed consent was obtained from all participants involved in the study during the first treatment visit in the drug dependence care centres.

Data Availability Statement: The data that support the findings of this study are not publicly available but are available from the corresponding author (M.G.B) upon reasonable request.

Acknowledgments: We thank Gail Craigie for editorial assistance and Carlos García Forero for his valuable comments during the analysis of the article.

Conflicts of Interest: M.T. is a co-author of this paper and member of the Recent Advances in Dual Disorders (Addiction and Other Mental Disorder) Special Issue of the Journal of Clinical Medicine. The rest of the authors declare no conflict of interest. The funders had no role in the design of the study; in the collection, analyses, or interpretation of data; in the writing of the manuscript, or in the decision to publish the results.

Appendix A

Table A1. Baseline sociodemographic and clinical information routinely collected by survey in outpatient drug dependence care centres in Barcelona.

Sociodemographic Variables	
Sex	Male
	Female
Age	
Residence area	
Educational level	Cannot read or write
	Unfinished primary education
	Completed primary education
	Elementary school or ESO
	Upper secondary school, BUP, COU, intermediate professional training
	University bachelor's degree of 3 years
	University bachelor's degree of 4 or 5 years
	Other higher education degrees
Cohabitation	Alone
	Alone with children
	With parents
	With a partner
	With a partner and children
	With friends
	Other

Table A1. Cont.

Sociodemographic Variables	
Employment status	Employee with indefinite contract or self-employed Employee with a temporary contract Unpaid work for the family Unemployed without having worked before Unemployed having worked before Permanent disability or retired Student Only housework Other
Legal history	Yes No
Clinical variables	
Treatment initiation	Self-initiative Family or friends' recommendation Drug dependence care referral Primary care referral Emergency department or hospital referral Social services referral Legal services referral Prison or similar Company, service of a company Other drug dependence services Other
Primary substance of use	
Secondary substance of use	
Third substance of use	
Fourth substance of use	
Substance use frequency	Every day 4 or 6 days per week 2 or 3 days per week Once a week Less than once a week No consumption
Substance use in years	
Previous substance use treatment	Yes, related to the current primary substance of use Yes, related to a different primary substance of use Yes, related to the current primary substance of use and for other substances No, never
Previous psychiatric treatment	Yes No
Medical history	Yes No
Psychiatric history	Yes No
Family history of substance use	Yes No

Table A1. Cont.

Sociodemographic Variables	
Self-perceived health	Excellent Good Regular Bad
Treatment centre	

Table A2. Assessment of the proportional hazards assumption of the final Cox regression model (model 4).

		Rho	Chi-Square	p-Value
DDSI-IV result	No dual disorder	.	.	.
	Dual disorder	−0.04967	1.01	0.314 *
Substance of use	Cocaine only	.	.	.
	Alcohol only	−0.07545	2.39	0.122 *
	Alcohol + stimulants	−0.01408	0.08	0.7767 *
	Alcohol or cocaine + cannabis	−0.02338	0.23	0.635 *
Sex	Female	.	.	.
	Male	−0.00478	0.01	0.924 *
Age	>45 years	.	.	.
	18–44 years	0.00698	0.02	0.887 *
Living arrangements	With others	.	.	.
	Alone	−0.03802	0.60	0.439 *
	Homeless or Institutionalised	0.03603	0.53	0.468 *
	Missing values	−0.04295	0.75	0.388 *
Previous psychiatric treatment	Yes	.	.	.
	No	−0.10596	4.49	0.034
	Missing values	−0.03373	0.46	0.498 *
Physician/Psychiatrist visits		0.34088	47.90	<0.001
Psychologist visits		0.17575	14.19	<0.001
Social worker visits		0.05082	1.57	0.210 *

*, indicates that the Cox proportional hazard assumption (p-Value > 0.05) was observed.

References

1. World Health Organization. *Lexicon of Alcohol and Drug Terms*; World Health Organization: Geneva, Switzerland, 1994.
2. Regier, D.A.; Farmer, M.E.; Rae, D.S.; Locke, B.Z.; Keith, S.J.; Judd, L.L.; Goodwin, F.K. Comorbidity of mental disorders with alcohol and other drug abuse. Results from the Epidemiologic Catchment Area (ECA) Study. *JAMA* **1990**, *264*, 2511–2518. [CrossRef] [PubMed]
3. Kessler, R.C.; McGonagle, K.A.; Zhao, S. Lifetime and 12-month prevalence of DSM-III-R psychiatric disorders in the United States. Results from the National Comorbidity Survey. *Arch. Gen. Psychiatry* **1994**, *51*, 8–19. [CrossRef] [PubMed]
4. Compton, W.M.; Thomas, Y.F.; Stinson, F.S.; Compton, W.M.; Thomas, Y.F.; Stinson, F.S.; Grant, B.F. Prevalence, correlates, disability, and comorbidity of DSM-IV drug abuse and dependence in the United States. *Arch. Gen. Psychiatry* **2007**, *64*, 566–576. [CrossRef] [PubMed]
5. Megnin-Viggars, O.; Brown, M.; Marcus, E.; Stockton, S.; Pilling, S. *Severe Mental Illness and Substance Misuse (Dual Diagnosis): Community Health and Social Care Services*; Public Health and Social Care Centre at the National Institute for Health and Care Excellence (NICE): London, UK, 2015.
6. Torrens, M.; Mestre-Pintó, J.-I.; Domingo-Salvany, A. *Comorbidity of Substance Use and Mental Disorders in Europe*; European Monitoring Centre for Drugs and Drug Addiction; Publications Office of the European Union: Luxembourg, 2015. [CrossRef]
7. Hamilton, I. The 10 most important debates surrounding dual diagnosis. *Adv. Dual Diagn.* **2014**, *7*, 118–128. [CrossRef]
8. Kessler, R.C.; Üstün, T.B. The World Mental Health (WMH) Survey Initiative version of the World Health Organization (WHO) Composite International Diagnostic Interview (CIDI). *Int. J. Methods Psychiatr. Res.* **2004**, *13*, 93–121. [CrossRef] [PubMed]

9. Navarro-Mateu, F.; Morán-Sánchez, I.; Alonso, J.; Tormo, M.J.; Pujalte, M.L.; Garriga, A.; Aguilar-Gaxiola, S.; Navarro, C. Cultural adaptation of the Latin American version of the World Health Organization Composite International Diagnostic Interview (WHO-CIDI) (v 3.0) for use in Spain. *Gac. Sanit.* **2013**, *27*, 325–331. [CrossRef]
10. Torrens, M.; Martin-Santos, R.; Samet, S. Importance of clinical diagnoses for comorbidity studies in substance use disorders. *Neurotox. Res.* **2006**, *10*, 253–261. [CrossRef]
11. Torrens, M.; Gilchrist, G.; Domingo-Salvany, A. Psychiatric comorbidity in illicit drug users: Substance-induced versus independent disorders. *Drug Alcohol Depend.* **2011**, *113*, 147–156. [CrossRef]
12. Herrero, M.J.; Domingo-Salvany, A.; Torrens, M.; Brugal, M.T.; The ITINERE Investigators. Psychiatric comorbidity in young cocaine users: Induced versus independent disorders. *Addiction* **2008**, *103*, 284–293. [CrossRef]
13. Rounsaville, B.; Anton, S.; Carroll, K.; Budde, D.; Prusoff, B.A.; Gawin, F. Psychiatric diagnoses of treatment-seeking cocaine abusers. *Arch. Gen. Psychiatry* **1991**, *48*, 43–51. [CrossRef]
14. Arias, F.; Szerman, N.; Vega, P.; Mesias, B.; Basurte, I.; Morant, C.; Ochoa, E.; Poyo, F.; Babin, F. Cocaine abuse or dependency and other psychiatric disorders. Madrid study on dual pathology. *Rev. Psiquiatr Salud Ment.* **2013**, *6*, 121–128. [CrossRef] [PubMed]
15. Carrà, G.; Bartoli, F.; Clerici, M.; el-Guebaly, N. Psychopathology of dual diagnosis: New trumpets and old uncertainties. *J. Psychopathol.* **2015**, *21*, 390–399.
16. Kranzler, H.R.; Tinsley, J.A. (Eds.) *Dual Diagnosis and Psychiatric Treatment. Substance Abuse and Comorbid Disorders*, 2nd ed.; CRC Press: New York, NY, USA, 2004. [CrossRef]
17. Guitart, A.; Espelt, A.; Astellano, Y.; Suelves, J.M.; Villalbí, J.R.; Brugal, M.T. Injury-Related Mortality Over 12 Years in a Cohort of Patients with Alcohol Use Disorders: Higher Mortality Among Young People and Women. *Alcohol Clin. Exp. Res.* **2015**, *39*, 1158–1165. [CrossRef] [PubMed]
18. Szerman, N.; Lopez-Castroman, J.; Arias, F.; Morant, C.; Babín, F.; Mesías, B.; Basurte, I.; Vega, P.; Baca-García, E. Dual Diagnosis and Suicide Risk in a Spanish Outpatient Sample. *Subst. Use Misuse* **2012**, *47*, 383–389. [CrossRef] [PubMed]
19. Magura, S.; Laudet, A.; Mahmood, D.; Rosenblum, A.; Knight, E. Adherence to Medication Regimens and Participation in Dual-Focus Self-Help Groups. *Psychiatr. Serv.* **2002**, *53*, 310–316. [CrossRef]
20. Wolpe, P.R.; Gorton, G.; Serota, R.; Sanford, B. Predicting Compliance of Dual Diagnosis Inpatients With Aftercare Treatment. *Psychiatr. Serv.* **2006**, *44*, 45–49. [CrossRef]
21. Brown, C.; Bennett, M.; Li, L.; Bellack, A.S. Predictors of initiation and engagement in substance abuse treatment among individuals with co-occurring serious mental illness and substance use disorders. *Addict. Behav.* **2011**, *36*, 439–447. [CrossRef]
22. Roncero, C.; Szerman, N.; Terán, A.; Pino, C.; Vazquez, J.M.; Velasco, E.; Garcia Dorado, M.; Casas, M. Professionals' perception on the management of patients with dual disorders. *Patient Prefer. Adherence* **2016**, *10*, 1855–1868. [CrossRef]
23. Herbeck, D.M.; Fitek, D.J.; Svikis, D.S.; Montoya, I.D.; Marcus, S.C.; West, J.C. Treatment compliance in patients with comorbid psychiatric and substance use disorders. *Am. J. Addict.* **2005**, *14*, 195–207. [CrossRef]
24. Magura, S.; Rosenblum, A.; Fong, C. Factors associated with medication adherence among psychiatric outpatients at substance abuse risk. *Open Addict. J.* **2011**, *4*, 58–64. [CrossRef]
25. Daigre, C.; Perea-Ortueta, M.; Berenguer, M.; Esculies, O.; Sorribes-Puertas, M.; Palma-Alvarez, R.; Martínez-Luna, N.; Ramos-Quiroga, J.A.; Grau-López, L. Psychiatric factors affecting recovery after a long term treatment program for substance use disorder. *Psychiatry Res.* **2019**, *276*, 283–289. [CrossRef] [PubMed]
26. Parés-Badell, O.; Barbaglia, G.; Robinowitz, N.; Majó, X.; Torrens, M.; Espelt, A.; Bartroli, M.; Gotsens, M.; Brugal, M.T. Integration of harm reduction and treatment into care centres for substance use: The Barcelona model. *Int. J. Drug Policy* **2020**, *76*, 102614. [CrossRef] [PubMed]
27. World Health Organization. *The ICD-10 Classification of Mental and Behavioural Disorders: Clinical Descriptions and Diagnostic Guidelines*; World Health Organization: Geneva, Switzerland, 1992.
28. Mestre-Pintó, J.I.; Domingo-Salvany, A.; Martín-Santos, R.; Torrens, M.; PsyCoBarcelona Group. Dual Diagnosis Screening Interview to Identify Psychiatric Comorbidity in Substance Users: Development and Validation of a Brief Instrument. *Eur. Addict. Res.* **2014**, *20*, 41–48. [CrossRef]
29. Mestre-Pintó, J.-I.; Torrens, M.D.; Domingo-Salvany, A.D. Evaluación de una Entrevista de Cribado para la Detección de Comorbilidad Psiquiátrica en Sujetos Consumidores de Sustancias de Abuso—Dipòsit Digital de Documents de la UAB. Universitat Autònoma de Barcelona. 2011. Available online: https://ddd.uab.cat/record/127412/ (accessed on 24 April 2022).
30. Von Elm, E.; Altman, D.; Gøtzsche, P.; Mulrow, C.D.; Pocock, S.J.; Poole, C.; Schlesselman, J.J.; Egger, M.; STROBE Initiative. Strengthening the Reporting of Observational Studies in Epidemiology (STROBE): Explanation and elaboration. *Int. J. Surg.* **2014**, *12*, 1500–1524. [CrossRef]
31. Observatorio Español de las Drogas y las Toxicomanias. *Indicador: Admisiones a Tratamiento por Consumo de Sustancias Psicoactivas*; Plan Nacional Sobre Drogas; Ministerio de Sanidad: Madrid, Spain, 2013.
32. European Monitoring Centre for Drugs and Drug Addiction. *Treatment Demand Indicator (TDI) Standard Protocol 3.0. Guidelines for Reporting Data on People Entering Drug Treatment in European Countries*; Publications Office of the European Union: Luxembourg, 2012. [CrossRef]
33. Araos, P.; Vergara-Moragues, E.; Pedraz, M.; Pavon-Moron, F.J.; Campos Cloute, R.; Calado, M.; Ruiz, J.; García-Marchena, N.; Ben Hirsch-Gornemann, M.; Torrens, M.; et al. Comorbilidad psicopatológica en consumidores de cocaína en tratamiento ambulatorio. Psychopathological comorbidity in cocaine users in outpatient treatment. *Adicciones* **2014**, *26*, 15–26. [CrossRef] [PubMed]

34. Langås, A.M.; Malt, U.F.; Opjordsmoen, S. Substance use disorders and comorbid mental disorders in first-time admitted patients from a catchment area. *Eur. Addict. Res.* **2011**, *18*, 16–25. [CrossRef]
35. Arias, F.; Szerman, N.; Vega, P.; Mesias, B.; Basurte, I.; Morant, C.; Ochoa, E.; Poyo, F.; Babin, F. Alcohol abuse or dependence and other psychiatric disorders. Madrid study on the prevalence of dual pathology. *Ment. Health Subst. Use* **2013**, *6*, 339–350. [CrossRef]
36. Dedeu, T.; Bolibar, B.; Gené, J.; Pareja, C. *Building Primary Care in a Changing Europe: Case Studies*; Kringos, D.S., Boerma, W.G.W., Hutchinson, A., Eds.; European Observatory on Health Systems and Policies: Copenhagen, Denmark, 2015.
37. Roncero, C.; Rodríguez-Cintas, L.; Barral, C.; Fuste, G.; Daigre, C.; Ramos-Quiroga, J.A.; Casas, M. Treatment adherence to treatment in substance users referred from Psychiatric Emergency service to outpatient treatment. *Actas Españolas de Psiquiatría* **2012**, *40*, 63–69. [CrossRef]
38. Di Matteo, M. Social support and patient adherence to medical treatment: A meta-analysis. *Heal. Psychol.* **2004**, *23*, 207–218. [CrossRef]
39. Tracy, E.; Biegel, D. Personal social networks and dual disorders: A literature review and implications for practice and future research. *J. Dual Diagn.* **2006**, *2*, 59–88. [CrossRef]
40. Laudet, A.B.; Magura, S.; Vogel, H.S.; Knight, E. Support, mutual aid and recovery from dual diagnosis. *Commun. Ment. Health J.* **2000**, *36*, 457–476. [CrossRef] [PubMed]
41. Villalbí, J.R.; Espelt, A.; Sureda, X.; Bosque-Prous, M.; Teixidó-Compañó, E.; Puigcorbé, S.; Franco, M.; Brugal, M.T. The urban environment of alcohol: A study on the availability, promotion and visibility of its use in the neighborhoods of Barcelona. *Adicciones* **2019**, *31*, 33–40. [CrossRef] [PubMed]
42. Shortt, N.K.; Rind, E.; Pearce, J.; Mitchell, R.; Curtis, S. Alcohol Risk Environments, Vulnerability, and Social Inequalities in Alcohol Consumption. *Ann. Am. Assoc. Geogr.* **2018**, *108*, 1210–1227. [CrossRef]
43. Mori-Gamarra, F.; Moure-Rodríguez, L.; Sureda, X.; Carbia, C.; Royé, D.; Montes-Martínez, A.; Cadaveira, F.; Caamaño-Isorna, F. Alcohol outlet density and alcohol consumption in Galician youth. *Gac. Sanit.* **2020**, *34*, 15–20. [CrossRef] [PubMed]
44. Timko, C.; Ilgen, M.; Haverfield, M.; Shelley, A.; Breland, J.Y. Polysubstance use by psychiatry inpatients with co-occurring mental health and substance use disorders. *Drug Alcohol Depend.* **2017**, *180*, 319–322. [CrossRef] [PubMed]
45. Connor, J.P.; Gullo, M.J.; White, A.; Kelly, A.B. Polysubstance use: Diagnostic challenges, patterns of use and health. *Curr. Opin. Psychiatry* **2014**, *27*, 269–275. [CrossRef]
46. Weitzman, E.R.; Ziemnik, R.E.; Huang, Q.; Levy, S. Alcohol and Marijuana Use and Treatment Nonadherence Among Medically Vulnerable Youth. *Pediatrics* **2015**, *136*, 450–457. [CrossRef]
47. Madoz-Gúrpide, A.; Vicent, V.G.; Fuentes, E.L. Variables predictivas del alta terapéutica entre pacientes con patología dual grave atendidos en una comunidad terapéutica de drogodependencias con unidad psiquiátrica. *Adicciones* **2013**, *25*, 300–308. [CrossRef]

Suicidality as a Predictor of Overdose among Patients with Substance Use Disorders

Viviana E. Horigian [1,*], Renae D. Schmidt [1], Dikla Shmueli-Blumberg [2], Kathryn Hefner [2], Judith Feinberg [3], Radhika Kondapaka [2], Daniel J. Feaster [1], Rui Duan [1], Sophia Gonzalez [1], Carly Davis [1], Rodrigo Marín-Navarrete [4] and Susan Tross [5]

1. Department of Public Health Sciences, University of Miami Miller School of Medicine, 1120 Northwest 14th Street, Miami, FL 33136, USA
2. The Emmes Company, LLC, 401 N. Washington St., Suite 700, Rockville, MD 20850, USA
3. Departments of Behavioral Medicine and Psychiatry & Medicine/Infectious Diseases, West Virginia University School of Medicine, 930 Chestnut Ridge Road, Morgantown, WV 26505, USA
4. Division of Research and Translational Education, Centros de Integración Juvenil A.C., San Jerónimo Avenue 372, Jardines del Pedregal, Mexico City 01900, Mexico
5. Department of Psychiatry, Columbia University, 1051 Riverside Drive, New York, NY 10032, USA
* Correspondence: vhorigian@med.miami.edu; Tel.:+1-(305)-243-4305

Abstract: Increasing rates of overdose and overdose deaths are a significant public health problem. Research has examined co-occurring mental health conditions, including suicidality, as a risk factor for intentional and unintentional overdose among individuals with substance use disorder (SUD). However, this research has been limited to single site studies of self-reported outcomes. The current research evaluated suicidality as a predictor of overdose events in 2541 participants who use substances enrolled across eight multi-site clinical trials completed within the National Drug Abuse Treatment Clinical Trials Network between 2012 to 2021. The trials assessed baseline suicidality with the Concise Health Risk Tracking Self-Report (CHRT-SR). Overdose events were determined by reports of adverse events, cause of death, or hospitalization due to substance overdose, and verified through a rigorous adjudication process. Multivariate logistic regression was performed to assess continuous CHRT-SR score as a predictor of overdose, controlling for covariates. CHRT-SR score was associated with overdose events ($p = 0.03$) during the trial; the likelihood of overdose increased as continuous CHRT score increased (OR 1.02). Participants with lifetime heroin use were more likely to overdose (OR 3.08). Response to the marked rise in overdose deaths should integrate suicide risk reduction as part of prevention strategies.

Keywords: substance use disorders; dual disorders; co-occurring disorders; suicidality; overdose

1. Introduction

Increasing rates of overdose and overdose deaths are significant public health problems in the US [1]. While opioids have been the leading cause of overdose and overdose deaths, recent evidence suggests increases in overdose deaths due to stimulants [1,2]. Studies also suggest that among individuals who use substances, concurrent use of multiple substances is " ... the norm rather than the exception" [3]. Research also indicates that individuals might shift their substance use preferences across their lifespan [4]. It is important to understand and address the social determinants of health and to identify factors and underlying conditions that put individuals at risk for overdose and other adverse outcomes.

The frequent co-occurrence of mental health conditions among individuals with substance use disorder (SUD) is often termed "dual disorders" [5]. Mental health conditions are highly prevalent in individuals seeking treatment for substance use disorders [6]. Major depression (50–60%) [7,8], post-traumatic stress disorder (PTSD) (47%) [9], and anxiety (31.2%) [10] are common among persons with opioid use disorder (OUD), and a majority report suffering from insomnia [11]. Similarly, mental health conditions are highly prevalent in persons with stimulant use disorders, with 35.7 to 41.6% having a lifetime history of major depression [8] and between 23 to 42% with lifetime history of PTSD [12]. Depressive symptoms along with other mental health conditions have been associated with nonfatal overdoses among individuals with SUD, drawing attention to the importance of early identification and treatment for these co-occurring conditions [6,13,14].

Suicide is the 10th leading cause of death in the United States and is a contributor to premature mortality [15]. With the goal of better understanding and preventing opioid overdose and overdose fatalities, recent literature has drawn attention to the distinction between intentional and unintentional overdoses among opioid users [2,16]. Suicidal thoughts might increase the risk of non-fatal overdose and potentially elevate the risk for future intentional overdose or unintentional overdose. Because suicidal ideation and intent may underlie many overdose events [17], studies have shed light on the importance of further characterizing overdose events with the final goal of deploying specific prevention strategies to individuals with suicidal risk and intent [16,18,19]. While these are important contributions that have brought attention to suicidality as an overdose risk factor, these analyses have been limited to single-site or single system studies, have focused on small samples of OUD patients with self-reported intentionality and outcomes, and have been constrained by patient recall.

The co-occurrence of mental health and substance use disorders increases suicidal ideation and behavior [20]. The identification of suicidality is therefore clinically relevant, particularly among persons with dual disorders [21–23]. The Concise Health Risk Tracking SR (CHRT-SR) [24] is a self-reported measure that—unlike other clinical assessments for suicide [25,26]—assesses other important associated symptoms related to suicide propensity aside from ideation and intent. These include pessimism, lack of social support, helplessness, and despair. The CHRT-SR has proven to have excellent psychometric properties in patients with major depression [24], bipolar disorders [27,28], and stimulant use disorders [29]. Early identification at treatment entry, whether the individual is driven by suicidal thoughts and intent or by hopelessness and despair, expands the opportunities for intervention and could prevent fatalities.

The objective of this study is to evaluate whether suicidality at treatment entry is a baseline predictor of overdose events in patients with SUD, using data from the National Drug Abuse Treatment Clinical Trials Network (CTN) [30] multi-protocol platform and its associated NIDA Data Share website. We predict that those with higher baseline suicidality assessment scores, indicative of suicidal propensity, ideation, and/or intent, will be more likely to have an overdose event than those with lower scores.

2. Methods

The study uses data collected from eight randomized clinical trials that were implemented within the CTN, a network that provides an infrastructure in which the National Institute on Drug Abuse (NIDA), medical and specialty treatment providers, academic centers, researchers, and patients cooperatively develop, validate, refine, and deliver new treatment options for patients with SUD [30]. There are 16 CTN research sites termed 'nodes' in the U.S. that conduct clinical trials across diverse settings and populations. For this study, we analyzed data that was approved for public release or that was publicly available on NIDA Data Share website (https://datashare.nida.nih.gov/ (accessed on 15 February 2022)). Data Share is an electronic environment that allows access to data from completed trials to promote new research using secondary analyses [31].

2.1. Participants

We analyzed data from eight multicenter CTN trials that included 2543 participants [32–39]. Only 2541 participants were included in the analysis (2 participants were excluded due to missing data). Included studies: (1) were completed in the last 10 years (2012–2021), (2) used the CHRT-SR as a measure to assess suicidality of patients at baseline, prior to treatment, and (3) captured overdose events via the adverse event form, death form, and/or hospital utilization form. Trial characteristics are described in Table 1. While each of these eight multisite trials secured approval from their respective Institutional Review Board, the current study only used de-identified data and therefore was exempt from ethical review.

Table 1. Selected CTN Trial Characteristics.

Trial	Study Title	Study Type	Sample Size	Main Target Substance	Recruitment Setting	Intervention Period/Follow Up Period
CTN 0037 [32,40]	Stimulant Reduction Intervention Using Dosed Exercise (STRIDE)	2-arm RCT	302	Stimulants (Cocaine and Methamphetamine)	Residential substance use treatment programs	12 weeks/ 36 weeks
CTN 0049 [33,41]	Project HOPE: Hospital Visit as Opportunity for Prevention and Engagement for HIV-Infected Drug Users	3-arm RCT	801 *	Any substance	Inpatient, Hospitalized, enrolled at bedside	26 weeks/ 52 weeks
CTN 0051 [34,42]	Extended-Release Naltrexone vs. Buprenorphine for Opioid Treatment (X:BOT)	2-arm comparative effectiveness RCT	570	Opioids	Community based treatment programs	24 weeks/ 36 weeks
CTN 0053 [35,43]	Achieving Cannabis Cessation: Evaluating N-Acetylcysteine Treatment (ACCENT)	Double-blind, placebo controlled 2-arm RCT	302	Cannabis	Multicenter, "treatment-seeking cannabis-dependent adults who submit positive urine cannabinoid testing during screening"	12 weeks/ 16 weeks
CTN 0054 [36,44]	Accelerated Development of Additive Pharmacotherapy Treatment (ADAPT)	2-stage pilot study	49	Methamphetamine	Outpatient, community treatment programs	8 weeks/ 9 weeks
CTN 0064 [37,45]	Linkage to Hepatitis C Virus (HCV) Care among HIV/HCV Co-infected Substance Users	2-arm RCT	113	Any substance	Follow up population of CTN 0049	26 weeks/ 52 weeks
CTN 0067 [38,46]	Comparing Treatments for HIV-Infected Opioid Users in an Integrated Care Effectiveness Study (CHOICES) Scale-Up	2-arm RCT	116	Opioids	Primary Care	24 weeks/ 24 weeks
CTN 0068 [39,47]	Accelerated Development of Additive Pharmacotherapy Treatment (ADAPT-2) for Methamphetamine Use Disorder	Double-blind, placebo controlled 2-arm RCT with adaptive design	403	Methamphetamine	Adults 18–65 were recruited from communities near the trial sites with the use of ads and direct referrals	12 weeks/ 16 weeks

RCT: Randomized Controlled Trial. * The CTN 0049 population assessed in this analysis includes only those unduplicated patients ($N = 688$ of 801 total) who were not re-randomized to CTN 0064 ($N = 113$).

2.2. Independent Variable: Suicidality

The independent variable analyzed as the predictor was the baseline suicidality score as measured by the 12-item CHRT-SR [24] that evaluates suicide propensity, ideation, and intent. Items assess signs and symptoms, including characteristics such as pessimism, lack of social support, helplessness, and despair; the last three items assess active suicidal ideation and behavior. Responses are measured by a 5-point Likert scale ranging from strongly disagree (1) to strongly agree (5), with total scores ranging from 12 to 60. The CHRT-SR was also used to create a binary indicator of suicidality if a participant responded "Yes" to any of the three following items indicative of suicidal thoughts: "I have been having thoughts of killing myself", "I have thoughts about how I might kill myself", or "I have a plan to kill myself". The Cronbach's alpha for CHRT-SR was acceptable for all trials (CTN0037: 0.86; CTN0049: 0.91; CTN0051: 0.87; CTN0053: 0.89; CTN0054: 0.87; CTN0064: 0.90; CTN0067: 0.86; CTN0068: 0.89).

2.3. Dependent Variable and Adjudication Process: Overdose Events

An overdose event during the study period, the outcome of interest, was defined as a binary outcome (Present: yes/Absent: no). Responses were determined through a review of the dataset for: (1) MedDRA-Preferred Terms captured in Adverse Event forms, (2) primary cause of death reported on death form, or (3) hospital utilization due to overdose reported on hospitalization forms. Through a rigorous adjudication process, a panel of experts consisting of a subgroup of study co-authors (VEH, RDS, DB, KH, JF, ST) followed explicit steps and key terms recommended by a CTN medical monitor (RK) as they reviewed the recorded adverse events, deaths, and hospitalizations. The key recommended term for adverse event forms was "overdose", but related terms such as acute amphetamine toxidrome, respiratory depression and drug intoxication were considered where the term overdose was not recorded but suspected. For these overdose suspected cases, the medical monitor reviewed narratives from the study forms for an indication of involved substances which were then discussed by the panel to reach consensus on the adjudication of the outcome. For the 2 trials where both the hospitalization and death forms were used (CTN 0049 [33,41] and CTN 0064 [37,45]), the panel reviewed all causes for hospitalization (primary discharge diagnosis) and the primary cause of death as recorded in the database. Deaths due to overdose were listed as "Drug Use/Overdose" or "Substance Use". Key terms used to search the hospitalization events included "Overdose", "Abuse", "Intoxication", and "Detox"; however, all primary discharge diagnoses were considered individually by the panel.

2.4. Covariates

The panel used a process of consensus to decide on the pertinent covariates to include in the model, and the measures that should be used in each trial to ascertain the variables/covariates of interest. Decisions were made based on the literature and standard practice. Demographic covariates considered across the protocols included age, gender, and race/ethnicity.

Given the correlation between depression and suicidality, the prevalence of baseline depression was also assessed by creating a binary indicator of depression using the instrument that had been part of each trial's procedures. Depression measures included the 9-item Patient Health Questionnaire (PHQ-9 [26]: CTN0067 [38,46], CTN0068 [39,47]), the 18-item Brief Symptom Inventory (BSI-18 [48]: CTN0049 [33,41], CTN0064 [37,45]), the Addiction Severity Index Lite (ASI Lite [49];CTN0037 [32,40], CTN0051 [34,42]), the Medical and Psychiatric History (CTN0054 [36,44]), and the Hospital Anxiety and Depression Scale (HADS [50]: CTN0053 [35,43]). Because lifetime heroin use [51], recent alcohol and benzodiazepine use [52], and past psychiatric history [53], increase risk of overdose, these factors were also included as covariates in the model. Each of these covariates was assessed by creating binary variables of each distinct instrument or question across the 8 trials. The assessment of lifetime use of heroin included the Addiction Severity Index Lite (ASI Lite [49]: 0037 [32,40], 0049 [33,41], 0051 [34,42], 0064 [37,45], 0067 [38,46]) and the Alcohol and Substance History (0054 [36,44], 0068 [39,47]). One trial, CTN 0054, did not assess lifetime use of heroin. Recent alcohol and benzodiazepine use was determined by creating a binary indicator using each trial's instrument to assess this variable. The assessment of alcohol and benzodiazepine use was determined by the ASI Lite (0037 [32,40], 0049 [33,41], 0051 [34,42], 0064 [37,45], 0067 [38,46]), and the DSM-5 checklist [54] (CTN0054 [36,44], CTN0053 [35,43], CTN0068 [39,47]). Psychiatric history exclusive of depression was determined as a binary indicator, using each trial's instrument to assess this variable. The assessment of psychiatric history included the Medical History Form (0051 [34,42], 0054 [36,44], 0067 [38,46], 0068 [39,47]), ASI Lite (CTN 0037 [32,40]), Additional Psychiatric Diagnosis Form (CTN0064 [37,45]), and the Mini International Neuropsychiatric Interview, version 6.0 (MINI 6.0 [55]: 0053 [35,43]). For participants in CTN0049, psychiatric diagnosis was considered via two instruments. First, the team reviewed the Initial Hospital Admission form, and included patients as having a history of psychiatric diagnosis if the primary diagnosis during admission and/or any comorbid diagnoses included terms or conditions such as "suicidal ideation", "psychosis", "schizophrenia", "bipolar disorder", "PTSD", "hallucinations", "mood disorder" and "altered mental state". Second, if CTN0049 participants reported that they saw a professional for the primary purpose of getting help for psychological or emotional issues in the past 6 months (Service Utilization Detail Form [33,41]), they were also included as having a history of a mental health diagnosis.

Because these trials were diverse in the study treatments, settings, targeted substance use disorders and specific populations, we included trial as a covariate to account for this variability. Treatment arm (experimental or control) was also included to account for the difference in treatments within trials.

2.5. Analytic Plan

Descriptive statistics, including mean and standard deviation for continuous variables and frequencies and proportions for categorical variables, were calculated across trials and among participants with and without suicidality and with and without overdose events. A multivariate logistic regression, using a generalized estimating equation, analyzed continuous CHRT-SR score at baseline as a predictor of binary overdose event (present/not present), while controlling for covariates. Adjusted odds ratios and 95% confidence intervals were calculated. For all analyses, two-tailed p-values less than 0.05 were considered statistically significant. All analyses were performed using SAS version 9.4 [56].

3. Results

A total of 2541 participants were included in this analysis. The majority of participants were male (67.4%) and the mean age was 39.4 years (SD 11.4); 38.3% were Black, 41.3% White, and 14.4% Hispanic. Recent use of alcohol and benzodiazepines was reported by 60.0% and 15.8%, respectively, and 39.0% reported lifetime use of heroin. With regard to co-occurring mental health conditions, 51.6% scored in the depressed range at baseline, and 50.2% indicated that they had at least one preexisting psychiatric diagnosis. The mean baseline CHRT-SR score was 23.9 (SD 8.5; min 11, max 59). A total of 122 (4.8%) either agreed or strongly agreed with the last three items in the CHRT-SR scale and were categorized as suicidal at baseline. Among those who were suicidal, there was a higher proportion of Black/African American (45.1%), followed by White (38.5%) and Hispanic (13.1%) populations. Seventy-five participants (3.0%) had at least one overdose event during their study participation. Of these 49.3% were white, 26.7% were Black/African American and 20.0% were Hispanic. Of those participants who reported suicidal thoughts and intent, only 6 (4.9%) had an overdose event.

Demographic characteristics of the participants can be found in Table 2, and proportions of gender and of race/ethnicity overall, among those who were suicidal, and among those with an overdose event can be found in Figures 1 and 2. Demographic information by study can be found in the primary outcomes' publications [32–39]. Total participants in analyses varied slightly due to occasional missing data.

Table 2. Participant characteristics overall, by suicidal yes/no, by overdose yes/no.

		Overall (N = 2541) Mean (Standard Deviation) or N (%)	Suicidal * (N = 122) M (SD) or N (%)	Non-Suicidal (N = 2418) M (SD) or N (%)	Mean CHRT-SR Score M (SD)	Yes Overdose (N = 75) M (SD) or N (%)	No Overdose (N = 2466) M (SD) or N (%)
Age		39.4 (11.4)	42.4 (10.5)	39.2 (11.5)	-	39.1 (11.8)	39.4 (11.4)
Sex	Female	829 (32.6%)	28 (23.0%)	800 (33.1%)	23.8 (8.3)	22 (29.3%)	806 (32.7%)
	Male	1712 (67.4%)	94 (77.0%)	1618 (66.9%)	23.9 (8.6)	53 (70.7%)	1659 (67.3%)
Race/Ethnicity	Black/Af Am	972 (38.3%)	55 (45.1%)	916 (37.9%)	23.5 (8.6)	20 (26.7%)	951 (38.6%)
	Hispanic	366 (14.4%)	16 (13.1%)	350 (14.5%)	24.0 (8.4)	15 (20.0%)	351 (14.2%)
	Other	153 (6.0%)	4 (3.3%)	149 (6.2%)	25.0 (8.0)	3 (4.0%)	150 (6.1%)
	White	1050 (41.3%)	47 (38.5%)	1003 (41.5%)	23.9 (8.6)	37 (49.3%)	1013 (41.1%)
Treatment Arm Assignment	Experimental	1310 (51.6%)	64 (52.5%)	1245 (51.5%)	24.0 (8.5)	45 (60.0%)	1265 (51.3%)
	Control	1231 (48.5%)	58 (47.5%)	1173 (48.5%)	23.7 (8.6)	30 (40.0%)	1200 (48.7%)
Depressed	Yes	1310 (51.6%)	112 (91.8%)	1197 (49.5%)	27.0 (8.7)	37 (49.3%)	1273 (51.7%)
	No	1230 (48.4%)	10 (8.2%)	1220 (50.5%)	20.5 (6.9)	38 (50.7%)	1191 (48.3%)
History of Psychiatric Diagnosis	Yes	1276 (50.2%)	75 (61.5%)	1200 (49.6%)	25.2 (8.7)	42 (56.0%)	1233 (50.0%)
	No	1265 (49.8%)	47 (38.5%)	1218 (50.4%)	22.5 (8.1)	33 (44.0%)	1232 (50.0%)
Recent Alcohol Use	Yes	1523 (60.0%)	72 (60.0%)	1450 (60.0%)	23.5 (8.6)	37 (49.3%)	1485 (60.3%)
	No	1016 (40.0%)	48 (40.0%)	968 (40.0%)	24.4 (8.4)	38 (50.7%)	978 (39.7%)
Recent Benzo Use	Yes	400 (15.8%)	19 (15.8%)	381 (15.8%)	25.2 (8.6)	18 (24.0%)	382 (15.5%)
	No	2139 (84.2%)	101 (84.2%)	2037 (84.2%)	23.6 (8.5)	57 (76.0%)	2081 (84.5%)
Lifetime Heroin Use	Yes	992 (39.0%)	41 (33.6%)	951 (39.3%)	25.4 (8.0)	53 (70.7%)	939 (38.1%)
	No	1245 (49.0%)	74 (60.7%)	1170 (48.4%)	23.8 (8.9)	21 (28.0%)	1223 (49.6%)
	Missing	304 (12.0%)	7 (5.7%)	297 (12.3%)	19.1 (7.0)	1 (1.3%)	303 (12.3%)
Suicidal	Yes	122 (4.8%)	122 (4.8%)	-	39.8 (7.9)	6 (8.0%)	116 (4.7%)
	No	2418 (95.2%)	-	2418 (95.2%)	23.1 (7.8)	69 (92.0%)	2348 (95.2%)
Overdose	Yes	75 (3.0%)	6 (4.9%)	69 (2.9%)	25.8 (8.8)	75 (3.0%)	-
	No	2465 (97.0%)	116 (95.1%)	2348 (97.1%)	23.8 (8.5)	-	2465 (97.1%)
CHRT-SR Score		23.9 (8.5)	39.8 (7.8)	23.1 (7.8)	-	25.8 (8.8)	23.8 (8.5)

* One participant is missing from the suicidal total due to missing responses to the last 3 items on CHRT.

Preliminary results of model fit revealed that age, gender, and race/ethnicity were not significant in the model, and therefore dropped from the final model. Results of logistic regression show that the continuous CHRT-SR score was associated ($p = 0.03$) with overdose events and the likelihood of overdose increased as the continuous CHRT-SR score increased (OR 1.02; 95% CI = 1.00–1.04). Depression, recent use of alcohol or benzodiazepines, history of psychiatric disorders, and treatment arm were not associated with higher odds of overdose, but lifetime use of heroin was associated ($p < 0.01$) with increased odds of overdose (OR 3.08; 95% CI = 1.93–4.92). Model results can be found in Table 3.

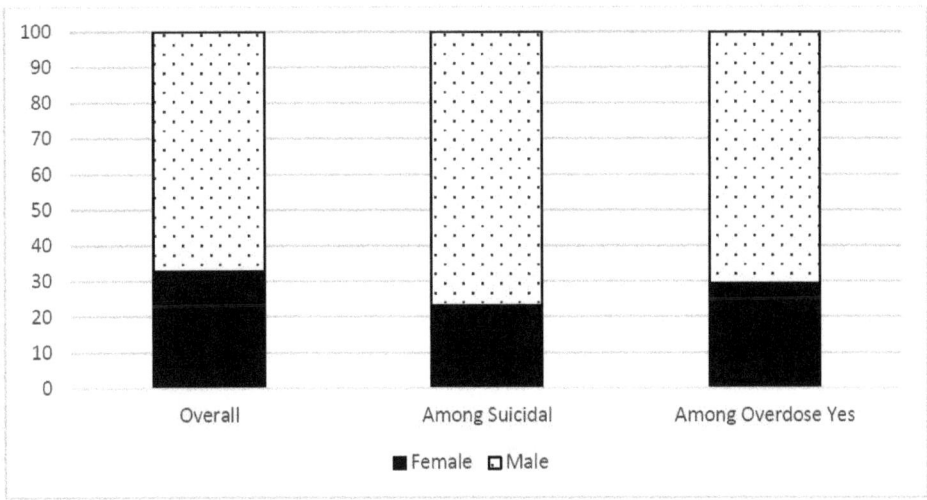

Figure 1. Proportion of Female/Male overall, among those who are suicidal, and among those with an overdose event.

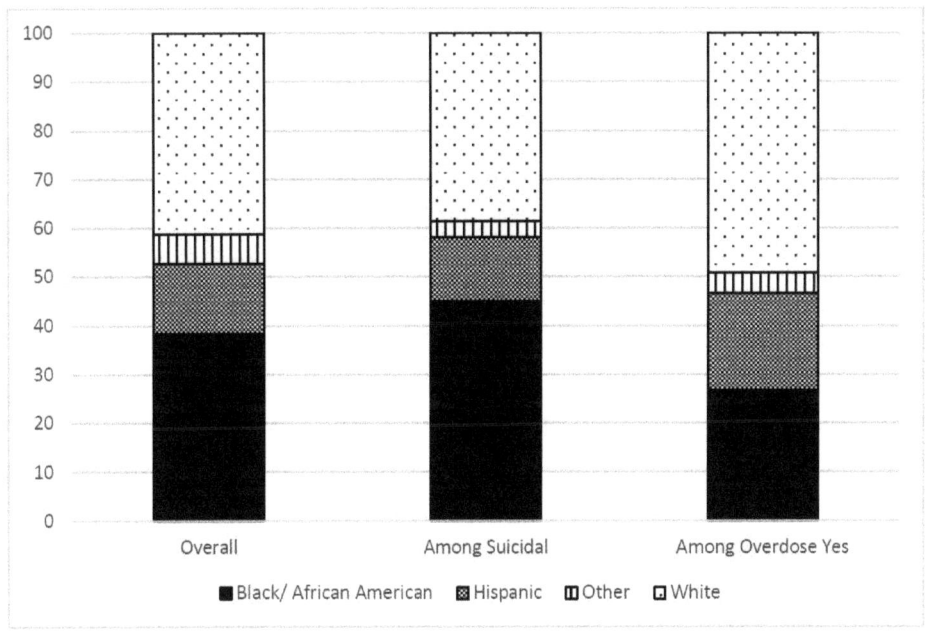

Figure 2. Proportion of Race/Ethnicity overall, among those who are suicidal, and among those with an overdose event.

Table 3. Results of logistic regression/generalized estimating equation assessing CHRT-SR as a continuous predictor of overdose.

		Odds Ratio	95% Confidence Limits		p-Value
CHRT-SR Score		1.02	1.00	1.04	0.03
Depressed	Yes	0.76	0.32	1.83	0.54
	No	0	0	0	
Recent Alcohol Use	Yes	0.81	0.63	1.05	0.11
	No	0	0	0	
Recent Benzo Use	Yes	1.40	0.77	2.54	0.27
	No	0	0	0	
Lifetime Heroin Use	Missing	0.19	0.11	0.32	<0.01
	Yes	3.08	1.93	4.92	<0.01
	No	0	0	0	
History of Psychiatric Diagnosis	Yes	0.85	0.65	1.11	0.23
	No	0	0	0	
Treatment Arm	Experimental	1.48	0.81	2.70	0.20
	Control	0	0	0	.

4. Discussion

Results of this study demonstrate that suicide propensity, ideation and intent, as assessed by the continuous CHRT-SR score, were associated with overdose events amongst patients seeking treatment in eight clinical trials for SUD. Increases in the total score of CHRT-SR were associated with a higher likelihood of experiencing an overdose event. To our knowledge this is the first study exploring the relationship of suicidality and overdose events in a substance-using, treatment-seeking population.

Surprisingly, only 4.8% of the sample endorsed suicidal ideation or intent at baseline. This is possibly explained by the fact that most studies excluded actively suicidal patients at enrollment. Suicidal ideation and intent have not been previously documented systematically during treatment in patients with SUD or dual disorders. Rather, assessments have been based on suicide mortality in these populations. Esang and Ahmed [57] reported an increased risk of suicide in patients with substance use and psychiatric conditions. Increased opioid overdose risk has been described in patients with OUD [58]. Studies assessing suicidal intent after an overdose report highly variable prevalence of suicidal ideation. For example, while one study documented that 58.0% of patients with OUD who overdosed indicated a desire to die [18], another reported only 6.6% of opioid overdose survivors firmly expressed their intent to die [16]. In addition, these retrospective studies relied on patients' self-reports, where reconstruction of the feelings, thoughts, and desire prior to the overdose event might be misconstrued or be prone to recall bias. Suicidal ideation and intent have been documented in prior studies of patients with acute major depression with non-psychotic features. Based on the type of assessment used, the prevalence of suicidal thoughts and intent ranged from 10.7% to 19.0% at baseline [59]. The prevalence of suicidal ideation or intent documented in our study is therefore lower than that observed in patients in treatment for major depression. Of note, the prevalence of depression in our sample was 51.6%, and 50.2% of the participants reported a previous psychiatric history. While the association between depression and SUD in our sample was high, other studies have demonstrated even higher levels of depression in patients with SUD [60].

Results from this study confirm that lifetime heroin use is associated with an increased likelihood of an overdose event. Brandt and colleagues [58] and Stover and colleagues [19] have demonstrated increased risk of opioid overdose events in patients with a history of heroin use. Surprisingly, and in contrast with the literature, neither depression nor recent alcohol or benzodiazepine use were associated with overdose events in our study. This might be explained by the variability in the approach to the assessment of depression across trials, or that participants were only experiencing mild depressive disorders, and therefore, the association with increased overdose was not observed as expected.

Consistent with the literature, overdose events were more frequent in the White population (49.3%), followed by Black/African American (26.7%) and Hispanic (20.0%) populations, whereas suicidality was more frequent in Black/African American (45.1%), followed by White (38.5%) and Hispanic (13.1%) populations. Gicquelais and colleagues [16] found that active or passive suicidal intent was more prevalent in Whites (86.3%) followed by multiracial individuals (9.3%), whereas only 4.3% of the Black/African American sample intended to die. In our study, the choice of substance used may have accounted for the racial/ethnic differences we found. However, this is speculative, given that most of the information on the overdose was self-reported at the time of documentation and was inconsistently documented in the narrative of overdose events, preventing identification of specific substances involved.

The present study has several strengths. First, it provides an examination across multiple sites and multiple studies expanding on prior single site examinations of suicidality and overdose. Second, it expands on the use of large datasets to rapidly answer practical clinical questions and furthers the understanding of mental health conditions and their association with adverse substance use outcomes.

This study also presents several limitations. First, the design of this study only allowed for examination of associations and not causation. Second, the population enrolled across these eight clinical trials is representative of individuals seeking treatment for SUD who agreed to participate in a research study. Therefore, our results might not be generalizable to the entire population of persons with SUD and other co-occurring mental health conditions. It is noteworthy that while the panel of experts ascertained outcomes using a binary yes/no approach for each of the covariates, the measures used to evaluate these variables differed across trials and may have had slightly different meanings. However, the tradeoff of this heterogeneity might be mitigated by the large sample size accrued across multiple sites and conducted over 10 years. Finally, heroin use was not assessed in one of the trials and is reported as missing data in our results.

This study highlights the relevance of assessing suicidality at baseline for patients entering treatment. As drug overdose deaths continue to rise in the U.S. and worldwide and suicide remains a leading cause of death, particularly in patients with comorbid substance abuse and mental health disorders, multi-pronged approaches covering prevention, early detection, and intervention are needed. Integration of suicide risk reduction should be included as part of an overall prevention strategy in response to the steep climb in overdose fatalities. Entry into treatment for SUD and other co-occurring mental health conditions presents an invaluable opportunity to re-set, evaluate suicide risk, and employ early prevention plans.

Author Contributions: V.E.H. formulated the research question and drafted the first version of the manuscript. D.S.-B., K.H., J.F., S.T., V.E.H. and R.D.S. reviewed and decided on measures for all covariates across trials. D.J.F. provided methodological guidance and approach for the model created for data analysis. R.D.S. drafted the methods section and performed the analyses, with support of R.D. R.K. serves as the medical monitor at the Emmes company and provided guidance to the expert panel. D.S.-B., K.H., J.F., S.T., R.K., V.E.H. and R.D.S. are the expert panel members who adjudicated the outcomes. R.M.-N. guided on journal fit and contributed to revisions to the manuscript. S.G. and C.D. conducted literature searches and background review and contributed to the referencing system. All authors have read and agreed to the published version of the manuscript.

Funding: Research reported in this publication was supported by the National Institute on Drug Abuse of the National Institutes of Health under Award Numbers UG1DA013720, 2UG1DA049436, U54GM104942, UG1DA013035-09, 2UG1DA049436-01, 75N95019D00013/N01DA-19-2250 (NIDA DSC contract to The Emmes Company, LLC), and 75N95020D00012/N01DA-20-2251 (NIDA CCC contract to The Emmes Company, LLC). The content is solely the responsibility of the authors and does not necessarily represent the official views of the National Institutes of Health.

Institutional Review Board Statement: Each of the 8 multisite trials secured approval from their respective Institutional Review Board. However, the current study only used de-identified data and therefore was exempt from ethical review.

Informed Consent Statement: Not applicable.

Data Availability Statement: CTN trial data is publicly available on NIDA Data Share: https://datashare.nida.nih.gov/ (accessed on 15 February 2022). CTN 0064, CTN 0067 and 0068 data has been approved for upload onto NIDA Data Share and will be publicly available soon.

Acknowledgments: We would like to acknowledge the Principal Investigators from the 8 CTN trials: Madhukar Trivedi (CTN0037, CTN0068); Lisa Metsch (CTN0049, CTN0064), John Rotrosen (CTN0051); Edward Nunes (CTN0051); Kevin Gray (CTN0053); Walter Ling (CTN0054); Larissa Mooney (CTN0054); and Todd Korthuis (CTN0067) for their support for this study. We also want to acknowledge The Emmes company for provision of coordination, regulatory oversight and data management and analysis for all the trials covered by this work. Finally, we would like to acknowledge the Center for the National Drug Abuse Treatment Clinical Trials Network, Betty Tai and her team for the support of the Comorbidity Special Interest Group from which this analysis was developed.

Conflicts of Interest: The authors declare no conflict of interest.

References

1. O'Donnell, J.; Tanz, L.J.; Gladden, R.M.; Davis, N.L.; Bitting, J. Trends in and Characteristics of Drug Overdose Deaths Involving Illicitly Manufactured Fentanyls—United States, 2019–2020. *MMWR Morb. Mortal. Wkly. Rep.* **2021**, *70*, 1740–1746. [CrossRef]
2. Han, B.; Compton, W.M.; Jones, C.M.; Einstein, E.B.; Volkow, N.D. Methamphetamine Use, Methamphetamine Use Disorder, and Associated Overdose Deaths Among US Adults. *JAMA Psychiatry* **2021**, *78*, 1329–1342. [CrossRef]
3. Ellis, M.S.; Kasper, Z.A.; Cicero, T.J. Polysubstance use trends and variability among individuals with opioid use disorder in rural versus urban settings. *Prev. Med.* **2021**, *152*, 106729. [CrossRef]
4. Compton, W.M.; Valentino, R.J.; DuPont, R.L. Polysubstance use in the U.S. opioid crisis. *Mol. Psychiatry* **2021**, *26*, 41–50. [CrossRef]
5. WHO. *Lexicon of Alcohol and Drug Terms*; World Health Organization: Geneva, Switzerland, 1994.
6. Vekaria, V.; Bose, B.; Murphy, S.M.; Avery, J.; Alexopoulos, G.; Pathak, J. Association of co-occurring opioid or other substance use disorders with increased healthcare utilization in patients with depression. *Transl. Psychiatry* **2021**, *11*, 265. [CrossRef]
7. Tormohlen, K.N.; Mojtabai, R.; Seiwell, A.; McGinty, E.E.; Stuart, E.A.; Tobin, K.E.; Troiani, V. Co-Occurring Opioid Use and Depressive Disorders: Patient Characteristics and Co-Occurring Health Conditions. *J. Dual Diagn.* **2021**, *17*, 296–303. [CrossRef]
8. Conway, K.P.; Compton, W.; Stinson, F.S.; Grant, B.F. Lifetime comorbidity of DSM-IV mood and anxiety disorders and specific drug use disorders: Results from the National Epidemiologic Survey on Alcohol and Related Conditions. *J. Clin. Psychiatry* **2006**, *67*, 247–257. [CrossRef]
9. Meier, A.; Lambert-Harris, C.; McGovern, M.P.; Xie, H.; An, M.; McLeman, B. Co-occurring prescription opioid use problems and posttraumatic stress disorder symptom severity. *Am. J. Drug Alcohol Abuse* **2014**, *40*, 304–311. [CrossRef]
10. Liu, S.; Nwabueze, C.; Pan, Y.; Walter, S.M.; Su, B.; Xu, C.; Winstanley, E.L.; Wang, K. Polysubstance Use, Mood Disorders, and Chronic Conditions With Anxiety in Opioid Patients. *West. J. Nurs. Res.* **2021**. [CrossRef] [PubMed]
11. Chakravorty, S.; Vandrey, R.G.; He, S.; Stein, M.D. Sleep Management Among Patients with Substance Use Disorders. *Med. Clin. N. Am.* **2018**, *102*, 733–743. [CrossRef]
12. Saunders, E.C.; Lambert-Harris, C.; McGovern, M.P.; Meier, A.; Xie, H. The Prevalence of Posttraumatic Stress Disorder Symptoms among Addiction Treatment Patients with Cocaine Use Disorders. *J. Psychoact. Drugs* **2015**, *47*, 42–50. [CrossRef] [PubMed]
13. Keen, C.; Kinner, S.A.; Young, J.T.; Jang, K.; Gan, W.; Samji, H.; Zhao, B.; Krausz, M.; Slaunwhite, A. Prevalence of co-occurring mental illness and substance use disorder and association with overdose: A linked data cohort study among residents of British Columbia, Canada. *Addiction* **2022**, *117*, 129–140. [CrossRef] [PubMed]
14. Keen, C.; Young, J.T.; Borschmann, R.; Kinner, S.A. Non-fatal drug overdose after release from prison: A prospective data linkage study. *Drug Alcohol Depend.* **2020**, *206*, 107707. [CrossRef]
15. Hedegaard, H.; Curtin, S.C.; Warner, M. Suicide Mortality in the United States, 1999–2019. *NCHS Data Brief* **2020**, 1–8. [CrossRef]
16. Gicquelais, R.E.; Jannausch, M.; Bohnert, A.S.B.; Thomas, L.; Sen, S.; Fernandez, A.C. Links between suicidal intent, polysubstance use, and medical treatment after non-fatal opioid overdose. *Drug Alcohol Depend.* **2020**, *212*, 108041. [CrossRef]
17. Bohnert, A.S.B.; Walton, M.A.; Cunningham, R.M.; Ilgen, M.A.; Barry, K.; Chermack, S.T.; Blow, F.C. Overdose and adverse drug event experiences among adult patients in the emergency department. *Addict. Behav.* **2018**, *86*, 66–72. [CrossRef]

18. Connery, H.S.; Taghian, N.; Kim, J.; Griffin, M.; Rockett, I.R.H.; Weiss, R.D.; Kathryn McHugh, R. Suicidal motivations reported by opioid overdose survivors: A cross-sectional study of adults with opioid use disorder. *Drug Alcohol Depend.* **2019**, *205*, 107612. [CrossRef]
19. Stover, A.N.; Rockett, I.R.H.; Smith, G.S.; LeMasters, T.; Scott, V.G.; Kelly, K.M.; Winstanley, E.L. Distinguishing clinical factors associated with unintentional overdose, suicidal ideation, and attempted suicide among opioid use disorder in-patients. *J. Psychiatr. Res.* **2022**, *153*, 245–253. [CrossRef]
20. Bohnert, A.S.B.; Ilgen, M.A. Understanding Links among Opioid Use, Overdose, and Suicide. *N. Engl. J. Med.* **2019**, *380*, 71–79. [CrossRef]
21. Abroms, M.; Sher, L. Dual Disorders and Suicide. *J. Dual Diagn.* **2016**, *12*, 148–149. [CrossRef]
22. Ponizovsky, A.M.; Rosca, P.; Haklai, Z.; Goldberger, N. Trends in dual diagnosis of severe mental illness and substance use disorders, 1996–2010, Israel. *Drug Alcohol Depend.* **2015**, *148*, 203–208. [CrossRef]
23. Szerman, N.; Lopez-Castroman, J.; Arias, F.; Morant, C.; Babin, F.; Mesias, B.; Basurte, I.; Vega, P.; Baca-Garcia, E. Dual diagnosis and suicide risk in a Spanish outpatient sample. *Subst. Use Misuse* **2012**, *47*, 383–389. [CrossRef]
24. Trivedi, M.H.; Wisniewski, S.R.; Morris, D.W.; Fava, M.; Gollan, J.K.; Warden, D.; Nierenberg, A.A.; Gaynes, B.N.; Husain, M.M.; Luther, J.F.; et al. Concise Health Risk Tracking scale: A brief self-report and clinician rating of suicidal risk. *J. Clin. Psychiatry* **2011**, *72*, 757–764. [CrossRef]
25. Posner, K.; Brown, G.K.; Stanley, B.; Brent, D.A.; Yershova, K.V.; Oquendo, M.A.; Currier, G.W.; Melvin, G.A.; Greenhill, L.; Shen, S.; et al. The Columbia-Suicide Severity Rating Scale: Initial validity and internal consistency findings from three multisite studies with adolescents and adults. *Am. J. Psychiatry* **2011**, *168*, 1266–1277. [CrossRef]
26. Kroenke, K.; Spitzer, R.L.; Williams, J.B. The PHQ-9: Validity of a brief depression severity measure. *J. Gen. Intern. Med.* **2001**, *16*, 606–613. [CrossRef]
27. Villegas, A.C.; DuBois, C.M.; Celano, C.M.; Beale, E.E.; Mastromauro, C.A.; Stewart, J.G.; Auerbach, R.P.; Huffman, J.C.; Hoeppner, B.B. A longitudinal investigation of the Concise Health Risk Tracking Self-Report (CHRT-SR) in suicidal patients during and after hospitalization. *Psychiatry Res.* **2018**, *262*, 558–565. [CrossRef]
28. Ostacher, M.J.; Nierenberg, A.A.; Rabideau, D.; Reilly-Harrington, N.A.; Sylvia, L.G.; Gold, A.K.; Shesler, L.W.; Ketter, T.A.; Bowden, C.L.; Calabrese, J.R.; et al. A clinical measure of suicidal ideation, suicidal behavior, and associated symptoms in bipolar disorder: Psychometric properties of the Concise Health Risk Tracking Self-Report (CHRT-SR). *J. Psychiatr. Res.* **2015**, *71*, 126–133. [CrossRef]
29. Sanchez, K.; Killian, M.O.; Mayes, T.L.; Greer, T.L.; Trombello, J.M.; Lindblad, R.; Grannemann, B.D.; Carmody, T.J.; Rush, A.J.; Walker, R.; et al. A psychometric evaluation of the Concise Health Risk Tracking Self-Report (CHRT-SR)- a measure of suicidality-in patients with stimulant use disorder. *J. Psychiatr. Res.* **2018**, *102*, 65–71. [CrossRef]
30. NIDA. About the CTN. Available online: https://nida.nih.gov/about-nida/organization/cctn/ctn/about-ctn (accessed on 20 April 2022).
31. NIDA. Data Share Website: Home. Available online: https://datashare.nida.nih.gov/ (accessed on 20 May 2022).
32. Trivedi, M.H.; Greer, T.L.; Rethorst, C.D.; Carmody, T.; Grannemann, B.D.; Walker, R.; Warden, D.; Shores-Wilson, K.; Stoutenberg, M.; Oden, N.; et al. Randomized Controlled Trial Comparing Exercise to Health Education for Stimulant Use Disorder: Results From the CTN-0037 STimulant Reduction Intervention Using Dosed Exercise (STRIDE) Study. *J. Clin. Psychiatry* **2017**, *78*, 1075–1082. [CrossRef]
33. Metsch, L.R.; Feaster, D.J.; Gooden, L.; Matheson, T.; Stitzer, M.; Das, M.; Jain, M.K.; Rodriguez, A.E.; Armstrong, W.S.; Lucas, G.M.; et al. Effect of Patient Navigation With or Without Financial Incentives on Viral Suppression Among Hospitalized Patients With HIV Infection and Substance Use: A Randomized Clinical Trial. *JAMA* **2016**, *316*, 156–170. [CrossRef]
34. Lee, J.D.; Nunes, E.V., Jr.; Novo, P.; Bachrach, K.; Bailey, G.L.; Bhatt, S.; Farkas, S.; Fishman, M.; Gauthier, P.; Hodgkins, C.C.; et al. Comparative effectiveness of extended-release naltrexone versus buprenorphine-naloxone for opioid relapse prevention: A multicentre, open-label, randomised controlled trial. *Lancet* **2018**, *391*, 309–318. [CrossRef]
35. Gray, K.M.; Sonne, S.C.; McClure, E.A.; Ghitza, U.E.; Matthews, A.G.; McRae-Clark, A.L.; Carroll, K.M.; Potter, J.S.; Wiest, K.; Mooney, L.J.; et al. A randomized placebo-controlled trial of N-acetylcysteine for cannabis use disorder in adults. *Drug Alcohol Depend.* **2017**, *177*, 249–257. [CrossRef] [PubMed]
36. Mooney, L.J.; Hillhouse, M.P.; Thomas, C.; Ang, A.; Sharma, G.; Terry, G.; Chang, L.; Walker, R.; Trivedi, M.; Croteau, D.; et al. Utilizing a Two-stage Design to Investigate the Safety and Potential Efficacy of Monthly Naltrexone Plus Once-daily Bupropion as a Treatment for Methamphetamine Use Disorder. *J. Addict. Med.* **2016**, *10*, 236–243. [CrossRef] [PubMed]
37. Metsch, L.R.; Feaster, D.J.; Gooden, L.K.; Masson, C.; Perlman, D.C.; Jain, M.K.; Matheson, T.; Nelson, C.M.; Jacobs, P.; Tross, S.; et al. Care Facilitation Advances Movement Along the Hepatitis C Care Continuum for Persons With Human Immunodeficiency Virus, Hepatitis C, and Substance Use: A Randomized Clinical Trial (CTN-0064). *Open Forum Infect. Dis.* **2021**, *8*, ofab334. [CrossRef]
38. Korthuis, P.T.; Cook, R.R.; Lum, P.J.; Waddell, E.N.; Tookes, H.; Vergara-Rodriguez, P.; Kunkel, L.E.; Lucas, G.M.; Rodriguez, A.E.; Bielavitz, S.; et al. HIV clinic-based extended-release naltrexone versus treatment as usual for people with HIV and opioid use disorder: A non-blinded, randomized non-inferiority trial. *Addiction* **2022**, *117*, 1961–1971. [CrossRef]
39. Trivedi, M.H.; Walker, R.; Ling, W.; Dela Cruz, A.; Sharma, G.; Carmody, T.; Ghitza, U.E.; Wahle, A.; Kim, M.; Shores-Wilson, K.; et al. Bupropion and Naltrexone in Methamphetamine Use Disorder. *N. Engl. J. Med.* **2021**, *384*, 140–153. [CrossRef]

40. NIDA. Protocol NIDA-CTN-0037: Stimulant Reduction Intervention Using Dosed Exercise (STRIDE). Available online: http://ctndisseminationlibrary.org/protocols/ctn0037.htm (accessed on 10 July 2022).
41. NIDA. Protocol NIDA-CTN-0049: Project HOPE Hospital Visit as Oopportunity for Prevention and Engagement for HIV-Infected Drug Users. Available online: http://ctndisseminationlibrary.org/protocols/ctn0049.htm (accessed on 10 July 2022).
42. NIDA. Protocol NIDA-CTN-0051: Extended-Release Naltrexone vs. Buprenorphine for Opioid Treatment (X:BOT). Available online: http://ctndisseminationlibrary.org/protocols/ctn0051.htm (accessed on 10 July 2022).
43. NIDA. Protocol NIDA-CTN-0053: Achieving Cannabis Cessation- Evaluating N-Acetylcysteine Treatment (ACCENT). Available online: http://ctndisseminationlibrary.org/protocols/ctn0053.htm (accessed on 10 July 2022).
44. NIDA. Protcol NIDA-CTN-0054: Accelerated Development of Additive Pharmacotherapy Treatment (ADAPT) for Methamphetamine Use Disorder. Available online: http://ctndisseminationlibrary.org/protocols/ctn0054.htm (accessed on 10 July 2022).
45. NIDA. Protocol NIDA-CTN-0064: Linkage to Hepatitis C Virus (HCV) Care Among HIV/HCV Co-infected Substance Users. Available online: http://ctndisseminationlibrary.org/protocols/ctn0064.htm (accessed on 10 July 2022).
46. NIDA. Protocol NIDA-CTN-0067: Comparing Treatments for HIV-Positive Opioid Users in an Integrated Care Effectiveness Study (CHOICES: Scale-Up. Available online: http://ctndisseminationlibrary.org/protocols/ctn0067.htm (accessed on 10 July 2022).
47. NIDA. Protocol NIDA-CTN-0068: Accelerated Development of Additive Pharmacotherapy Treatment (ADAPT-2) for Methamphetamine Use Disorder. Available online: http://ctndisseminationlibrary.org/protocols/ctn0068.htm (accessed on 10 July 2022).
48. Derogatis, L. *Brief Symptom Inventory (BSI) 18: Administration, Scoring, and Procedures Manual*, 3rd ed.; National Computer Systems: Minneapolis, MN, USA, 2000.
49. McLellan, A.T.; Kushner, H.; Metzger, D.; Peters, R.; Smith, I.; Grissom, G.; Pettinati, H.; Argeriou, M. The Fifth Edition of the Addiction Severity Index. *J. Subst. Abuse Treat.* **1992**, *9*, 199–213. [CrossRef]
50. Zigmond, A.S.; Snaith, R.P. The hospital anxiety and depression scale. *Acta Psychiatr. Scand.* **1983**, *67*, 361–370. [CrossRef]
51. Siegler, A.; Tuazon, E.; Bradley O'Brien, D.; Paone, D. Unintentional opioid overdose deaths in New York City, 2005–2010: A place-based approach to reduce risk. *Int. J. Drug Policy* **2014**, *25*, 569–574. [CrossRef]
52. Riley, E.D.; Evans, J.L.; Hahn, J.A.; Briceno, A.; Davidson, P.J.; Lum, P.J.; Page, K. A Longitudinal Study of Multiple Drug Use and Overdose Among Young People Who Inject Drugs. *Am. J. Public Health* **2016**, *106*, 915–917. [CrossRef]
53. Zedler, B.; Xie, L.; Wang, L.; Joyce, A.; Vick, C.; Brigham, J.; Kariburyo, F.; Baser, O.; Murrelle, L. Development of a Risk Index for Serious Prescription Opioid-Induced Respiratory Depression or Overdose in Veterans' Health Administration Patients. *Pain Med.* **2015**, *16*, 1566–1579. [CrossRef] [PubMed]
54. Association, A.P. *Diagnostic and Statistical Manual of Mental Disorders (DSM-5) Fifth Edition*, 5th ed.; American Psychiatric Association: Washington, DC, USA, 2013.
55. Sheehan, D.V.; Lecrubier, Y.; Sheehan, K.H.; Amorim, P.; Janavs, J.; Weiller, E.; Hergueta, T.; Baker, R.; Dunbar, G.C. The Mini-International Neuropsychiatric Interview (M.I.N.I.): The development and validation of a structured diagnostic psychiatric interview for DSM-IV and ICD-10. *J. Clin. Psychiatry* **1998**, *59* (Suppl. 20), 22–33. [PubMed]
56. SAS Institute Inc. *SAS® OnDemand for Academics: User's Guide*; SAS Institute Inc.: Cary, NC, USA, 2014.
57. Esang, M.; Ahmed, S. A Closer Look at Substance Use and Suicide. *Am. J. Psychiatry* **2018**, *13*, 6–8. [CrossRef]
58. Brandt, L.; Hu, M.; Liu, Y.; Castillo, F.; Odom, G.; Balise, R.; Feaster, D.; Nunes, E.; Luo, S. *Risks of Overdose Events for Patients Undergoing Opioid Use Disorder Treatment*; The College on Problems of Drug Dependence: Minneapolis, MN, USA, 2022.
59. De La Garza, N.; Rush, A.J.; Killian, M.O.; Grannemann, B.D.; Carmody, T.J.; Trivedi, M.H. The Concise Health Risk Tracking Self-Report (CHRT-SR) assessment of suicidality in depressed outpatients: A psychometric evaluation. *Depress. Anxiety* **2019**, *36*, 313–320. [CrossRef]
60. Mohamed, I.I.; Ahmad, H.E.K.; Hassaan, S.; Hassan, S. Assessment of anxiety and depression among substance use disorder patients: A case-control study. *Middle East Curr. Psychiatry* **2020**, *27*, 22. [CrossRef]

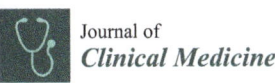

Article

Dual Disorders in the Consultation Liaison Addiction Service: Gender Perspective and Quality of Life

Teresa Ferrer-Farré [1,2,†], Fernando Dinamarca [3,4,†], Joan Ignasi Mestre-Pintó [1,4], Francina Fonseca [1,3,4,*] and Marta Torrens [2,3,4]

1. Department of Experimental and Health Sciences (CEXS), Universitat Pompeu Fabra, 08002 Barcelona, Spain; teresaff95@gmail.com (T.F.-F.); jmestre@imim.es (J.I.M.-P.)
2. Department of Psychiatry and Legal Medicine, Universitat Autònoma de Barcelona, 08290 Cerdanyola del Vallès, Spain; mtorrens@parcdesalutmar.cat
3. Institute of Neuropsychiatry and Addictions, Parc de Salut Mar, 08003 Barcelona, Spain; fdinamarca@psmar.cat
4. Addiction Research Group, IMIM-Institut Hospital del Mar d'Investigacions Mèdiques, 08003 Barcelona, Spain
* Correspondence: mffonseca@psmar.cat
† These authors contributed equally to this work.

Abstract: Dual disorders (DD) and gender differences comprise an area of considerable concern in patients with substance use disorder (SUD). This study aims to describe the presence of DD among patients with SUD admitted to a general hospital and attended by a consultation liaison addiction service (CLAS), in addition to assessing its association with addiction severity and quality of life from a gender perspective, between 1 January and 30 September 2020. The dual diagnosis screening interview (DDSI), the severity of dependence scale (SDS), and the WHO well-being index were used to evaluate the patients. In the overall sample, DD prevalence was 36.8%, (women: 53.8% vs. men: 32.7%, NS). In both genders the most prevalent DD was depression (33.8%, women: 46.2% vs. men: 30.9%, $p = 0.296$). Women presented more panic disorders (46.2% vs. 12.7%, $p = 0.019$) and generalized anxiety (38.5% vs. 10.9%, $p = 0.049$) than men. When DD was present, women had worse quality of life than men (21.7 vs. 50 points, $p = 0.02$). During lockdown period 77 patients were attended to and 13 had COVID-19 infection, with no differences in relation to sociodemographic and consumption history variables. The study confirms a high prevalence of DD among patients with SUD admitted to a general hospital for any pathology, and its being associated with worse quality of life, particularly in women.

Keywords: dual diagnosis; substance use disorders; consultation liaison service; quality of life; gender

1. Introduction

Dual disorder (DD) is the coexistence in the same patient of a substance use disorder (SUD) and another psychiatric condition [1]. Whilst not a new phenomenon, it is gaining importance due to its marked prevalence and complexity with respect to the clinical approach of such patients.

Several studies show that, compared with patients with only SUD, DD patients require a greater number of emergency room admissions and hospitalizations in psychiatry services. They also present higher suicide rates and more risky behaviour associated with mortality and infectious diseases, such as HIV and hepatitis viruses [2,3]. Moreover, in addition to more frequent episodes of violent behaviour, such patients have greater social problems (higher unemployment rates) [4]. Consequently, DD patients present a greater risk of addiction chronicity and severity, their treatment is more difficult and expensive, and they have a worse prognosis than those with only one psychiatric disorder (SUD or other) [5,6].

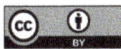

It has also been observed that DD patients have a worse perceived quality of life (QoL) than those with only SUD, a little-studied parameter that is gaining relevance as an indicator of the results of the treatments offered [7–10].

To date, studies carried out to determine DD prevalence in mental health units and addiction services have reported a high incidence in both cases [11–13]. To the best of our knowledge, however, no studies have been performed analysing this prevalence in patients admitted to a general hospital, beyond the emergency room, for any health reason besides SUD. Furthermore, in recent years, interest in gender perspective in the study of addictions has increased [14]. Gender plays a crucial role in determining vulnerability, clinical presentation, and treatment outcomes in patients with SUD. Women are more vulnerable than men in the addiction process, since they progress more quickly from the first substance contact to their addiction (telescoping effect), requiring less dose and time of use to reach a greater degree of addiction severity [14–16]. Women with SUD present more medical and psychiatric comorbidities than their male counterparts [17]. In women with SUD (compared to men with SUD) a higher prevalence of infections (HIV, HCV, etc.) has been observed, and in terms of DD, the most common psychiatric disorders are depression, anxiety, and post-traumatic stress disorders (PTSD). Finally, a higher incidence of gender-based violence and history of sexual abuse has been detected among women with SUD, leading them to being more susceptible to psychiatric illness and a resulting worse perceived QoL than SUD men [18–20].

The objective of the present study was to analyse DD prevalence among patients with SUD admitted to a general hospital for any health problem, whether related to their addiction or not. They were attended by a consultation liaison addiction service (CLAS), which assessed addiction severity and perceived QoL in addition to a gender perspective. The study was interrupted by the COVID-19 lockdown; consequently, as a secondary objective, we compared the characteristics of patients attending CLAS during those months who were unable to receive face-to-face interview assessment.

2. Materials and Methods

2.1. Participants

The study sample was made up of patients with an SUD diagnosis according to DSM 5 criteria [21] admitted to a general hospital (Hospital del Mar) for any health problem, whether directly related to their addiction or not, and attended by the CLAS. Patient recruitment of patients was carried out between 1 January and 30 September 2020.

2.2. Inclusion and Exclusion Criteria

Inclusion criteria were: (1) patients with any SUD diagnosis admitted and assessed by the CLAS at Hospital del Mar; (2) being over 18 years of age; and (3) speaking/understanding Spanish. Exclusion criteria were: (1) documented mental retardation/moderate-severe neurocognitive impairment, with prior neuropsychological evaluation or assessed in the psychopathological examination and the Spanish version of the Montreal Cognitive Assessment 26 (MOCA 26) test [22] (a score 10–17 indicating moderate neurocognitive deterioration, and less than 10 severe neurocognitive deterioration); (2) acute confusional disorder (according to psychopathological examination); (3) not speaking/understanding Spanish; and (4) the patient's clinical condition hindering evaluation. If any of the exclusion criteria were transitory (such as delirium or intoxication), the interview was carried out once the condition had improved.

2.3. Assessment Instruments

For DD screening, a dual diagnostic screening interview (DDSI) was used [23]. DDSI is an instrument that assesses the following mental conditions: panic disorder, generalized anxiety disorder, specific phobia, social phobia, agoraphobia, depression, dysthymia, mania, psychosis, attention deficit hyperactivity disorder (ADHD), and PTSD. The diagnoses obtained with the DDSI are lifetime psychiatric diagnoses.

QoL was evaluated with the WHO well-being index [24]. This self-administered tool consists of 5 questions that refer to the physical–emotional state of the patient in the previous 2 weeks. The total score obtained ranges from 0 to 100 points, and the higher the score the greater the well-being.

Addiction severity was measured with the Spanish version of the Severity of Dependence Scale (SDS) [25,26], The self-administered SDS consists of 5 questions referring to substance use in the previous year. The total score ranges from 0 to 15 points, a higher score indicates a greater degree of dependence on the substance in question.

2.4. Procedure

The CLAS at Hospital del Mar receives daily requests for interventions with patients who present an SUD concomitantly to their cause of admission. As part of standard procedure, clinical and sociodemographic data are collected in a database and include details of substance use and comorbidities (including serological status of HIV and hepatitis viruses). Patients who met the inclusion criteria were informed and, if they agreed to participate, an independent researcher conducted the study. DDSI was performed first followed by the WHO Well-being Index and the SDS. The total time of the evaluation was a maximum of 25–30 min.

Due to the COVID-19 lockdown (from 10 March 2020 to 22 June 2020) the independent researcher had no face-to-face access to the patients. Basic sociodemographic and clinical data gathered from the CLAS in this period were analysed.

2.5. Analysis of Data

A descriptive analysis of variables was carried out and possible differences by gender from the interviews were analysed. To do so, the mean, median, standard deviation, range, and frequency were calculated according to the nature of each variable. Kolmogorov–Smirnov normality tests were performed and, consequently, non-parametric tests were used. For the comparison of means between groups the Mann–Whitney and Wilcoxon U tests and Chi-square for categorical variables were employed. All calculations were carried out using the IBM (IBM Corp. Released 2013. IBM SPSS Statistics for Windows, Version 22.0. Armonk, NY, USA: IBM Corp.).

2.6. Ethics

Patients who met the inclusion criteria were informed of the characteristics of the study and the confidentiality of data processing. Prior to the interview they were asked to sign an informed consent. There was no impact on the patients' usual treatment. The study was approved by the Parc de Salut Mar Clinical Research Ethics Committee (SEIC-PSMAR); CEIm project number: 2019/8970/I.

3. Results

During the entire period of study, a total of 233 patients were admitted by the CLAS. In the lockdown period (from 10 March 2020 to 22 June 2020) 77 patients were only attended by the liaison team and were included for a separate analysis. Of the 156, a total of 104 were candidates, and 68 patients completed the assessment interviews and were included for the principal objective (see Figure 1). There were no differences in gender proportion or other sociodemographic variables of the included patients versus the non-included ones.

3.1. Sociodemographic Characteristics

The characteristics of the 68 patients that completed the interview are shown in Table 1. Women (n = 13) represented 19% of the sample. Mean age was 50.99 years (SD = 11.67) and there were no differences between genders. Neither were there gender differences found with respect to civil status, employment situation, living conditions, and criminal records (Table 1).

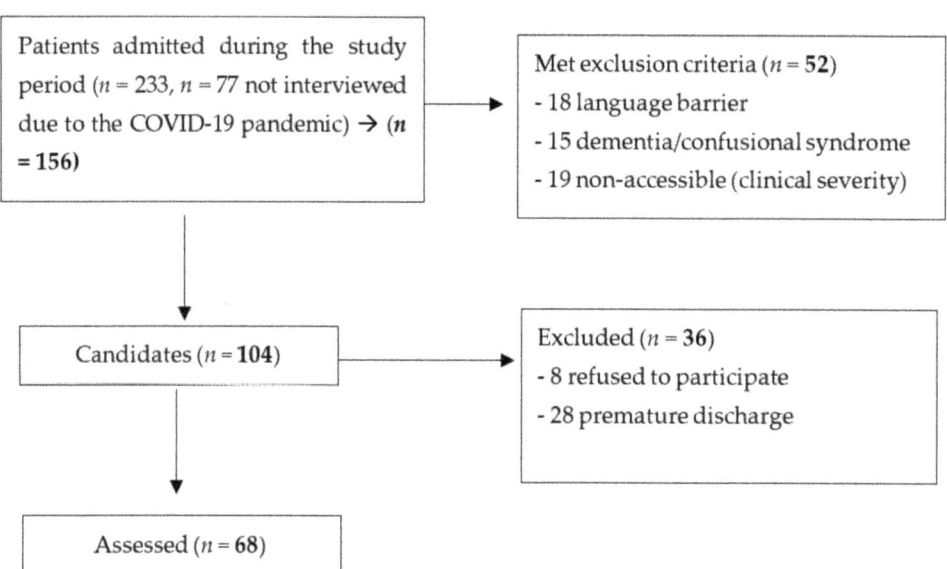

Figure 1. Flowchart for study enrolment.

Table 1. Demographic characteristics of the sample stratified by gender.

	Women n = 13	Men n = 55	Participants n = 68	
	n (%)	n (%)	n (%)	p
Age (mean ± SD) years	47.92 ± 10.15	51.71 ± 11.97	50.99 ± 11.67	0.310
Civil status				
Single	5 (41.7)	23 (43.4)	28 (41.1)	0.433
Married/partner	3 (25)	13 (24.5)	16 (23.5)	
Others	5 (38.4)	19 (34.5)	24 (35.2)	
Origin				0.217
National	11 (84.6)	37 (67.3)	48 (70.6)	
Employment situation				
Employed	1 (8.3)	7 (12.7)	8 (11.7)	0.740
Unemployed	8 (66.7)	25 (45.4)	33 (48.5)	
Retired	4 (25)	11 (20)	15 (22.1)	
Others	0	12 (21.8)	12 (17.6)	
Living with				
Nobody	0	13 (23.6)	13 (19.7)	0.336
Family	9 (69.2)	21 (38.1)	30 (45.5)	
Homeless	3 (23.1)	13 (23.6)	16 (24.2)	
Others	1 (7.7)	8 (15.5)	9 (13.2)	
Criminal records				0.559
No	8 (72.7)	35 (67.3)	43 (63.2)	

SD: Standard deviation.

3.2. Clinical Characteristics

The clinical characteristics of the 68 patients are shown in Table 2. Regarding the main drug of use, alcohol was present in 47.1% of the patients, followed by opiates (38.2%) and cocaine (10.3%), with no differences by gender.

Table 2. Clinical characteristics of the sample, stratified by gender.

		Women (n = 13)	Men (n = 55)	Participants (n = 68)	
		n%	n%	n%	p
Main drug:	Opiates	5 (38.5)	21 (38.2)	26 (38.2)	
	Alcohol	6 (46.2)	26 (47.3)	32 (47.1)	
	Cocaine	2 (15.4)	5 (9.1)	7 (10.3)	0.896
	Amphetamines	0	2 (3.6)	2 (3)	
	Tobacco	0	1 (1.8)	1 (1.5)	
Commencement age of main drug ($\bar{x} \pm$ SD), years		23 ± 8.26	17.83 ± 5.91	18.71 ± 6.59	**0.018**
Total abstinence time ($\bar{x} \pm$ SD), months		18.73 ± 24.50	25.31 ± 37.28	24.15 ± 35.27	0.903
Time since last consumption of the main drug ($\bar{x} \pm$ SD), months		6.08 ± 20.76	3.98 ± 14.30	4.37 ± 15.54	0.850
Patients previously involved in an addiction treatment		10 (76.9)	30 (55.6)	40 (58.9)	0.159
Age at first addiction treatment ($\bar{x} \pm$ SD) years		35.75 ± 13.26	34.39 ± 14.9	34.74 ± 14.29	0.572
HIV antibodies positive		3 (23.1)	10 (18.2)	13 (19.1)	0.702
Ab HCV serology positive		4 (30.8)	16 (29.1)	20 (29.4)	0.954
Ab core HBV serology positive		4 (30.8)	10 (18.2)	14 (20.6)	0.601
Ag surface HBV positive		0	2 (3.6)	2 (2.9)	0.728
Chronic liver disease		5 (38.5)	19 (34.5)	24 (35.3)	0.909

SD: standard deviation, SUD: substance use disorder, HIV: human immunodeficiency viruses, HBV: hepatitis B virus, HCV: hepatitis C virus, Ag. Antigen, Ab. Antibody. Bold numbers represent statistically significant results.

The mean commencement age of the main substance was 18.71 years, which was lower in men than women (17.83 vs. 23 years, $p = 0.018$). The mean of total abstinence time was 24.15 months, without differences by gender. More than half the sample (58.9%) had been previously involved in addiction treatment without differences between men and women. There were no differences between genders regarding HIV and hepatitis B and C virus infections (HBV and HCV).

3.3. Dual Disorder Assessment

Of the 68 patients interviewed, 25 (36.8%) had positive screening for DD; depression was the most prevalent (33.8%) followed by psychosis and panic (both 19.1%) (Table 3).

Prevalence of DD was 32.7% in men and 53.8% in women. In the former, the most common psychiatric disorder was depression (30.9%), followed by psychosis (16.4%), mania and PTSD (both 14.5%). While in the latter, the most frequent psychiatric disorders were depression and panic (both 46.2%), followed by generalized anxiety (38.5%).

Panic disorder and generalized anxiety were greater for women than men ($p = 0.019$ $p = 0.049$ for generalized anxiety, respectively) (Table 3).

When analysing DD with other clinical variables, a greater proportion of patients with HIV antibodies was observed (36% vs. 9.3%; $p = 0.02$). No differences were found for the other clinical and sociodemographic variables.

Table 3. Prevalence of DD amongst patients that completed the interview, stratified by gender.

Psychiatric Diagnoses	Women n = 13 n (%)	Men n = 55 n (%)	Participants n = 68 n (%)	p
Dual Disorder	7 (53.8)	18 (32.7)	25 (36.8)	0.156
Panic	6 (46.2)	7 (12.7)	13 (19.1)	**0.019**
Generalized anxiety	5 (38.5)	6 (10.9)	11 (16.2)	**0.049**
Simple phobia	3 (23.1)	3 (5.5)	6 (8.8)	0.104
Social phobia	1 (7.7)	4 (7.3)	5 (7.4)	0.958
Agoraphobia	1 (7.7)	2 (3.6)	3 (4.4)	0.522
Dysthymia	3 (23.1)	4 (7.3)	7 (10.3)	0.092
Depression	6 (46.2)	17 (30.9)	23 (33.8)	0.296
Mania	3 (23.1)	8 (14.5)	11 (16.2)	0.174
Psychosis	4 (30.8)	9 (16.4)	13 (19.1)	0.445
ADHD	3 (23.1)	6 (10.9)	9 (13.2)	0.479
PTSD	1 (7.7)	8 (14.5)	9 (13.2)	0.512

DD: Dual Disorder, ADHD: attention deficit hyperactivity disorder, PTSD: post-traumatic stress disorder. Patients can present more than one psychiatric diagnosis. Bold numbers represent statistically significant results.

3.4. Dual Disorder and Quality of Life

Considering only patients with DD (18 men and 7 women), the QoL index was higher for men ($\bar{x}$:50 points vs. $\bar{x}$:21.7 points, respectively, $p = 0.02$). This difference did not change when the comparison was made excluding patients with HIV antibodies that could bias results. No gender differences were detected in non-DD patients (Table 4).

Table 4. Total scores of WHO and SDS in DD vs. non-DD patients.

	DD	Women (n = 13)	Men (n = 55)	Total (n = 68)	p
WHO ($\bar{x} \pm$ SD)	No	62 ± 23.83	52.32 ± 30.9	53.67 ± 30.03	0.404
	Yes	21.71 ± 21.52	50 ± 31.02	42.08 ± 31.0	**0.020**
SDS ($\bar{x} \pm$ SD)	No	4.5 ± 3.27	6.92 ± 4.14	6.58 ± 4.08	0.146
	Yes	10.14 ± 3.72	7.39 ± 4.65	8.16 ± 4.52	0.145

WHO: WHO well-being Index; SDS: Severity of Dependence Scale; SD: standard deviation. Bold numbers represent statistically significant results.

3.5. Dual Disorder and Severity of Addiction

According to SDS, the mean severity of dependence was 6.58 points (SD = 4.08) in non-DD patients and 8.16 points (SD = 4.52) in DD ones, without differences in gender (Table 4).

3.6. Sociodemographic and Clinical Characteristics of Patients Attended during Lockdown Period

During the lockdown period 77 patients were attended by the CLAS and could not be included for interview assessment. No differences were found in relation to gender proportion and all the clinical and sociodemographic variables analysed in this study (Tables S1 and S2). Of these patients, 13 (16.8%) were diagnosed with COVID-19 infection.

4. Discussion

The prevalence of DD among patients with SUD admitted to the general hospital was around 37% and depression was the most frequent psychiatric disorder in both genders, representing more than a third of the sample. This prevalence is described for the first time in a CLAS of a general hospital. Other studies had reported a depression incidence of 10–15% in general hospital inpatients [27,28], but not in SUD patients.

Although in our study women tended to have more DD than men (53.8% vs. 32.7%), differences were not significant, probably related to their low number. This is in contrast with other studies, where women with SUD presented more DD than men [28,29]. Depression was the most common DD in both genders, while panic and generalized anxiety were more frequent in women. We could not confirm results of other studies [14–18], except for a higher prevalence of anxiety disorders in women compared to men. We think a possible explanation, besides the small sample size, could be an under-diagnosis or lower self-report of consumption, specifically in women, that limit their seeking consultation.

Regarding the self-perceived QoL, there are several communications that associate worse QoL with the presence of addiction and other mental health problems [7,8,10]. In our sample there were no differences between patients with and without DD, when separating by gender; however, in women, the QoL self-perception was significantly worse, which could not be explained by other analysed sociodemographic and clinical factors. We observed that the presence of HIV antibodies was associated with more DD but not with worse QoL. QoL has been proposed as a neglected factor that could play a critical role in sustaining remission [30], according to these results; therefore, women with DD had a more difficult path to recovery.

In relation to addiction severity, there was a tendency for it to be worse in women and in patients with DD, although such differences were non-significant.

The COVID-19 pandemic changed conditions for everybody, including patients and clinicians. We analysed the data of patients that could not be interviewed by the study researcher and observed no marked differences with respect to the other participants, with the exception of 13 diagnosed with COVID-19. Nevertheless, other factors, such as isolation and the infection itself, could have had different implications in the psychopathology and well being of these patients; therefore, it will be crucial to look forward prospectively.

Regarding the limitations of the study, it should be noted that the sample was small, especially the number of women, which could be associated with some bias and limit external validity; women are usually underrepresented in addiction research and it is essential to design the projects with gender perspective. In addition, due to the COVID-19 pandemic, the interviews ceased for a few months, which also led to the final sample being smaller than expected. Nevertheless, we adapted to this situation by adding an additional objective. There were no differences in gender proportion or sociodemographic variables of included patients versus non-included ones; the sample therefore should be representative. In addition, the comorbid diagnosis has been obtained with a screening tool and not by a structured interview. For this reason, although there is a high sensitivity, there would be less specificity to obtain diagnosis; however, previous studies validating the DDSI screening tool have found acceptable specificity for the majority of diagnoses [23].

Patients with more severe clinical conditions were excluded as they were unable to complete the assessment, and also those diagnosed with COVID-19 infection. It is thus possible that the QoL and addiction severity scores might have been worse.

In addition, there could have been a selection bias since only those patients that general medicine deemed necessary were assessed. There may have been others in which the SUD was considered less important, either because the patients did not report it, were abstinent, or it was simply not detected. This might also explain why the number of women with SUD was much lower than that of men [31]. Regarding women, it would also have been useful to obtain information about their backgrounds, for instance, if they were mothers, had suffered gender violence and/or sexual abuse and so on, and observe whether such factors were more prevalent in patients with DD. More stigma is associated with addicted women than men which could be a reason not to seek help during hospital admission.

5. Conclusions

In this study, patients were assessed by a psychiatry liaison service specializing in addiction. The study provides some insights into the characteristics of in-ward patients with an SUD and reinforces the need of an individualized approach.

Our findings suggest a high prevalence of DD amongst patients that were attended by the addiction liaison service of a general hospital. Furthermore, parameters such as QoL and addiction severity were worse when DD was present, especially in the group of women. Such results support the importance of routinely exploring substance consumption in hospitalized patients, and assessing the presence of dual pathologies, as they can play a role not only in medical pathology, but also in QoL, and particularly in women. More studies will be necessary to determine the implications of these differences in order to elucidate specific needs.

Supplementary Materials: The following are available online at https://www.mdpi.com/2077-0383/10/23/5572/s1, Table S1. Sociodemographic characteristics of participant patients vs. lockdown period patients. Table S2. Clinical characteristics of participant patients vs. lockdown period patients.

Author Contributions: M.T., F.D. and F.F. were responsible for the study concept and design. M.T., F.D. and T.F.-F. designed the protocol. M.T. and F.D. supervised the data research and conduct of the study. T.F.-F. conducted the interviews and wrote the first draft. J.I.M.-P., T.F.-F. and F.D. analysed and interpreted findings. T.F.-F. and F.D. wrote the initial draft of the manuscript. M.T., F.F. and F.D. supervised and revised the manuscript. All authors have read and agreed to the published version of the manuscript.

Funding: This work was supported by grants from the Instituto de Salud Carlos III–ISCIII Red de Trastornos Adictivos 2016 (RD16/0017/0010), and the Generalitat de Catalunya (2017SGR-530).

Institutional Review Board Statement: The study was approved by the Parc de Salut Mar Clinical Research Ethics Committee (SEIC-PSMAR); CEIm project number: 2019/8970/I. It does not involve psychological or pharmacological intervention, and participation is totally voluntary. The project was carried out in accordance with the principles of the protection of rights and human dignity, as stated in the Declaration of Helsinki and according to current regulations. It follows law 14/2007 on Biomedical Research. The information was treated confidentially, complying with organic law 15/1999 of 13 December 1999.

Informed Consent Statement: The participants were informed in writing about the study, the objectives, its voluntary nature, and any other matter that requires to be specified, as stated in the informed consent.

Data Availability Statement: Data are available upon request. Please contact the corresponding author if they are required.

Conflicts of Interest: The authors declare that they have no conflict of interest.

References

1. World Health Organization. *Lexicon of Alcohol and Drug Terms*; World Health Organization: Geneva, Switzerland, 1994.
2. Durvasula, R.; Miller, T.R. Substance abuse treatment in persons with HIV/AIDS: Challenges in managing triple diagnosis. *IJBM* **2014**, *40*, 43–52. [CrossRef] [PubMed]
3. Adan, A.; Torrens, M. Special issue: Diagnosis and management of addiction and other mental disorders (Dual Disorders). *J. Clin. Med.* **2021**, *10*, 1307. [CrossRef] [PubMed]
4. Torres, G.N.; Cristóbal, J.P.; Martín, J.R. Dual Diagnosis: A Theoretical Approximation from Review of Literature. *J. Drug Abuse* **2019**, *5*, 4.
5. Volkow, N.D.; Torrens, M.; Poznyak, V.; Sáenz, E.; Busse, A.; Kashino, W.; Krupchanka, D.; Kestel, D.; Campello, G.; Gerra, G. Managing dual disorders: A statement by the Informal Scientific Network, UN Commission on Narcotic Drugs. *World Psychiatry* **2020**, *19*, 396–397. [CrossRef]
6. Torrens, M.; Mestre-Pintó, J.; Montanari, L.; Vicente, J.; Domingo-Salvany, A. Patología dual: Una perspectiva europea. *Adicciones* **2017**, *29*, 3–5. [CrossRef]
7. Chahua, M.; Sanchez-Niubo, A.; Torrens, M.; Sordo, L.; Bravo, M.; Brugal, M.; Domingo-Salvany, A. Quality of life in a community sample of young cocaine and/or heroin users: The role of mental disorders. *Qual. Life Res.* **2015**, *24*, 2129–2137. [CrossRef]

8. Lozano, O.M.; Rojas, A.J.; Fernandez, F. Psychiatric comorbidity and severity of dependence on substance users: How it impacts on their health-related quality of life? *J. Ment. Health* **2017**, *26*, 119–126. [CrossRef]
9. Abdel-Baki, A.; Ouellet-Plamondon, C.; Salvat, É.; Grar, K.; Potvin, S. Symptomatic and funcional outcomes of substance use disorder persistence 2 years after admission to a first-episode psychosis program. *Psychiatry Res.* **2017**, *247*, 113–119. [CrossRef]
10. Adan, A.; Marquez-Arrico, J.; Gilchrist, G. Comparison of health-related quality of life among men with different co-existing severe mental disorders in treatment for substance use. *Health Qual. Life Outcomes* **2017**, *15*, 209. [CrossRef]
11. Torrens, M.; Mestre-Pintó, J.J.; Domingo-Salvany, A. *Comorbidity of Substance Use and Mental Disorders in Europe*; EMCDDA, Publications Office of the European Union: Luxembourg, 2015; ISBN 978-92-9168-834-0.
12. Mancheño, J.J.; Navas, S.; Gutiérrez, M.L.; Rosa, A.; Cáceres, M.P.; Lozano, O.M. Analysis of the profiles of patients with dual pathology attending addiction centers, mental health centers, and a coordinated service. *Ann. Psychol.* **2019**, *35*, 233–241.
13. García-Carretero, M.A.; Novalbos-Ruiz, J.P.; Robles-Martínez, M.; Jordán-Quintero, M.A.; O'Ferrall-González, C. Psychopathological profile and prevalence of dual pathology on patients with alcoholic dependence undergoing outpatient treatment. *Actas Esp. Psiquiatr.* **2017**, *45*, 1–11.
14. Fonseca, F.; Robles-Martínez, M.; Tirado-Muñoz, J.; Alías-Ferri, M.; Mestre-Pintó, J.I.; Coratu, A.M.; Torrens, M. A gender perspective of addictive disorders. *Curr. Addict. Rep.* **2021**, *8*, 89–99. [CrossRef]
15. McHugh, R.K.; Votaw, V.R.; Sugarman, D.E.; Greenfield, S.F. Sex and gender differences in substance use disorders. *Psychol. Rev.* **2018**, *66*, 12–23. [CrossRef]
16. Frem, Y.; Torrens, M.; Domingo-Salvany, A.; Gilchrist, G. Gender differences in lifetime psychiatric and substance use disorders among people who use substances in Barcelona, Spain. *Adv. Dual Diagn.* **2017**, *10*, 45–56. [CrossRef]
17. Gilchrist, G.; Blánquez, A.; Torrens, M. Psychiatric, Behavioural and Social Risk Factors for HIV Infection among Female Drug Users. *AIDS Behav.* **2011**, *10*, 3–10. [CrossRef]
18. Tirado-Muñoz, J.; Gilchrist, G.; Fischer, G.; Taylor, A.; Moskalewicz, J.; Giammarchi, C.; Köchl, B.; Munro, A.; Dąbrowska, K.; Shaw, A.; et al. Psychiatric comorbidity and intimate partner violence among women who inject drugs in Europe: A cross-sectional study. *Arch. Womens Ment. Health* **2017**, *21*, 259–269. [CrossRef]
19. Caldentey, C.; Tirado-Muñoz, J.; Ferrer, T.; Fonseca, F.; Rossi, P.; Mestre-Pintó, J.I.; Torrens, M. Violencia de género en mujeres con consumo de sustancias ingresadas en el hospital general: Cribado y prevalencia. *Adicciones* **2017**, *29*, 172–179. [CrossRef]
20. Weaver, T.L.; Gilbert, L.; El-Bassel, N.; Resnick, H.S.; Noursi, S. Identifying and intervening with substance-using women exposed to intimate partner violence: Phenomenology, comorbidities, and integrated approaches within primary care and other agency Settings. *J. Womens Health* **2015**, *24*, 51–56. [CrossRef]
21. American Psychiatric Association. Diagnostic and Statistical Manual of Mental Disorders. 2013. Available online: https://doi.org/10.1176/appi.books.9780890425596 (accessed on 25 November 2021).
22. Ojeda, N.; Del Pino, R.; Ibarretxe-Bilbao, N.; Schretlen, D.J.; Pena, J. Test de evaluacion cognitiva de Montreal: Normalizacion y estandarizacion de la prueba en poblacion española [Montreal Cognitive Assessment Test: Normalization and standardization for Spanish population]. *Rev Neurol.* **2016**, *63*, 488–496.
23. Mestre-Pintó, J.I.; Domingo-Salvany, A.; Martín-Santos, R.; Torrens, M.; PsyCoBarcelona Group. Dual Diagnosis Screening Interview to Identify Psychiatric Comorbidity in Substance Users: Development and Validation of a Brief Instrument. *Eur. Addict. Res.* **2014**, *20*, 41–48. [CrossRef]
24. World Health Organization (WHO). Use of Well-Being Measures in Primary Health Care/ TheDepCare Project. 1998. Available online: https://www.euro.who.int/__data/assets/pdf_file/0016/130750/E60246.pdf (accessed on 25 November 2021).
25. Gossop, M.; Darke, S.; Griffiths, P.; Hando, J.; Powis, B.; Hall, W.; Strang, J. The Severity of Dependence Scale (SDS): Psychometric properties of the SDS in English and Australian samples of heroin, cocaine and amphetamine users. *Addiction* **1995**, *90*, 607–614. [CrossRef] [PubMed]
26. González-Saiz, F.; de Las Cuevas, C.; Barrio, G.; Domingo-Salvany, A. Versión española consensuada de la Severity of Dependence Scale (SDS) [Spanish version of the Severity of Dependence Scale (SDS)]. *Med. Clin.* **2008**, *131*, 797–798. [CrossRef]
27. Walker, J.; Burke, K.; Wanat, M.; Fisher, R.; Fielding, J.; Mulick, A.; Puntis, S.; Sharpe, J.; Esposti, M.D.; Harriss, E.; et al. The prevalence of depression in general hospital inpatients: A systematic review and meta-analysis of interview-based studies. *Psychol. Med.* **2018**, *48*, 2285–2298. [CrossRef] [PubMed]
28. Campuzano-Cortina, C.; Feijoó-Fonnegra, L.M.; Manzur-Pineda, K.; Palacio-Muñoz, M.; Rendón-Fonnegra, J.; Montoya, L.; Berrouet, M.C.; Restrepo, D. Comorbidity between depressive symptoms and substance use in-patients hospitalized for non-psychiatric diseases. *Rev. Colomb. Psiquiatr. (Engl. Ed.)* **2021**, *50*, 130–137. [CrossRef]
29. Farré, A.; Tirado-Muñoz, J.; Torrens, M. Dual Depression: A Sex Perspective. *Addict. Disord. Their Treat.* **2017**, *16*, 180–186. [CrossRef]
30. Laudet, A.B.; Becker, J.B.; White, W.L. Don't wanna go through that madness no more: Quality of life satisfaction as predictor of sustained remission from illicit drug misuse. *Subst. Use Misuse* **2009**, *44*, 227–252. [CrossRef]
31. McHugh, R.K.; Wigderson, S.; Greenfield, S.F. Epidemiology of substance use in reproductive-age women. *Obstet. Gynecol. Clin. N. Am.* **2014**, *41*, 177–189. [CrossRef]

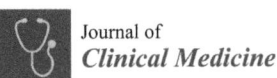

Article

Differential Effects of Patient Navigation across Latent Profiles of Barriers to Care among People Living with HIV and Comorbid Conditions

Sharleen M. Traynor [1], Renae D. Schmidt [2,*], Lauren K. Gooden [3], Tim Matheson [4], Louise Haynes [5], Allan Rodriguez [6], Michael Mugavero [7], Petra Jacobs [8], Raul Mandler [9], Carlos Del Rio [10], Adam W. Carrico [2], Viviana E. Horigian [2], Lisa R. Metsch [3] and Daniel J. Feaster [2]

[1] Clinical Trials Research Associate Program, Durham Technical Community College, Durham, NC 27703, USA
[2] Department of Public Health Sciences, University of Miami Miller School of Medicine, 1120 Northwest 14th Street, Miami, FL 33136, USA
[3] Sociomedical Sciences Mailman School of Public Health, Columbia University, 722 West 168th Street, New York, NY 10032, USA
[4] Center on Substance Use and Health, San Francisco Department of Public Health, San Francisco, CA 94102, USA
[5] Department of Psychiatry and Behavioral Science, Medical University of South Carolina, Charleston, SC 29425, USA
[6] Division of Infectious Diseases, University of Miami Miller School of Medicine, Miami, FL 33136, USA
[7] Department of Medicine, Division of Infectious Diseases, University of Alabama at Birmingham, 1900 University Blvd # 229, Birmingham, AL 35233, USA
[8] Center for Clinical Trials Network, National Institute on Drug Abuse, Rockville, MD 20892, USA
[9] Division of Therapeutics and Medical Consequences, National Institute on Drug Abuse, National Institutes of Health, Bethesda, MD 20892, USA
[10] Division of Infectious Diseases, Emory University, Atlanta, GA 30322, USA
* Correspondence: rds174@miami.edu; Tel.: +1-(952)-270-5051

Citation: Traynor, S.M.; Schmidt, R.D.; Gooden, L.K.; Matheson, T.; Haynes, L.; Rodriguez, A.; Mugavero, M.; Jacobs, P.; Mandler, R.; Del Rio, C.; et al. Differential Effects of Patient Navigation across Latent Profiles of Barriers to Care among People Living with HIV and Comorbid Conditions. *J. Clin. Med.* **2023**, *12*, 114. https://doi.org/10.3390/jcm12010114

Academic Editor: Icro Maremmani

Received: 2 November 2022
Revised: 29 November 2022
Accepted: 10 December 2022
Published: 23 December 2022

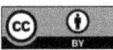

Copyright: © 2022 by the authors. Licensee MDPI, Basel, Switzerland. This article is an open access article distributed under the terms and conditions of the Creative Commons Attribution (CC BY) license (https://creativecommons.org/licenses/by/4.0/).

Abstract: Engaging people living with HIV who report substance use (PLWH-SU) in care is essential to HIV medical management and prevention of new HIV infections. Factors associated with poor engagement in HIV care include a combination of syndemic psychosocial factors, mental and physical comorbidities, and structural barriers to healthcare utilization. Patient navigation (PN) is designed to reduce barriers to care, but its effectiveness among PLWH-SU remains unclear. We analyzed data from NIDA Clinical Trials Network's CTN-0049, a three-arm randomized controlled trial testing the effect of a 6-month PN with and without contingency management (CM), on engagement in HIV care and viral suppression among PLWH-SU (n = 801). Latent profile analysis was used to identify subgroups of individuals' experiences to 23 barriers to care. The effects of PN on engagement in care and viral suppression were compared across latent profiles. Three latent profiles of barriers to care were identified. The results revealed that PN interventions are likely to be most effective for PLWH-SU with fewer, less severe healthcare barriers. Special attention should be given to individuals with a history of abuse, intimate partner violence, and discrimination, as they may be less likely to benefit from PN alone and require additional interventions.

Keywords: HIV; substance use; patient navigation; co-occurring disorders; barriers to care; social determinants of health; syndemic framework

1. Introduction

Despite major progress in the effectiveness and availability of antiretroviral therapy (ART), considerable challenges in the treatment of people living with HIV (PLWH) remain. There are significant gaps in the HIV care continuum, with the greatest deficits seen in retaining individuals in care and achieving viral suppression. Of the 1.1 million individuals living with HIV in the U.S., the Centers for Disease Control and Prevention (CDC) estimates that only 49% are continuously engaged or retained in HIV care and 53% have reached viral suppression [1]. One population that is particularly difficult to engage in care comprises people living with HIV who report substance use (PLWH-SU). In a 2018 review examining predictors of outcomes along the HIV care continuum, substance use was the most commonly cited risk factor associated with poor retention [2]. Compared to PLWH who report no substance use, those who use substances are less likely to access antiretroviral therapy, less likely to adhere to medication plans, and more likely to fall out of care [3]. Psychiatric comorbidities were also found to be predictors of poor retention in HIV care [4,5], and co-occurring diagnoses or "dual disorders"—the presence of both a substance use disorder and at least one psychiatric disorder [6]—among PLWH further complicate clinical management and deter retention in treatment [7]. This can lead to uncontrolled infection, which contributes to ongoing disease transmission. The need for interventions to improve engagement of this high-risk population in HIV care remains a national public health priority [8].

To understand why PLWH-SU do not engage in care, it is necessary to recognize the challenges they face in accessing care. This requires a thorough examination of multi-level factors, including social determinants of health, associated with access to and retention in HIV care. Data from the 2016 sample of the Medical Monitoring Project, a nationally representative sample of all adults diagnosed with HIV in the U.S., showed that 42% of respondents had household incomes below the federal poverty threshold and 43% were unemployed [9]. These factors have consistently been shown to severely limit the resources available to obtain healthcare [10–12]. Additionally, 22% and 26% of respondents reported symptoms of depression and anxiety, respectively, both of which are associated with lowered healthcare utilization and poor adherence to treatment plans [9,13–15]. Other barriers to HIV treatment identified through both qualitative and quantitative studies include housing instability [11,16–19], food insecurity [16,20,21], transportation [18,22], substance use [2,23,24], intimate partner violence (IPV) [25,26], perceived stigma [23], discrimination [27], clinic location and hours [24], service availability [26], and privacy concerns [24,28]. Self-perceived barriers to care, including financial, structural, and logistical barriers, as well as concerns about personal health or service delivery, have been associated with higher rates of mortality among PLWH [29]. For PLWH-SU, their substance use presents additional barriers to care, such as stigma, incarceration, and difficulty maintaining scheduled treatment regimens [30–33].

One intervention specifically designed to help individuals overcome barriers to care is patient navigation (PN). PN is a patient-centered intervention that identifies strategies to eliminate barriers to care and guides individuals through the healthcare system. It employs a strengths-based case management approach [34] and motivational interviewing [35] to empower individuals to manage their healthcare. Examples of activities involved in PN include helping individuals obtain health insurance, scheduling medical appointments, arranging transportation or childcare services, and providing assistance in applying for social services [36]. Screening for social determinants of health, such as housing, is another critical navigation activity [37]. PN may be combined with other tools such as contingency management (CM), which offers financial incentives for completing various activities of a treatment plan. The use of incentives has been specifically useful for engaging people who use drugs and/or alcohol [38,39]. PN strategies can help individuals with layered and complex mental health and/or addictions overcome barriers to obtaining services from various, and often fragmented, systems [40,41].

Although PN was initially developed to help predominantly underrepresented minority women access breast cancer screening and treatment services, it is now used for a variety of patient populations [42,43]. Among PLWH, results of studies assessing the effect of PN on HIV care have been mixed. Some studies have shown that PN is efficacious for linking individuals to care and improving steps along the HIV care continuum [34,44–46], while others reported no effect [47,48]. These conflicting results have raised questions about the effectiveness of PN and warrant additional research to determine for which populations and in what circumstances PN is most beneficial [49]. The effectiveness of PN has been difficult to establish, in part because PN is classified as a "complex intervention." This means that it consists of several core components, targets multiple behaviors, and is often tailored to meet specific conditions [50,51]. The many sources of variation make it difficult to determine which aspects of the intervention are most beneficial. In the case of PN, intervention activities are highly dependent on the specific barriers encountered by each individual. Therefore, it is possible that PN works better for certain patients than for others, depending on the type and number of barriers experienced.

It is also possible that the combination of healthcare barriers, stemming from social determinants of health and other individual and interpersonal factors, may influence the effectiveness of an intervention such as PN on HIV care. Because many PLWH face multiple, concurrent barriers, there is a growing number of studies supporting the use of a syndemics framework for describing factors that influence HIV infection. The syndemics approach suggests that there is an overlap of interrelated factors that drives risk for multiple, co-occurring conditions [52]. Previous studies have identified several syndemic conditions known to occur among PLWH; these include mental illness, violence, homelessness, and socioeconomic disadvantage [53,54]. Previous research has shown that PLWH have an average of two to four syndemic conditions, but some may experience as many as eight conditions [55]. Studies have also shown that these concomitant syndemic factors act synergistically to produce poor health outcomes. For example, research on the interplay among psychosocial factors, substance use, and HIV risk-taking suggests that psychological problems and substance use interact to not only negatively impact retention in care [2], but are also associated with increased risky behaviors [56]. The clustering of risk factors creates a syndemic vulnerability that places individuals at increased risk for HIV acquisition, high-risk sexual behaviors, sexually transmitted infections, and more frequent substance use [52,57].

Additional work has been done to examine syndemic vulnerability as it relates to the HIV care continuum. Glynn et al. (2019) found that among PLWH in Miami, Florida, the odds of having low ART adherence (<80%) and unsuppressed viral load increased for every syndemic condition experienced [55]. This finding supported previous work showing that a higher number of syndemic factors is associated with poor medication adherence and lower odds of viral suppression [58,59]. In 2015, Mizuno et al. (2015) examined syndemic factors specifically among persons who inject drugs and found similar results [57]. All outcomes along the HIV care continuum worsened as the number of psychosocial risk factors increased.

Despite the insights of this previous research, it is limited, in that syndemic barriers to care are measured as a sum of the number of syndemic factors an individual experiences. This composite-score approach places equal weight on the influence of each risk factor and suggests that simply minimizing the number of barriers can lead to improved outcomes. It is possible, however, that the pattern of factors an individual faces is more important than simply the number of barriers. Some syndemic factors may be more significant barriers to treatment than others. Some barriers may be more likely to cluster together than other barriers, creating subgroups of individuals characterized by different combinations of healthcare barriers. Thus, examining patterns of experienced barriers and the impact of these patterns on subsequent health outcomes may provide an improved understanding of how individuals respond to interventions designed to address healthcare barriers.

The current study has two main objectives. The first objective is to describe subgroups of PLWH-SU that share common patterns of barriers to care. The second objective is to analyze how subgroup membership influences the association between PN interventions and HIV outcomes. The data for this study come from CTN-0049, a randomized, controlled trial that studied PN in a sample of 801 hospitalized PLWH-SU who had uncontrolled HIV [60]. The trial tested the effect of a 6-month PN intervention, offered with and without CM, on engagement in care and viral suppression at 6 and 12 months. The results showed that the PN and PN+CM interventions were effective for engaging participants in care at 6 months, and PN+CM was effective for viral suppression at 6 months. Although these effects were not maintained through the 12-month follow-up period, CTN-0049 provides a unique opportunity to explore factors that contributed to the short-term success of the intervention. The data from this study may help characterize the populations likely to benefit from PN; this characterization can inform future adjustments to the intervention, maximize its effectiveness, and result in a more efficient allocation of resources.

2. Materials and Methods

2.1. CTN-0049 Overview

The CTN-0049 study was a randomized, controlled trial supported by the National Institute on Drug Abuse's National Drug Abuse Treatment Clinical Trials Network and has been described in detail elsewhere [61]. Briefly, the purpose of CTN-0049 was to determine the effect of a structured PN intervention, delivered with or without CM, on HIV health outcomes among hospitalized PLWH-SU with advanced HIV disease. Participants were recruited between July 2012 and January 2014 from 11 U.S. hospitals with both a high HIV inpatient census and a high prevalence of substance use among patients. Patients were eligible for enrollment if they had a clinical indication that they were out of HIV care and had evidence of substance use in the past 12 months. A total of 801 participants were randomized to one of three treatment groups: (1) PN, (2) PN+CM, or (3) treatment as usual (TAU). Those randomized to one of the PN groups were offered up to 11 PN sessions over a 6-month intervention period. During sessions, navigators used a strengths-based case management approach to assist patients to coordinate care with clinicians, review their health information, address personal challenges, and provide direct psychosocial support. Those in PN+CM also received financial incentives for target behaviors, including session attendance, completion of paperwork, HIV clinic visits, SUD treatment visits, negative substance use specimens, blood draws, and active ART prescriptions. Participants in the TAU group did not interact with the patient navigators, and received the standard treatment provided at their hospital for linking hospitalized patients to outpatient HIV care and substance-use-disorders treatment, which at most hospitals was written referral. Patients were followed up at 6 months ($n = 761$) and 12 months ($n = 752$) post-randomization and assessed for HIV viral load and other outcomes; however, no differences in rates of HIV viral suppression or death among the three groups at 12 months were revealed.

2.2. Measures

2.2.1. Main Outcomes

This study examined how different barrier profiles influenced the effect of PN interventions on four separate outcomes—engagement in HIV care at 6 months, engagement in HIV care at 12 months, viral suppression at 6 months, and viral suppression at 12 months. Engagement in care was measured as a binary variable. Participants were considered "in care" if they self-reported affirmative responses to two questions: "During the past 6 months, did you go to any hospital clinic, hospital outpatient department, community clinic or neighborhood health center for medical care, for example, to care for your HIV/AIDS or other physical problems?" and "If Yes, were any of these HIV primary care visits?" HIV viral load was clinically measured from blood drawn at the 6 and 12-month study visits, or as abstracted from medical records if patients did not attend these visits. The outcome was treated as a binary variable, with a viral load ≤ 200 copies/mL defined as "suppressed" and a viral load > 200 copies/mL defined as "unsuppressed".

2.2.2. Demographics

Demographic variables were collected at baseline and used in the analysis as follows: age (in years; continuous), race (Black/White; binary), ethnicity (Hispanic/non-Hispanic; binary), and gender (male/female; binary). Education was measured as a categorical variable with these options: middle school or less, some high school/no diploma, high school diploma/GED, junior college, technical/trade/vocational school, some college, college graduate, or graduate/professional school. Categories of race, ethnicity, gender, and education were established in the primary outcomes paper for CTN-0049 [60]. Southern/non-southern residence was a binary variable determined by the study site location [61]. Sites in Atlanta, Baltimore, Birmingham, Dallas, and Miami were considered southern sites. Sites in Boston, Chicago, Los Angeles, New York, Philadelphia, and Pittsburg were considered non-southern sites.

2.2.3. Psychiatric History

Participants were classified as having a psychiatric history if either of two criteria were met: (1) an initial hospital intake (at time of enrollment) with a primary diagnosis and/or any comorbid diagnoses that included terms or conditions such as "suicidal ideation", "psychosis", "schizophrenia", "bipolar disorder", "PTSD", "hallucinations", "mood disorder", and "altered mental state," or (2) participant self-report that they "saw a professional for the primary purpose of getting help for psychological or emotional issues in the past 6 months".

2.2.4. Barriers to Care

An analysis of barriers to care was guided by a socioecological framework described by Mugavero et al. (2013) to examine engagement in HIV care across multiple levels of healthcare access [62]. Building upon earlier models of healthcare utilization, this framework categorizes healthcare utilization factors into four categories: (1) Individual factors, which may include demographics, personal health beliefs, past experiences, and coping skills; (2) Relationship factors, which may include connections with family, friends, and medical providers; (3) Community/health system factors, which may include community-level poverty, social norms, and the local health service infrastructure; and (4) Policy factors, which may include treatment guidelines, service coordination, and funding. This study specifically examined 23 barriers to care at the first two levels (individual and relationship factors) and health system factors at the third level. Addressing community factors and policy-level barriers was beyond the scope of this research. All measures were assessed at baseline.

I. Alcohol use severity—This was measured on a continuous scale using the Alcohol Use Disorders Identification Test (AUDIT) [63]. This is a 10-item questionnaire assessing the frequency of alcohol consumption, alcohol dependence, and harmful consequences of alcohol use. Each item was scored on a scale from 0 to 4, with a total score range from 0 to 40. A sample question is, "How often during the last year have you failed to do what was normally expected of you because of drinking?" (0 = never, 1 = less than monthly, 2 = monthly, 3 = weekly, 4 = daily or almost daily). Higher scores represent greater alcohol use severity.

II. Drug use severity—This was measured on a continuous scale using a short version of the Drug Abuse Screening Test, the DAST-10 [64,65]. This is a 10-item questionnaire with "yes" or "no" response options for each item. A sample item is, "Have you had 'blackouts' or 'flashbacks' as a result of drug use?" All items with a "yes" response represent 1 point on a total scale from 0 to 10. Greater scores represent greater drug use severity.

III. Food insecurity—This was measured on a continuous scale using the Household Food Security Access Scale [66]. This is a 9-item questionnaire assessing various food insecurity domains, such as quantity, quality, and uncertainty experienced in the past 4 weeks. Each item was scored from 0 to 3 based on the frequency of experiencing each domain. For example, "In the past four weeks, did you worry that your household would not have enough food? How often did this happen?" (0 = never, 1 = rarely, 2 = sometimes, 3 = often). Total scores ranged from 0 to 27, with higher scores representing greater food insecurity.

IV. History of abuse—This was measured as a binary variable. Participants who reported any history (either as a child or an adult) of being beaten, physically attacked or abused, raped, or sexually abused were scored a 1. Others were scored a 0.

V. History of IPV—This was measured as a binary variable and was based on 4 "yes/no" items from a previously published IPV screening tool [67]. A sample question is,

"Have you ever been in a relationship where a sexual partner threw, broke, or punched things?" Participants who answered affirmatively to any of the items were scored a 1. Others were scored a 0.

VI. Recent incarceration—This was measured as a binary variable and was based on participant self-report of being incarcerated in the past 6 months.
VII. Housing insecurity—This was measured as a binary variable. Participants who self-reported being homeless or living in a shelter, transitional housing, hotel, group home, or other residential facility in the last 6 months were scored a 1. Others were scored a 0.
VIII. Language barriers—This was measured as a binary variable and was based on participant self-report as to whether English was their second language.
IX. Lack of health insurance—This was measured as a binary variable and was based on participant self-report of current health insurance status.
X. Lack of a case manager—This was measured as a binary variable and was based on participant response to the question, "During the past 6 months, did you receive any help from case managers or social service workers with things like obtaining health care or legal services, housing, or easing money problems?"
XI. Lack of transportation—This was measured as a binary variable based on participant self-report about how they got to their most recent medical appointment. If participants indicated that they drove themselves, they were scored a 0. Others who, for example reported taking public transportation, being taken by somebody else, or walking, were scored a 1.
XII. Low access to healthcare—This was measured as a continuous variable using a 6-item instrument that was adapted from an instrument assessing medical care for low-income persons with HIV [10]. Each response was scored on a scale from 0 to 4, for a total score range from 0 to 24. Higher scores represented lower access to care, and in some cases, items were reverse-scored to maintain this pattern. A sample item is, "I am able to get medical care whenever I need it" (0 = strongly agree, 1 = somewhat agree, 3 = uncertain, 4 = somewhat disagree, 5 = strongly disagree).
XIII. Low health literacy—This was measured as a continuous variable using a brief 3-item health literacy screening tool [68]. Each response was scored on a scale from 0 to 4, for a total score range from 0 to 12. Items were reverse-scored so that higher scores represented lower health literacy. A sample question is, "How confident are you filling out medical forms by yourself?" (0 = extremely, 1 = quite a bit, 2 = somewhat, 3 = a little bit, 4 = not at all).
XIV. Low income—This was measured as a binary variable based on participant self-report of income level according to categories of income range. Participants with incomes less than $10,000/year were considered low-income. This cut point was chosen based on poverty thresholds determined by the 2014 U.S. Census Bureau, which was $12,071 for a single person [69].
XV. Low readiness for substance use treatment—This was measured as a continuous variable using 4 items derived from a previously published treatment readiness instrument. [70]. Each item was scored on a scale from 1 to 5, for a total score range from 4 to 20 Items were reverse-scored so that higher scores represented lower readiness for treatment. A sample item is, "You want to be in a treatment program" (1 = strongly agree, 2 = agree, 3 = undecided, 4 = disagree, 5 = strongly disagree).
XVI. Low perceived health status—This was measured as a continuous variable using the SF-12 instrument, a 12-item short form health survey [71]. Ten items were scored on a scale from 1 to 5, and two items were scored on a scale from 1 to 3, for a total score range from 12 to 56. Items were scored so that higher scores represented lower perceived health. A sample item is, "Does your health now limit you in moderate activities such as moving a table, pushing a vacuum cleaner, bowling, or playing golf?" (1 = no, not at all, 2 = yes, limited a little, 3 = yes, limited a lot).
XVII. Low social support—This was measured as a continuous variable based on responses to 5 items adapted from a social support instrument for HIV-infected individuals

measuring support over the last 4 weeks [72]. Each item was scored on a scale from 1 to 5, for a total score range from 5 to 25. Lower scores represented lower social support. A sample item is, "How often was someone to love and make you feel wanted available to you during the past 4 weeks if you needed it?" (1 = none of the time, 2 = a little of the time, 3 = some of the time, 4 = most of the time, 5 = all of the time).

XVIII. Medical mistrust—This was measured as a continuous variable using the Group-Based Medical Mistrust Scale [73]. Each of the 12-items were scored on a scale from 1 to 5, for a total score range from 12 to 60. Higher scores represented greater medical mistrust, and some items were reverse-scored to maintain this pattern. A sample item is, "Doctors and health care workers sometimes hide information from patients who belong to my ethnic group" (1 = strongly disagree, 2 = disagree, 3 = neither agree nor disagree, 4 = agree, 5 = strongly agree).

XIX. History of discrimination—This was measured as a binary variable. Participants who self-reported that they had ever experienced discrimination, been prevented from doing something, been hassled, or made to feel inferior in a healthcare setting because of their gender, sexual orientation, race, ethnicity, HIV status, or drug use were scored a 1. Others were scored a 0.

XX. Social conflict—This was measured as a continuous variable based on responses to 3 items adapted from a Conflictual Social Interactions instrument measuring conflict over the last 4 weeks [72]. Each item was scored on a scale from 1 to 5, for a total score range from 5 to 15. Higher scores represented greater social conflict. A sample item is, "During the past 4 weeks, how much of the time have you had serious disagreements with your family about things that were important to you?" (1 = none of the time, 2 = a little of the time, 3 = some of the time, 4 = most of the time, 5 = all of the time).

XXI. Psychological distress—This was measured as a continuous variable using the 18-item Brief Symptom Inventory to assess depression, anxiety, and somatization [74]. Each item was scored on a scale of 0 to 4 with higher scores representing greater psychological distress. The three domains were combined into a single score for a total score range of 0 to 72. A sample item is, "In the past 7 days, how much were you distressed by feeling lonely?" (0 = not at all, 1 = a little bit, 2 = moderately, 3 = quite a bit, 4 = extremely).

XXII. Negative attitudes toward substance use treatment—This was measured as a continuous variable using a 4-item subscale of the Treatment Attitude Profile [75]. Each item was scored on a scale of 1 to 5, for a total score range from 4 to 20. Higher scores represented greater negative attitudes toward treatment. A sample item is, "Substance use treatment programs have too many rules and regulations for me" (1 = strongly disagree, 2 = disagree, 3 = undecided, 4 = agree, 5 = strongly agree).

XXIII. Unemployment—This was measured as a binary variable based on participant self-report that they were unemployed.

2.3. Statistical Analyses

First, a latent profile analysis (LPA) was conducted to identify subgroups of individuals with similar barriers to care. LPA is a latent variable modeling technique that identifies unobserved subgroups of individuals within a population based on responses to a set of observed variables; it assumes that individuals can be categorized by patterns of responses that relate to profiles of personal and/or environmental attributes [76]. LPA, rather than a Latent Class Analysis, was used in this analysis, as it can accommodate both categorical and continuous indicators [77].

The current study included the 23 barriers to care previously described. Profile solutions were evaluated based on several standard fit indices, including Akaike information criteria (AIC), adjusted Bayesian criteria (BIC), model entropy, Lo–Mendel–Rubin test, and the bootstrapped likelihood-ratio test. Additionally, the clinical meaningfulness, interpretability, and sample size of each class were considered in the selection of the final model. Latent profile plots were created to visualize differences between the profiles. Differences in latent profiles by gender, race, and southern/non-southern residence were assessed using a likelihood-ratio test with a significance level of $\alpha = 0.05$.

Next, structural models were constructed to test how the relationship between the intervention groups (PN, PN+CM, and TAU) and the four distal outcomes of interest differed by profile. Model construction followed a 3-step approach [66,67]. In step 1, LPA was performed; age, gender, southern/non-southern residence, and treatment group were included as covariates using the auxiliary option in Mplus. In step 2, a new latent profile variable was created by incorporating the classification error obtained from the step 1 logits for classification probabilities. This classification method is preferred over other methods such as classify–analyze or pseudo-class draw approaches because it accounts for uncertainty in latent profile assignment and reduces bias [78]. In step 3, the distal outcome was regressed on the intervention variables, controlling for the covariates and comparing effects across the latent profiles. This process was repeated for each outcome. Odds ratios were used to interpret the effect of latent profile on each outcome.

3. Results

3.1. Characteristics of the Study Population

Select demographic, clinical, psychosocial, and healthcare access factors of the 801 study participants are summarized in Table 1. The sample was mostly male (67.4%), Black (82.5%), and Non-Hispanic (89.0%) with a mean age of 44.2 years. There were slightly more participants enrolled from southern sites (59.2%) than from northern sites. The average time since HIV diagnosis was 11.8 years. Most participants reported a history of being in HIV care (82.9%) and being on antiretroviral therapy (77.2%) at some point in their lives, but approximately two-thirds of the sample had a CD4 count of less than 200 cells/μL at enrollment. About one-third of participants reported injection drug use in the last 12 months, and 55.3% had a history of substance use treatment in the 6 months prior to enrollment. Approximately 22.0% of the study sample had a recorded psychiatric history. The overall baseline mean of psychological stress as measured by the BSI-18 was 22.5 (16.1 SD). Based on established BSI thresholds, there were 39 individuals with minor elevation, 17 with moderate elevation, and 11 with marked elevation [79].

Table 1. Characteristics of the CTN-0049 study sample ($n = 801$).

	Range	Treatment as Usual ($n = 264$)	Patient Navigation ($n = 266$)	Patient Navigation + Contingency Management ($n = 271$)
Demographics				
Age (years)	18–68	44.0 (10.1)	44.3 (9.9)	44.2 (10.0)
Male		184 (69.7%)	179 (67.3%)	177 (65.3%)
Black race		216 (81.8%)	226 (85.0%)	219 (80.8%)
Hispanic ethnicity		35 (13.3%)	28 (10.5%)	25 (9.2%)
Education (high school grad or more)		167 (63.3%)	149 (56.0%)	166 (61.3%)
Southern U.S. residence		155 (58.7%)	158 (59.4%)	161 (59.4%)
Clinical Characteristics				
Baseline CD4 count (cells/μL)	0–1482	152.6 (150.4)	157.5 (168.4)	171.3 (172.3)
Years since HIV diagnosis	0–32	12.1 (8.9)	12.1 (11.0)	11.2 (8.3)
Ever in HIV care		227 (86.3%)	219 (82.6%)	218 (80.4%)
History of antiretroviral therapy		208 (79.1%)	203 (76.3%)	207 (76.7%)
Injection drug use, last 12 months		85 (32.2%)	90 (33.8%)	85 (31.4%)
Substance use treatment, last 6 months		149 (56.6%)	152 (57.1%)	142 (52.4%)
Hepatitis C positive		87 (34.0%)	90 (34.0%)	81 (30.4%)
Psychiatric History		56 (7.0%)	67 (8.4%)	53 (6.6%)
Individual Barriers to Care				

Table 1. Cont.

	Range	Treatment as Usual (n = 264)	Patient Navigation (n = 266)	Patient Navigation + Contingency Management (n = 271)
Employed (full-time, part-time, temp)		34 (12.9%)	24 (9.0%)	35 (12.9%)
Low income (<$10,000/year)		166 (77.9%)	181 (80.4%)	171 (74.0%)
Uninsured		85 (32.6%)	88 (33.3%)	88 (32.6%)
Health literacy	0–12	9.2 (3.0)	9.0 (3.2)	8.8 (3.2)
Language barrier		37 (14.0%)	31 (11.7%)	31 (11.4%)
Access to healthcare	0–24	17.8 (4.7)	14.5 (5.0)	18.2 (4.7)
Perceived health status	0–55	33.3 (9.3)	33.8 (9.5)	33.9 (8.7)
Food insecurity	0–27	6.5 (8.2)	6.4 (8.1)	5.8 (7.3)
Housing insecurity		91 (34.5%)	106 (39.9%)	101 (37.3%)
Lack of transportation		199 (87.7%)	211 (92.1%)	229 (90.9%)
Psychosocial distress (BSI-18)	0–69	22.2 (16.1)	23.0 (16.4)	22.4 (15.8)
Alcohol use severity (AUDIT)	0–38	9.2 (9.5)	9.0 (9.7)	8.9 (9.5)
Substance use severity (DAST-10)	0–10	4.6 (2.9)	4.6 (3.0)	4.8 (2.9)
Negative treatment attitudes	4–20	10.7 (3.4)	10.7 (3.5)	10.7 (3.5)
Readiness for treatment	4–20	14.0 (4.4)	14.5 (3.8)	14.1 (4.4)
History of incarceration, last 6 months		16 (6.1%)	20 (7.5%)	15 (6.4%)
Relationship Barriers to Care				
Social support	0–25	14.7 (6.8)	14.6 (6.3)	14.7 (6.4)
Social conflict	0–15	6.9 (3.5)	6.6 (3.3)	6.8 (3.4)
Medical mistrust	12–60	29.1 (7.8)	28.9 (8.0)	28.1 (7.4)
History of discrimination	0–5	0.6 (1.2)	0.6 (1.1)	0.5 (1.0)
History of abuse		134 (50.8%)	129 (48.5%)	158 (58.3%)
History of intimate partner violence		145 (54.9%)	132 (49.6%)	151 (55.72%)
No case manager		188 (71.8%)	188 (70.7%)	182 (67.4%)

Range, mean (std dev) shown for continuous variables; n (%) shown for dichotomous variables. Abbreviations: BSI = Brief Symptom Inventory, AUDIT = Alcohol Use Disorders Identification Test, DAST = Drug Abuse Severity Test.

Many participants had achieved at least a high school education (60.2%), but most (77.4%) reported an annual income less than $10,000, and only 11.6% were employed. Most individuals reported unreliable transportation (90.3%), not having a case manager (70.0%), and low levels of social support (mean = 14.7 out of 25). Many participants, however, had health insurance (67.4%) and moderate to high levels of health literacy (mean = 9.0 out of 12). There were no differences in the distribution of baseline characteristics across treatment groups, which was expected due to randomized treatment assignment. The reliabilities of measurement scales are shown in Table 2. All scales had a Cronbach alpha > 0.70, indicating adequate reliability.

Table 2. Reliability of continuous scales used to measure barriers to care.

	Cronbach Alpha
Food insecurity	0.944
Intimate partner violence	0.829
Social support	0.861
Social conflict	0.746
Psychological Distress—(BSI-18)	0.916
Alcohol use severity (AUDIT)	0.864
Drug use severity (DAST-10)	0.824
Readiness for substance use treatment	0.835
Attitudes about substance use treatment	0.747
Perceived health status	0.856
Medical mistrust	0.849
Experienced discrimination	0.718
Health literacy	0.731
Access to care	0.725

Abbreviations: BSI = Brief Symptom Inventory, AUDIT = Alcohol Use Disorders Identification Test, DAST = Drug Abuse Severity Test.

3.2. LPA Results

Models of two to five profiles were considered for the LPA. The five-profile solution was ruled out because the best likelihood value could not be replicated after 2000 random starts. Among the remaining models, multiple fit statistics (Table 3) and interpretability indicated that a three-profile solution best fit the data. The sample-size adjusted BIC score (69,367.41) was lower in the three-profile solution than the two-profile solution (indicating a better fit), while maintaining a high entropy (0.863). The Lo–Mendell–Rubin adjusted likelihood-ratio test, however, showed that the four-profile solution did not significantly improve fit above the three-profile solution ($p = 0.166$). The three-profile solution also presented a logical substantive interpretation, adequate class distinction, and adequate sample sizes. Therefore, the three-profile solution was selected as the best model.

Table 3. Latent Profile Enumeration using 23 indicators of barriers to care.

Number of Profiles	Log-Likelihood	AIC	aBIC	Entropy	LMR-A p-Value	BLRT p-Value
1	−35,383.31	70,838.62	70,892.99	–	–	–
2	−34,802.32	69,724.63	69,815.25	0.802	<0.001	<0.001
3	−34,536.27	69,240.54	69,367.41	0.863	<0.001	<0.001
4	−34,426.40	69,068.80	69,231.91	0.892	0.166	<0.001

Abbreviations: AIC = Akaike information criteria, aBIC = adjusted Bayesian information criteria, LMR-A = Lo–Mendell–Rubin adjusted likelihood-ratio test, BLRT = bootstrapped likelihood-ratio test.

A comparison of the three profiles is described in Table 4 and displayed in Figure 1. Standardized means are shown for continuous variables, and proportions of item endorsement are shown for dichotomous variables. The first profile had relatively low barriers to care. Values for all barriers were the lowest for this profile except for lack of case management, low income, and not having insurance. This profile comprised half of study participants (50.3%) and was labeled "Lower Barriers (LB)." The second profile, which described 35.7% of the study sample, generally exhibited higher barriers to care compared to the first profile and was characterized by having a higher probability of reporting a history of abuse (67.3%) and intimate partner violence (65.6%). This profile was labeled "Higher Barriers with Abuse and Violence (HB-AV)." The third profile, which comprised 14.0% of the study sample, was quite close to the second, with similar values across most of the barriers. The main distinguishing features of this profile were an even higher likelihood of having a history of abuse (74.8%) and intimate partner violence (65.6%) and a high likelihood of having experienced discrimination (std mean = 5.41). This profile was labeled "Higher Barriers with Discrimination, Abuse and Violence (HB-DAV)." This three-profile solution was further analyzed for differences by key demographic characteristics including gender, race, and southern/non-southern residence (see Supplementary Materials.).

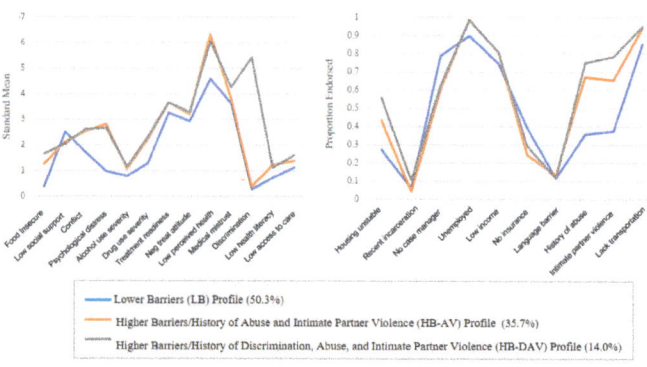

Figure 1. Visualization of Three-Class Latent Profile Analysis solution using 23 indicators of barriers to care.

Table 4. Standard means and proportions of continuous and categorical indicators by profile.

	Lower Barriers	Higher Barriers, Abuse and IPV	Higher Barriers, Discrimination, Abuse and IPV
Continuous Indicators		Standard Means	
Food insecurity	0.392	1.275	1.655
Social support (higher = more support)	2.528	2.132	2.043
Conflict	1.727	2.547	2.622
Psychological distress	0.995	2.827	2.674
Alcohol use severity	0.811	1.088	1.16
Drug use severity	1.302	2.249	2.33
Readiness for substance use treatment	3.276	3.659	3.659
Negative attitudes about drug treatment	2.945	3.216	3.277
Low perceived health status	4.602	6.334	6.042
Medical mistrust	3.637	3.835	4.263
History of discrimination	0.282	0.387	5.412
Low health literacy	0.751	1.244	1.125
Low access to care	1.154	1.404	1.617
Categorical Indicators		Proportion Endorsed	
Housing instability	27.4%	43.5%	55.6%
Recent incarceration (last 6 m)	6.4%	4.5%	10.6%
No case manager	78.7%	60.3%	62.3%
Unemployment	89.9%	98.7%	98.3%
Low income	74.5%	80.3%	80.6%
Uninsured	39.4%	24.7%	29.3%
Language barrier	11.8%	13.5%	11.7%
History of abuse	35.8%	67.3%	74.8%
History of intimate partner violence	37.7%	65.6%	78.2%
Lack of transportation	85.3%	94.3%	94.8%

3.3. Structural Model Results

Estimates for the final three-profile LPA are shown in Table 5. After controlling for race, gender, and southern/non-southern residence, structural models indicated that there were significant effects of the PN and PN+CM interventions on being engaged in care at 6 and 12 months and viral suppression at 6 months. However, these associations were only observed for certain profiles. The greatest effects were seen for the Lower Barrier (LB) profile, where the PN+CM group was associated with higher likelihood of being in care at 6 months ($\beta = 1.37$, OR = 3.94, $p < 0.001$), being virally suppressed at 6 months ($\beta = 0.687$, OR = 1.99, $p = 0.15$), and being in care at 12 months ($\beta = 0.881$, OR = 2.41, $p = 0.019$), compared to the TAU group. The PN-only group also had a significant effect on viral suppression at 6 months ($\beta = 0.610$, OR = 1.85, $p = 0.035$) and a marginally significant effect on being in care at 6 months ($\beta = 0.660$, OR = 1.93, $p = 0.054$), compared to the TAU group. The Higher Barriers with Abuse and Violence (HB-AV) profile had higher odds of being engaged in care for both the PN+CM group ($\beta = 1.25$, OR = 3.49, $p = 0.001$) and the PN group ($\beta = 0.981$, OR = 2.67, $p = 0.018$) compared to the TAU group, but there were no significant associations with the other distal outcomes of interest. The interventions did not have any significant effects for those with the Higher Barriers with Discrimination, Abuse, and Violence (HB-DAV) profile. Additionally, there were no significant intervention effects on viral suppression at 12 months for any of the latent profiles.

Table 5. Effect of patient navigation interventions on engagement in care and HIV viral suppression by latent profile.

	Lower Barriers (n = 403)			Higher Barriers, Abuse, IPV (n = 286)			Higher Barriers, Discrimination, Abuse, IPV (n = 112)		
	est.	s.e.	p-val	est	s.e.	p-val	est	s.e.	p-val
Engaged in care—6 months									
PN intervention	0.660	0.342	0.054	0.981	0.413	0.018	0.160	0.706	0.820
PN+CM intervention	1.370	0.387	<0.001	1.250	0.393	0.001	1.881	1.185	0.112
Race	−1.242	0.651	0.056	0.636	0.395	0.107	1.087	0.848	0.200
Age	−0.016	0.014	0.248	−0.010	0.018	0.566	−0.111	0.041	0.007
Gender	0.074	0.325	0.820	−0.209	0.334	0.532	−0.799	0.850	0.347
Southern U.S.	−0.928	0.357	0.009	−0.884	0.357	0.013	−0.426	0.758	0.574
In care at baseline	0.643	0.334	0.054	0.325	0.349	0.352	2.284	0.789	0.004
Viral suppression—6 months									
PN intervention	0.610	0.291	0.035	−0.357	0.392	0.363	−0.318	0.534	0.551
PN+CM intervention	0.687	0.282	0.015	0.337	0.340	0.321	−0.008	0.581	0.988
Race	−0.534	0.331	0.107	−0.704	0.362	0.052	−0.521	0.627	0.406
Age	−0.005	0.011	0.655	0.029	0.017	0.086	0.039	0.024	0.107
Gender	−0.398	0.283	0.160	−0.295	0.305	0.332	0.584	0.498	0.241
Southern U.S.	−0.679	0.236	0.004	0.027	0.297	0.927	−1.107	0.463	0.017
Suppressed at baseline	0.943	0.404	0.019	1.206	0.474	0.011	1.613	0.693	0.02
Engaged in care—12 months									
PN intervention	0.140	0.335	0.676	0.165	0.428	0.700	−0.358	0.584	0.540
PN+CM intervention	0.881	0.376	0.019	0.143	0.392	0.716	0.075	0.789	0.925
Race	−0.495	0.501	0.323	0.095	0.217	0.828	1.576	0.71	0.026
Age	−0.002	0.014	0.891	0.026	0.018	0.142	0.025	0.028	0.377
Gender	−0.225	0.313	0.473	−0.072	0.335	0.829	−0.581	0.627	0.355
Southern U.S.	−0.381	0.322	0.237	−0.577	0.343	0.093	0.634	0.558	0.256
In care at baseline	1.237	0.344	<0.001	0.186	0.34	0.584	0.832	0.542	0.125
Viral suppression—12 months									
PN intervention	0.406	0.282	0.151	−0.249	0.398	0.531	−0.264	0.565	0.640
PN+CM intervention	0.266	0.288	0.356	0.339	0.354	0.338	−0.619	0.614	0.313
Race	−0.927	0.333	0.005	−0.357	0.365	0.328	−1.476	0.722	0.041
Age	0.013	0.012	0.267	0.014	0.017	0.419	0.034	0.031	0.271
Gender	−0.087	0.268	0.746	0.178	0.305	0.559	0.389	0.517	0.451
Southern U.S.	−0.718	0.238	0.003	−0.674	0.309	0.029	−0.787	0.489	0.108
Suppressed at baseline	0.179	0.403	0.656	0.991	0.471	0.035	1.669	0.615	0.007

4. Discussion

This study provides important insights about the differential effects of PN interventions for engaging PLWH-SU in care. It suggests that PN, offered with or without CM, is most effective for individuals with relatively low levels of healthcare barriers. Of the three barrier profiles identified in this analysis, the LB group had the greatest response to PN, with higher 6- and 12-month rates of engagement in care and viral suppression than the TAU group. The positive intervention effects observed for the LB group may be explained by the absence of extreme healthcare barriers that would delay or compete with the need to engage in care. For example, if a patient has an overwhelming and immediate need to address an aspect of their wellbeing, such as a severe mental health condition or unstable housing, the patient may prioritize such a need over HIV care. The navigator would need to help resolve these other issues before the patient is ready to focus on HIV care. If, however, a patient is stable and does not require other assistance, the patient navigator can focus on linking the individual directly to care.

Conversely, individuals with a history of abuse, IPV, and discrimination are not likely to benefit from stand-alone PN interventions. In this analysis, the HB-AV group had only a partial response to the PN and PN+CM interventions. These individuals had higher odds of being engaged in care at 6 months, but these effects were not sustained at 12 months and did not lead to viral suppression. Finally, the HB-DAV group did not respond to either of the PN interventions. These results imply that PN (with or without CM) is not sufficient for all patient populations and underscore the importance of a thorough assessment of patients' needs when recommending behavioral interventions. In an era of precision medicine, the development of personalized interventions is becoming increasingly more valuable in prevention science.

These findings contribute to the current science of healthcare utilization among PLWH-SU by identifying high-risk barrier profiles. Specifically, a history of abuse, intimate partner violence, and/or discrimination are important indicators of a high overall level of healthcare barriers. In both profiles characterized by abuse and IPV, nearly all other barriers were present at higher rates compared to the profile without abuse and IPV. This is consistent with other work, most notably Singer's work on the SAVA syndemic of substance abuse, violence, and HIV/AIDS, indicating that these factors are likely to co-occur [25,26,53,69,80]. Individuals who experience IPV and/or abuse are more likely to suffer from depression and other psychiatric disorders [54] Substance use in this context further perpetuates violence and abuse. Healthcare personnel should be cognizant of these factors, incorporate screening for multiple conditions into practice, and be prepared to link patients to the appropriate programs or provide appropriate co-located services.

This study also provides insights about the potential impacts of trauma and abuse on the effectiveness of health interventions. PN interventions designed to engage PLWH-SU in care were not found to be effective for individuals with a history of IPV, physical or sexual abuse, or discrimination. This finding may be related to the possibility that individuals are still in abusive relationships at the time PN interventions are administered. Individuals in such situations may lack the resources and/or the autonomy to independently seek healthcare or suffer from fear or anxiety about being in a healthcare setting where the abuse may be discovered. Even if an individual is not actively in an abusive situation, the harms from past events may have lingering mental health effects that influence one's decision to seek care. Additionally, if a person experienced abuse or discrimination in a healthcare setting, this could deter that person from seeking care in the future. Thus, the identification of psychosocial barriers to care is an important part of a routine needs assessment, and it is especially important to determine if there is a history of abuse or IPV, with or without discrimination. Alternatives to PN, or PN delivered in combination with other interventions, may be required to result in positive health outcomes for these individuals.

Another noteworthy finding is that among the subgroups that had positive responses to the PN interventions, the effects were stronger when CM was added to PN, compared to PN alone. It could be that the combination of PN and CM interventions targets both intrinsic and extrinsic motivations for behavior change [70]. Alternatively, the financial incentives may have enhanced the effect of PN by encouraging individuals to attend more PN sessions [81]. Additional research is needed to evaluate the effect of this combined approach on this study's population and other patient populations.

The results of this study should be considered with the following limitations. First, there may have been some degree of measurement error associated with the barriers to care included in the analysis. All measures were self-reported and some of the barriers were measured indirectly. For example, information about transportation barriers was derived from responses about how participants got to their clinic appointment. A better way would be to specifically ask about transportation barriers to healthcare. Measurement tools designed specifically to evaluate barriers to HIV care, such as the Kalichman's Barriers to Medical Care instrument [82], should be considered for future studies. Second, this analysis considered only individual and relationship-level barriers to care. A more comprehensive examination that includes higher level barriers, such as system and policy factors, may reveal other distinct profiles that impact the response to interventions and should be explored in future analysis. Finally, the results of this work are limited to a specific population and may not be generalizable to other populations of PLWH. This study's population was a highly disadvantaged group of individuals with advanced HIV disease. This may have reduced the variability in observed healthcare barriers, as most of the CTN-0049 participants suffered from multiple barriers. Further research is needed to determine if similar barrier profiles exist in other populations.

Despite these limitations, this study has significant implications for public health practice. It underscores the importance of screening PLWH-SU for a history of abuse, IPV, and discrimination. Not only are they indicators of particularly vulnerable individuals, but they may also reduce the effectiveness of otherwise beneficial interventions. If these conditions are present, protocols should be initiated to make the appropriate referrals to mental health or social services. Screenings and follow-up assessments should be an ongoing part of interventions, not just part of the baseline evaluation. While this study was conducted in a U.S. population enrolled in a clinical trial, there may be important considerations for other PLWH populations with co-occurring drug use to identify and meet needs at the complex intersection of substance use and HIV services. A global review of studies assessing the integration of HIV and substance-use services showed that increased service integration can improve patient outcomes among this population across a variety of service models, both in and outside the U.S. [83]. Additionally, strategies to integrate treatment for mental health and substance use disorders among PLWH have been implemented in low-to-middle income countries [84]. Finally, this study builds on existing work by describing the complexities of how healthcare barriers group together. It suggests that, in addition to the number of barriers to care an individual faces, there are specific-barriers profiles that can differentially impact care. As a next step, it would be useful to conduct a direct comparison of latent variable approaches using barrier profiles with the composite-risk score method used in previous studies.

5. Conclusions

In summary, this research elucidated the complexities of engaging PLWH-SU in treatment. It identified distinct healthcare barrier profiles among PLWH-SU enrolled in CTN-0049, each with different responses to PN interventions. These results help to inform the use of PN programs and provide a more efficient target for PN resources by more narrowly defining the patient population for which PN is effective.

Supplementary Materials: The following supporting information can be downloaded at: https://www.mdpi.com/article/10.3390/jcm12010114/s1, Figure S1: Differences in 3-Class Latent Profile Analysis model by gender. Figure S2: Differences in 3-Class Latent Profile Analysis model by race. Figure S3: Differences in 3-Class Latent Profile Analysis model by southern/non-southern residence.

Author Contributions: Conceptualization, S.M.T., L.R.M. and D.J.F.; formal analysis, S.M.T. and D.J.F.; methodology, S.M.T., A.W.C. and D.J.F.; project administration, L.R.M. and D.J.F.; supervision, A.W.C., V.E.H., L.R.M. and D.J.F.; writing—original draft, S.M.T.; writing—review and editing, R.D.S., L.K.G., T.M., L.H., A.R., M.M., P.J., R.M., C.D.R., A.W.C., V.E.H., L.R.M. and D.J.F. All authors have read and agreed to the published version of the manuscript.

Funding: This work was supported by the National Institutes on Drug Abuse [U10DA013720 and UG1DA013720], the Miami CFAR [P30AI073961], the Emory Center for AIDS Research [P30AI050409] and the Center for HIV and Research in Mental Health [P30MH116867].

Institutional Review Board Statement: The parent study received approval from the respective Institutional Review Boards for each study site. However, the current study only used de-identified data and, therefore, was exempt from ethical review.

Informed Consent Statement: Not applicable.

Data Availability Statement: CTN 0049 trial data are publicly available on NIDA Data Share: https://datashare.nida.nih.gov/ (accessed on 7 September 2018).

Conflicts of Interest: The authors declare no conflict of interest.

Disclaimer: The authors are solely responsible for the content of this article, which does not necessarily represent the official views of the National Institute on Drug Abuse. Dr. Raul Mandler, an employee of the National Institute on Drug Abuse, is an author; he reviewed and approved the manuscript as a part of his authorship role as a Scientific Official.

References

1. CDC. Monitoring Selected National HIV Prevention and Care Objectives by Using HIV Surveillance Data—United States and 6 Dependent Areas. 2017. Available online: https://stacks.cdc.gov/view/cdc/79991 (accessed on 12 November 2019).
2. Bulsara, S.M.; Wainberg, M.L.; Newton-John, T.R.O. Predictors of Adult Retention in HIV Care: A Systematic Review. *AIDS Behav.* **2018**, *22*, 752–764. [CrossRef]
3. Weber, R.; Huber, M.; Battegay, M.; Stähelin, C.; Batanjer, E.C.; Calmy, A.; Bregenzer, A.; Bernasconi, E.; Schoeni-Affolter, F.; Ledergerber, B.; et al. Influence of noninjecting and injecting drug use on mortality, retention in the cohort, and antiretroviral therapy, in participants in the Swiss HIV Cohort Study. *HIV Med.* **2015**, *16*, 137–151. [CrossRef] [PubMed]
4. Tobias, C.R.; Cunningham, W.; Cabral, H.D.; Cunningham, C.O.; Eldred, L.; Naar-King, S.; Bradford, J.; Sohler, N.L.; Wong, M.D.; Drainoni, M.-L. Living with HIV but without medical care: Barriers to engagement. *AIDS Patient Care STDs* **2007**, *21*, 426–434. [CrossRef] [PubMed]
5. McMahon, J.H.; Moore, R.; Eu, B.; Tee, B.-K.; Chen, M.; El-Hayek, C.; Street, A.; Woolley, I.J.; Buggie, A.; Collins, D.; et al. Clinic Network Collaboration and Patient Tracing to Maximize Retention in HIV Care. *PLoS ONE* **2015**, *10*, e0127726. [CrossRef] [PubMed]
6. WHO. *Lexicon of Alcohol and Drug Terms*; World Health Organization: Geneva, Switzerland, 1994.
7. Zahari, M.M.; Hwan Bae, W.; Zainal, N.Z.; Habil, H.; Kamarulzaman, A.; Altice, F.L. Psychiatric and substance abuse comorbidity among HIV seropositive and HIV seronegative prisoners in Malaysia. *Am. J. Drug Alcohol Abuse* **2010**, *36*, 31–38. [CrossRef] [PubMed]
8. HHS. *National HIV/AIDS Strategy for the United States: Updated to 2020*; White House Office of National AIDS Policy, U.S. Department of Health & Human Services: Washington, DC, USA, 2015.
9. CDC. Behavioral and Clinical Characteristics of Persons with Diagnosed HIV Infection—Medical Monitoring Project, United States, 2017 Cycle (June 2017–May 2018). 2019. Available online: https://www.cdc.gov/hiv/pdf/library/reports/surveillance/cdc-hiv-surveillance-special-report-number-23.pdf (accessed on 12 November 2019).
10. Cunningham, W.E.; Hays, R.D.; Williams, K.W.; Beck, K.C.; Dixon, W.J.; Shapiro, M.F. Access to medical care and health-related quality of life for low-income persons with symptomatic human immunodeficiency virus. *Med. Care* **1995**, *33*, 739–754. [CrossRef]
11. Cunningham, W.E.; Andersen, R.M.; Katz, M.H.; Stein, M.D.; Turner, B.J.; Crystal, S.; Zierler, S.; Kuromiya, K.; Morton, S.C.; Clair, P.S.; et al. The impact of competing subsistence needs and barriers on access to medical care for persons with human immunodeficiency virus receiving care in the United States. *Med. Care* **1999**, *37*, 1270–1281. [CrossRef]
12. Lazar, M.; Davenport, L. Barriers to Health Care Access for Low Income Families: A Review of Literature. *J. Community Health Nurs.* **2018**, *35*, 28–37. [CrossRef]
13. Willie, T.C.; Overstreet, N.M.; Sullivan, T.P.; Sikkema, K.J.; Hansen, N.B. Barriers to HIV Medication Adherence: Examining Distinct Anxiety and Depression Symptoms among Women Living with HIV Who Experienced Childhood Sexual Abuse. *Behav. Med.* **2016**, *42*, 120–127. [CrossRef]
14. Mugavero, M.; Ostermann, J.; Whetten, K.; Leserman, J.; Swartz, M.; Stangl, D.; Thielman, N. Barriers to antiretroviral adherence: The importance of depression, abuse, and other traumatic events. *AIDS Patient Care STDs* **2006**, *20*, 418–428. [CrossRef]
15. ence, B.W.; Mills, J.; Bengtson, A.; Gaynes, B.N.; Breger, T.L.; Cook, R.L.; Moore, R.D.; Grelotti, D.J.; O'Cleirigh, C.; Mugavero, M.J. Association of Increased Chronicity of Depression with HIV Appointment Attendance, Treatment Failure, and Mortality Among HIV-Infected Adults in the United States. *JAMA Psychiatry* **2018**, *75*, 379–385.
16. Colasanti, J.; Stahl, N.; Farber, E.W.; Del Rio, C.; Armstrong, W.S. An Exploratory Study to Assess Individual and Structural Level Barriers Associated With Poor Retention and Re-engagement in Care Among Persons Living With HIV/AIDS. *J. Acquir. Immune Defic. Syndr.* **2017**, *74* (Suppl. S2), S113–S120. [CrossRef] [PubMed]
17. Riley, E.D.; Vittinghoff, E.; Koss, C.A.; Christopoulos, K.A.; Clemenzi-Allen, A.; Dilworth, S.E.; Carrico, A.W. Housing First: Unsuppressed Viral Load among Women Living with HIV in San Francisco. *AIDS Behav.* **2019**, *23*, 2326–2336. [CrossRef]
18. Sprague, C.; Simon, S.E. Understanding HIV care delays in the US South and the role of the social-level in HIV care engagement/retention: A qualitative study. *Int. J. Equity Health* **2014**, *13*, 28. [CrossRef] [PubMed]
19. Milloy, M.J.; Marshall, B.D.; Montaner, J.; Wood, E. Housing status and the health of people living with HIV/AIDS. *Curr. HIV/AIDS Rep.* **2012**, *9*, 364–374. [CrossRef] [PubMed]
20. Anema, A.; Vogenthaler, N.; Frongillo, E.A.; Kadiyala, S.; Weiser, S.D. Food insecurity and HIV/AIDS: Current knowledge, gaps, and research priorities. *Curr. HIV/AIDS Rep.* **2009**, *6*, 224–231. [CrossRef]
21. Spinelli, M.A.; Frongillo, E.A.; Sheira, L.A.; Palar, K.; Tien, P.C.; Wilson, T.; Merenstein, D.; Cohen, M.; Adedimeji, A.; Wentz, E.; et al. Food Insecurity is Associated with Poor HIV Outcomes among Women in the United States. *AIDS Behav.* **2017**, *21*, 3473–3477. [CrossRef]

22. Yehia, B.R.; Stewart, L.; Momplaisir, F.; Mody, A.; Holtzman, C.W.; Jacobs, L.M.; Hines, J.; Mounzer, K.; Glanz, K.; Metlay, J.P.; et al. Barriers and facilitators to patient retention in HIV care. *BMC Infect. Dis.* **2015**, *15*, 246. [CrossRef]
23. Quinn, K.G.; Reed, S.J.; Dickson-Gomez, J.; Kelly, J.A. An Exploration of Syndemic Factors That Influence Engagement in HIV Care Among Black Men. *Qual. Health Res.* **2018**, *28*, 1077–1087. [CrossRef]
24. Shubber, Z.; Mills, E.J.; Nachega, J.; Vreeman, R.; Freitas, M.; Bock, P.; Nsanzimana, S.; Penazzato, M.; Appolo, T.; Doherty, M.; et al. Patient-Reported Barriers to Adherence to Antiretroviral Therapy: A Systematic Review and Meta-Analysis. *PLoS Med.* **2016**, *13*, e1002183. [CrossRef]
25. Anderson, J.C.; Campbell, J.C.; Glass, N.E.; Decker, M.R.; Perrin, N.; Farley, J. Impact of intimate partner violence on clinic attendance, viral suppression and CD4 cell count of women living with HIV in an urban clinic setting. *AIDS Care* **2018**, *30*, 399–408. [CrossRef] [PubMed]
26. Machtinger, E.L.; Haberer, J.E.; Wilson, T.C.; Weiss, D.S. Recent trauma is associated with antiretroviral failure and HIV transmission risk behavior among HIV-positive women and female-identified transgenders. *AIDS Behav.* **2012**, *16*, 2160–2170. [CrossRef] [PubMed]
27. Taylor, B.S.; Fornos, L.; Tarbutton, J.; Muñoz, J.; Saber, J.A.; Bullock, D.; Villarreal, R.; Nijhawan, A.E. HIV Care Engagement in the South from the Patient and Provider Perspective: The Role of Stigma, Social Support, and Shared Decision-Making. *AIDS Patient Care STDs* **2018**, *32*, 368–378. [CrossRef]
28. Lin, D.; Zhang, C.Y.; He, Z.K.; Zhao, X.D. How does hard-to-reach status affect antiretroviral therapy adherence in the HIV-infected population? Results from a meta-analysis of observational studies. *BMC Public Health* **2019**, *19*, 789. [CrossRef]
29. Bassett, I.V.; Coleman, S.M.; Giddy, J.; Bogart, L.M.; Chaisson, C.E.; Ross, D.; Flash, M.J.E.; Govender, T.; Walensky, R.P.; Freedberg, K.A.; et al. Barriers to Care and 1-Year Mortality among Newly Diagnosed HIV-Infected People in Durban, South Africa. *J. Acquir. Immune Defic. Syndr.* **2017**, *74*, 432–438. [CrossRef]
30. Grau, L.E.; Griffiths-Kundishora, A.; Heimer, R.; Hutcheson, M.; Nunn, A.; Towey, C.; Stopka, T.J. Barriers and facilitators of the HIV care continuum in Southern New England for people with drug or alcohol use and living with HIV/AIDS: Perspectives of HIV surveillance experts and service providers. *Addict. Sci. Clin. Pract.* **2017**, *12*, 24. [CrossRef]
31. Kuchinad, K.E.; Hutton, H.E.; Monroe, A.K.; Anderson, G.; Moore, R.D.; Chander, G. A qualitative study of barriers to and facilitators of optimal engagement in care among PLWH and substance use/misuse. *BMC Res. Notes* **2016**, *9*, 229. [CrossRef]
32. Kamarulzaman, A.; Altice, F.L. Challenges in managing HIV in people who use drugs. *Curr. Opin. Infect. Dis.* **2015**, *28*, 10–16. [CrossRef]
33. Sionean, C.; Le, B.C.; Hageman, K.; Oster, A.M.; Wejnert, C.; Hess, K.L.; Paz-Bailey, G. HIV Risk, prevention, and testing behaviors among heterosexuals at increased risk for HIV infection–National HIV Behavioral Surveillance System, 21 U.S. cities, 2010. *MMWR. Surveill. Summ.* **2014**, *63*, 1–39.
34. Gardner, L.I.; Metsch, L.R.; Anderson-Mahoney, P.; Loughlin, A.M.; Del Rio, C.; Strathdee, S.; Sansom, S.L.; A Siegal, H.; E Greenberg, A.; Holmberg, S.D. Efficacy of a brief case management intervention to link recently diagnosed HIV-infected persons to care. *Aids* **2005**, *19*, 423–431. [CrossRef]
35. Miller, W.R.; Rollnick, S. *Motivational Interviewing: Helping People Change*; Guilford Press: New York, NY, USA, 2012.
36. Kelly, K.J.; Doucet, S.; Luke, A. Exploring the roles, functions, and background of patient navigators and case managers: A scoping review. *Int. J. Nurs. Stud.* **2019**, *98*, 27–47. [CrossRef] [PubMed]
37. Greene, G.J.; Reidy, E.; Felt, D.; Marro, R.; Johnson, A.K.; Phillips, G., II; Green, E.; Stonehouse, P. Implementation and evaluation of patient navigation in Chicago: Insights on addressing the social determinants of health and integrating HIV prevention and care services. *Eval. Program. Plan.* **2022**, *90*, 101977. [CrossRef] [PubMed]
38. Stitzer, M.L.; Hammond, A.S.; Matheson, T.; Sorensen, J.L.; Feaster, D.J.; Duan, R.; Gooden, L.; del Rio, C.; Metsch, L.R. Enhancing Patient Navigation with Contingent Incentives to Improve Healthcare Behaviors and Viral Load Suppression of Persons with HIV and Substance Use. *AIDS Patient Care STDs* **2018**, *32*, 288–296. [CrossRef] [PubMed]
39. Davis, D.R.; Kurti, A.N.; Skelly, J.M.; Redner, R.; White, T.J.; Higgins, S.T. A review of the literature on contingency management in the treatment of substance use disorders, 2009-2014. *Prev. Med.* **2016**, *92*, 36–46. [CrossRef]
40. Mullen, J.N.; Levitt, A.; Markoulakis, R. Supporting Individuals with Mental Health and/or Addictions Issues through Patient Navigation: A Scoping Review. *Community Ment. Health J.* **2022**. [CrossRef]
41. Bradford, J.B.; Coleman, S.; Cunningham, W. HIV System Navigation: An emerging model to improve HIV care access. *AIDS Patient Care STDs* **2007**, *21* (Suppl. S1), S49–S58. [CrossRef]
42. Freeman, H.P.; Rodriguez, R.L. History and principles of patient navigation. *Cancer* **2011**, *117* (Suppl. S15), 3539–3542. [CrossRef]
43. McBrien, K.A.; Ivers, N.; Barnieh, L.; Bailey, J.J.; Lorenzetti, D.L.; Nicholas, D.; Tonelli, M.; Hemmelgarn, B.; Lewanczuk, R.; Edwards, A.; et al. Patient navigators for people with chronic disease: A systematic review. *PLoS ONE* **2018**, *13*, e0191980. [CrossRef]
44. Myers, J.J.; Dufour, M.-S.K.; Koester, K.A.; Morewitz, M.; Packard, R.; Klein, K.M.; Estes, M.; Williams, B.; Riker, A.; Tulsky, J. The Effect of Patient Navigation on the Likelihood of Engagement in Clinical Care for HIV-Infected Individuals Leaving Jail. *Am. J. Public Health* **2018**, *108*, 385–392. [CrossRef]
45. Cunningham, W.E.; Weiss, R.E.; Nakazono, T.; Malek, M.A.; Shoptaw, S.J.; Ettner, S.L.; Harawa, N.T. Effectiveness of a Peer Navigation Intervention to Sustain Viral Suppression Among HIV-Positive Men and Transgender Women Released From Jail: The LINK LA Randomized Clinical Trial. *JAMA Intern. Med.* **2018**, *178*, 542–553. [CrossRef]

46. Metsch, L.R.; Pereyra, M.; Messinger, S.; Jeanty, Y.; Parish, C.; Valverde, E.; Cardenas, G.; Boza, H.; Tomar, S. Effects of a Brief Case Management Intervention Linking People with HIV to Oral Health Care: Project SMILE. *Am. J. Public Health* **2015**, *105*, 77–84. [CrossRef] [PubMed]
47. Wohl, D.A.; Scheyett, A.; Golin, C.E.; White, B.; Matuszewski, J.; Bowling, M.; Smith, P.; Duffin, F.; Rosen, D.; Kaplan, A.; et al. Intensive case management before and after prison release is no more effective than comprehensive pre-release discharge planning in linking HIV-infected prisoners to care: A randomized trial. *AIDS Behav.* **2011**, *15*, 356–364. [CrossRef] [PubMed]
48. Giordano, T.P.; Cully, J.; Amico, K.R.; Davila, J.A.; Kallen, M.A.; Hartman, C.; Wear, J.; Buscher, A.; Stanley, M. A Randomized Trial to Test a Peer Mentor Intervention to Improve Outcomes in Persons Hospitalized With HIV Infection. *Clin. Infect. Dis.* **2016**, *63*, 678–686. [CrossRef] [PubMed]
49. Mizuno, Y.; Higa, D.H.; Leighton, C.A.; Roland, K.B.; Deluca, J.B.; Koenig, L.J. Is HIV patient navigation associated with HIV care continuum outcomes? *Aids* **2018**, *32*, 2557–2571. [CrossRef]
50. Campbell, N.C.; Murray, E.; Darbyshire, J.; Emery, J.; Farmer, A.; Griffiths, F.; Guthrie, B.; Lester, H.; Wilson, P.; Kinmonth, A.L. Designing and evaluating complex interventions to improve health care. *BMJ* **2007**, *334*, 455–459. [CrossRef]
51. Kuhne, F.; Ehmcke, R.; Harter, M.; Kriston, L. Conceptual decomposition of complex health care interventions for evidence synthesis: A literature review. *J. Eval. Clin. Pract.* **2015**, *21*, 817–823. [CrossRef]
52. Singer, M.; Bulled, N.; Ostrach, B.; Mendenhall, E. Syndemics and the biosocial conception of health. *Lancet* **2017**, *389*, 941–950. [CrossRef]
53. Singer, M. A dose of drugs, a touch of violence, a case of AIDS: Conceptualizing the SAVA syndemic. *Free Inq. Create. Sociol.* **1996**, *24*, 99–110.
54. Meyer, J.P.; Springer, S.A.; Altice, F.L. Substance abuse, violence, and HIV in women: A literature review of the syndemic. *J. Women's Health* **2011**, *20*, 991–1006. [CrossRef]
55. Glynn, T.R.; Safren, S.A.; Carrico, A.W.; Mendez, N.A.; Duthely, L.M.; Dale, S.K.; Jones, D.L.; Feaster, D.J.; Rodriguez, A.E. High Levels of Syndemics and Their Association with Adherence, Viral Non-suppression, and Biobehavioral Transmission Risk in Miami, a U.S. City with an HIV/AIDS Epidemic. *AIDS Behav.* **2019**, *23*, 2956–2965. [CrossRef]
56. Klinkenberg, W.D.; Sacks, S.; HIV/AIDS Treatment Adherence HaOaCSG. Mental disorders and drug abuse in persons living with HIV/AIDS. *AIDS Care* **2004**, *16* (Suppl. S1), S22–S42. [CrossRef] [PubMed]
57. Mizuno, Y.; Purcell, D.W.; Knowlton, A.R.; Wilkinson, J.D.; Gourevitch, M.N.; Knight, K.R. Syndemic vulnerability, sexual and injection risk behaviors, and HIV continuum of care outcomes in HIV-positive injection drug users. *AIDS Behav.* **2015**, *19*, 684–693. [CrossRef] [PubMed]
58. Blashill, A.J.; Bedoya, C.A.; Mayer, K.H.; O'Cleirigh, C.; Pinkston, M.M.; Remmert, J.E.; Mimiaga, M.J.; Safren, S.A. Psychosocial Syndemics are Additively Associated with Worse ART Adherence in HIV-Infected Individuals. *AIDS Behav.* **2015**, *19*, 981–986. [CrossRef]
59. Friedman, M.R.; Stall, R.; Silvestre, A.J.; Wei, C.; Shoptaw, S.; Herrick, A.; Surkan, P.; Teplin, L.; Plankey, M.W. Effects of syndemics on HIV viral load and medication adherence in the multicentre AIDS cohort study. *AIDS* **2015**, *29*, 1087–1096. [CrossRef] [PubMed]
60. Metsch, L.R.; Feaster, D.J.; Gooden, L.; Matheson, T.; Stitzer, M.; Das, M.; Jain, M.K.; Rodriguez, A.E.; Armstrong, W.S.; Del Rio, C.; et al. Effect of Patient Navigation with or Without Financial Incentives on Viral Suppression among Hospitalized Patients with HIV Infection and Substance Use: A Randomized Clinical Trial. *Jama* **2016**, *316*, 156–170. [CrossRef]
61. Philbin, M.M.; Feaster, D.J.; Gooden, L.; Duan, R.; Das, M.; Jacobs, P.; Lucas, G.M.; Batey, D.S.; Nijhawan, A.; Metsch, L.R.; et al. The North-South Divide: Substance Use Risk, Care Engagement, and Viral Suppression Among Hospitalized Human Immunodeficiency Virus-Infected Patients in 11 US Cities. *Clin. Infect. Dis. Off. Publ. Infect. Dis. Soc. Am.* **2019**, *68*, 146–149. [CrossRef]
62. Mugavero, M.J.; Amico, K.R.; Horn, T.; Thompson, M.A. The state of engagement in HIV care in the United States: From cascade to continuum to control. *Clin. Infect. Dis.* **2013**, *57*, 1164–1171. [CrossRef]
63. Babor, T.F.; Higgins-Biddle, J.C.; Saunders, J.B.; Monteiro, M.G. *The Alcohol Use DIsorders Identification Test: Guidelines for Use in Primary Care*, 2nd ed.; World Health Organization: Geneva, Switzerland, 2001.
64. Skinner, H.A. The drug abuse screening test. *Addict. Behav.* **1982**, *7*, 363–371. [CrossRef]
65. Yudko, E.; Lozhkina, O.; Fouts, A. A comprehensive review of the psychometric properties of the Drug Abuse Screening Test. *J. Subst. Abuse. Treat.* **2007**, *32*, 189–198. [CrossRef]
66. Coates, J.; Swindale, A.; Bilinsky, P. *Household Food Insecurity Access Scale (HFIAS) for Measurement of Household Food Access: Indicator Guide (v.3)*; Food and Nutrition Technical Assistance Project, Academy for Educational Development: Washington, DC, USA, 2007.
67. Kalokhe, A.S.; Paranjape, A.; Bell, C.E.; Cardenas, G.A.; Kuper, T.; Metsch, L.R.; Del Rio, C. Intimate partner violence among HIV-infected crack cocaine users. *AIDS Patient Care STDs* **2012**, *26*, 234–240. [CrossRef]
68. Chew, L.D.; Bradley, K.A.; Boyko, E.J. Brief questions to identify patients with inadequate health literacy. *Fam. Med.* **2004**, *36*, 588–594. [PubMed]
69. Bureau, U.S.C. Poverty Thresholds. Available online: https://www.census.gov/data/tables/time-series/demo/income-poverty/historical-poverty-thresholds.html (accessed on 13 October 2019).
70. Simpson, D.D.; Joe, G.W. Motivation as a Predictor of Early Dropout from Drug-Abuse Treatment. *Psychother* **1993**, *30*, 357–368. [CrossRef]

71. Ware, J., Jr.; Kosinski, M.; Keller, S.D. A 12-Item Short-Form Health Survey: Construction of scales and preliminary tests of reliability and validity. *Med. Care* **1996**, *34*, 220–233. [CrossRef]
72. Fleishman, J.A.; Sherbourne, C.D.; Crystal, S.; Collins, R.L.; Marshall, G.N.; Kelly, M.; Bozzette, S.A.; Shapiro, M.F.; Hays, R.D. Coping, conflictual social interactions, social support, and mood among HIV-infected persons. HCSUS Consortium. *Am. J. Community Psychol.* **2000**, *28*, 421–453. [CrossRef]
73. Thompson, H.S.; Valdimarsdottir, H.B.; Winkel, G.; Jandorf, L.; Redd, W. The Group-Based Medical Mistrust Scale: Psychometric properties and association with breast cancer screening. *Prev. Med.* **2004**, *38*, 209–218. [CrossRef]
74. Derogatis, L.R.; Melisaratos, N. The Brief Symptom Inventory: An introductory report. *Psychol. Med.* **1983**, *13*, 595–605. [CrossRef]
75. Neff, J.A.; Zule, W.A. Predicting treatment-seeking behavior: Psychometric properties of a brief self-report scale. *Subst. Use Misuse* **2000**, *35*, 585–599. [CrossRef]
76. Collins, L.M.; Lanza, S.T. *Latent Class and Latent Transition Analysis: With Applications in the Social, Behavioral, and Health Sciences*; John Wiley & Sons: Hoboken, NJ, USA, 2009; Volume 718.
77. Muthen, L.K.; Muthen, B.O. *Mplus User's Guide*, 8th ed.; Muthen & Muthen: Los Angeles, CA, USA, 2017.
78. Bolck, A.; Croon, M.; Hagenaars, J. Estimating latent structure models with categorical variables: One-step versus three-step estimators. *Polit. Anal.* **2004**, *12*, 3–27. [CrossRef]
79. Recklitis, C.J.; Blackmon, J.E.; Chang, G. Validity of the Brief Symptom Inventory-18 (BSI-18) for identifying depression and anxiety in young adult cancer survivors: Comparison with a Structured Clinical Diagnostic Interview. *Psychol. Assess.* **2017**, *29*, 1189–1200. [CrossRef] [PubMed]
80. Leddy, A.M.; Weiss, E.; Yam, E.; Pulerwitz, J. Gender-based violence and engagement in biomedical HIV prevention, care and treatment: A scoping review. *BMC Public Health* **2019**, *19*, 897. [CrossRef]
81. Stitzer, M.; Matheson, T.; Cunningham, C.; Sorensen, J.L.; Feaster, D.J.; Gooden, L.; Hammond, A.S.; Fitzsimons, H.; Metsch, L.R. Enhancing patient navigation to improve intervention session attendance and viral load suppression of persons with HIV and substance use: A secondary post hoc analysis of the Project HOPE study. *Addict. Sci. Clin. Pract.* **2017**, *12*, 16. [CrossRef] [PubMed]
82. Kalichman, S.C.; Catz, S.; Ramachandran, B. Barriers to HIV/AIDS treatment and treatment adherence among African-American adults with disadvantaged education. *J. Natl. Med. Assoc.* **1999**, *91*, 439–446. [PubMed]
83. Haldane, V.; Cervero-Liceras, F.; Chuah, F.L.; Ong, S.E.; Murphy, G.; Sigfrid, L.; Watt, N.; Balabanova, D.; Hogarth, S.; Maimaris, W.; et al. Integrating HIV and substance use services: A systematic review. *J. Int. AIDS Soc.* **2017**, *20*, 21585. [CrossRef] [PubMed]
84. Parcesepe, A.M.; Mugglin, C.; Nalugoda, F.; Bernard, C.; Yunihastuti, E.; Althoff, K.; Jaquet, A.; Haas, A.D.; Duda, S.N.; Wester, C.W.; et al. Screening and management of mental health and substance use disorders in HIV treatment settings in low- and middle-income countries within the global IeDEA consortium. *J. Int. AIDS Soc.* **2018**, *21*, e25101. [CrossRef]

Disclaimer/Publisher's Note: The statements, opinions and data contained in all publications are solely those of the individual author(s) and contributor(s) and not of MDPI and/or the editor(s). MDPI and/or the editor(s) disclaim responsibility for any injury to people or property resulting from any ideas, methods, instructions or products referred to in the content.

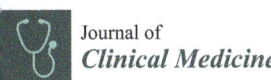

Article

Bridge Nodes between Personality Traits and Alcohol-Use Disorder Criteria: The Relevance of Externalizing Traits of Risk Taking, Callousness, and Irresponsibility

Ana De la Rosa-Cáceres [1], Marta Narvaez-Camargo [1], Andrea Blanc-Molina [1], Nehemías Romero-Pérez [1], Daniel Dacosta-Sánchez [1], Bella María González-Ponce [1], Alberto Parrado-González [1], Lidia Torres-Rosado [1], Cinta Mancheño-Velasco [1] and Óscar Martín Lozano-Rojas [1,2,*]

[1] Departamento de Psicología Clínica y Experimental, University of Huelva, 21071 Huelva, Spain; ana.delarosa@dpces.uhu.es (A.D.l.R.-C.); marta.narvaez885@alu.uhu.es (M.N.-C.); andrea.blanc@dpces.uhu.es (A.B.-M.); nehemias.romero@dpces.uhu.es (N.R.-P.); daniel.daco@dpces.uhu.es (D.D.-S.); bellamaria.gonzalez@dpces.uhu.es (B.M.G.-P.); alberto.parrado@dpces.uhu.es (A.P.-G.); lidia.torres@dpces.uhu.es (L.T.-R.); cinta.mancheno@dpces.uhu.es (C.M.-V.)
[2] Research Center for Natural Resources, Health and Environment, University of Huelva, 21071 Huelva, Spain
* Correspondence: oscar.lozano@dpsi.uhu.es

Abstract: Background: Personality disorders show strong comorbidities with alcohol-use disorder (AUD), and several personality traits have been found to be more frequent in people with AUD. This study analyzes which personality facets of those proposed in the Alternative Model of Personality Disorder (AMPD) of DSM-5 are associated with the diagnostic criteria of AUD. Methods: The sample was composed of 742 participants randomly selected from the Spanish population, and 243 patients attending mental health services. All participants were of legal age and signed an informed consent form. The instruments were administered to the community sample in an online format, and a psychologist conducted individual face-to-face interviews with the patients. AMPD facets were assessed through the Personality Inventory of DSM-5 Short-Form, and the AUD criteria through the Substance Dependence Severity Scale. A network analysis was applied to identify the personality facets mostly associated with the AUD criteria. Results: The network analysis showed the existence of three communities, grouping the AUD criteria, externalizing spectrum facets, and internalizing spectrum facets, respectively. Risk taking, callousness, and irresponsibility facets showed the strongest association with the AUD criteria, bridging externalizing personality traits with AUD criteria. Conclusions: The facets of risk taking, callousness, and irresponsibility should be accurately assessed in patients with AUD to differentiate between a possible primary personality disorder and a syndrome induced by alcohol addiction.

Keywords: alcohol-use disorders; personality disorders; externalizing; network analysis; antisocial personality disorder; borderline personality disorder

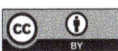

1. Introduction

Alcohol is the most widely consumed drug worldwide [1], yet only a fraction of alcohol consumers develop an alcohol-use disorder (AUD). Various factors have been suggested to increase the likelihood of developing AUDs, including genetic [2], social [3], neuropsychological [4], and psychopathological and personality traits [5].

Focusing on the latter, population-based studies show that comorbidity between AUD and PDs exceeds 40% [6], with the highest prevalence rates detected with antisocial, histrionic, and borderline personality disorders (PDs). Studies conducted with patient samples show that the prevalence rates of comorbid disorders are higher than those observed in the general population, noting that greater severity of AUD is associated with a higher probability of presenting these disorders [7]. A review conducted by Guy et al. [8] showed that in patients diagnosed with antisocial PD, lifetime AUD reached 76.7%, while among patients diagnosed with borderline PD the prevalence of AUD was 52.2%. In patients with AUD, studies have reported mixed prevalence rates. However, Trull et al. [9] estimate that in patients diagnosed with AUD, the general prevalence of PD exceeds 45%. Likewise, these authors point out that in AUD patients, Cluster B PD is more prevalent than clusters A and C.

The above evidence indicates that several personality traits are likely to be shared among individuals with AUD and PD. In this regard, numerous studies have been conducted using the Five-Factor Model (FFM) to determine which traits are characteristic of heavy alcohol users and those with AUD. For instance, a meta-analysis conducted by Malouff et al. [10] showed that low conscientiousness, low agreeableness, and high neuroticism were associated with alcohol consumption. A subsequent meta-analysis by Kotov et al. [11] also found that low conscientiousness and high neuroticism traits were more frequently found in people with AUD. However, no association was found with the agreeableness trait. Moreover, the meta-analysis by Hakulinen et al. [12] also agrees with previous studies by showing that lower agreeableness and conscientiousness and higher neuroticism are associated with heavy alcohol consumption. In addition, these authors also found that higher extraversion is associated with heavy alcohol consumption in a specific way; that is, the traits associated with the transition from moderate to heavy alcohol consumption were lower conscientiousness and higher extraversion. The latter trait, aligned with the detachment domain of the Alternative Model for Personality Disorders (AMPD), was found by Moraleda et al. [13] to be a distinctive trait of patients with AUD compared to those with other substance-use disorders. However, the described relationships between personality traits and AUD should be contextualized in those countries where alcohol consumption is widely accepted in the culture. Factors associated with disapproval of alcohol consumption, differences in family and interpersonal values, or attitudinal aspects that differ across cultures may mediate the relationships between personality traits and alcohol consumption [14].

Despite previous evidence suggesting that people with high alcohol consumption exhibit certain personality traits, the specific relationships between these traits and AUD are largely unknown. In this regard, network analysis could help to delve deeper into the relationships between personality traits and AUD. Although this type of technique has its origins in sociological studies, in the last decade it has been applied to the study of mental disorders [15]. Network analysis constitutes a set of techniques that allow the reciprocal relationships between symptoms or diagnostic criteria to be depicted in graphical form. Each symptom or diagnostic criterion is represented by a node, allowing for analysis of the interrelationships between these nodes [16,17]. Those nodes that are more densely related form substructures or clusters [18], which can be distinguished from other possible clusters. In addition, this technique allows us to determine which criteria or symptoms exert a greater influence on the others [19] and identify those nodes that are most strongly related to nodes of other distinct substructures. These nodes are considered useful for explaining comorbidity between various disorders, as shown by previous studies that have used network analysis to depict associations between AUD and internalizing traits [20].

Thus, the present study aimed to (1) examine the relationships between personality facets and AUD criteria according to their organization into different substructures in the network, as well as to test for invariance according to gender by comparing the structure, global strength, and edges between the networks of men and women; and (2) identify the bridge nodes between the different substructures identified, which could help to explain the comorbidity between PD and AUD.

2. Methods

2.1. Participants

The present study sample included 985 participants, composed of adults randomly selected from the general population ($n = 742$) and a sample of patients undergoing treatment at mental health services ($n = 243$).

The 742 adults in the community sample were selected by stratified random sampling, proportionally represented in the Spanish population according to age group, gender, and geographic area. The inclusion criteria for the community sample were being over 18 years old and not presenting any diagnosis of mental disorder. The 243 patients in the sample were being treated in public mental health services in the province of Huelva (Spain). The inclusion criteria for the patient sample were being over 18 years old and undergoing treatment in the mental health services during data collection. The exclusion criteria for both samples (patients and community) were (1) having been diagnosed with a medical or psychological disorder that disqualified them from taking the tests; and (2) not signing the informed consent form.

Sociodemographic characteristics of the total sample are presented in Table 1. Of the sample, 49.7% ($n = 490$) were female, with an age range of 18 to 80 years ($M = 44.93$; $SD = 14.6$). On the other hand, 24.26% of the sample met the diagnostic criteria for at least one mental disorder according to the Diagnostic and Statistical Manual of Mental Disorders, fifth edition (DSM-5). Table 2 shows the frequency and proportion of diagnoses for the patient sample ($n = 243$) and the whole sample ($n = 985$), with depressive disorders (38.68%) and anxiety disorders (36.21%) being the most frequent.

Table 1. Sociodemographic characteristics of participants.

Sociodemographic Characteristics	n	%
Gender		
Male	495	50.3
Female	490	49.7
Education level		
Did not complete primary education	17	1.7
Primary education	52	5.3
Secondary education	533	54.1
University studies	383	38.9
Employment status		
Employed	569	57.8
Unemployed	416	42.2

Table 2. Distribution of diagnoses in the patient sample.

	n	% Sample Patients ($n = 243$)	% All Sample ($n = 985$)
Neurodevelopmental Disorders	5	2.06	0.51
Schizophrenia Spectrum and Other Psychotic Disorders	21	8.64	2.13
Bipolar and Related Disorders	11	4.53	1.12
Depressive Disorders	94	38.68	9.54
Anxiety Disorders	88	36.21	8.93
Obsessive-Compulsive and Related Disorders	6	2.47	0.61
Trauma- and Stressor-Related Disorders	76	31.28	7.72
Dissociative Disorders	2	0.82	0.20
Somatic Symptom and Related Disorders	2	0.82	0.20
Feeding and Eating Disorders	4	1.65	0.41
Substance-Related and Addictive Disorders	10	4.12	1.02
Personality Disorders	25	10.29	2.54

2.2. Measures

The *Personality Inventory for DSM-5-Short Form* -PID-5-SF- [21] in its Spanish version [22]. The PID-5-SF assesses the 25 personality facets identified in the Alternative Model of Personality Disorder (AMPD) of the DSM-5: Anhedonia, Anxiousness, Attention Seeking, Callousness, Deceitfulness, Depressivity, Distractibility, Eccentricity, Emotional Lability, Grandiosity, Hostility, Impulsivity, Intimacy Avoidance, Irresponsibility, Manipulativeness, Perceptual Dysregulation, Perseveration, Restricted Affectivity, Rigid Perfectionism, Risk Taking, Separation Insecurity, Submissiveness, Suspiciousness, Unusual Beliefs and Experiences, and Withdrawal. These facets are organized into five higher-order domains: Negative Affect, Detachment, Antagonism, Disinhibition, and Psychoticism. The 25 facets are assessed through 100 Likert-response format items (four items per facet) from 0 ("*very false or often false*") to 3 ("*very true or often true*"). Higher scores indicate a greater presence of the facets.

This instrument has shown adequate test–retest reliability and internal consistency. Likewise, according to the Standards for Educational and Psychological Testing [23], evidence has been provided on its internal structure and relationship with other variables [22].

For the sample used in this study, Cronbach's Alpha coefficient values above 80 were found for 14 of the 25 facets; another nine facets showed internal consistency values above 0.70, and only two facets presented internal consistency values below this value (Callousness: $\alpha = 0.69$ and Irresponsibility: $\alpha = 0.63$).

Spanish version of the *Substance Dependence Severity Scale -SDSS- for DSM-5* [24,25]: The SDSS consists of a semistructured interview designed to assess the severity of dependence on one or more substances [26]. This instrument evaluates the diagnostic criteria established in the DSM-5, using an evaluation timeframe of 30 days prior to the interview.

The Spanish version of the SDSS has shown evidence of good psychometric properties in terms of reliability and validity [24,25]. In this study, only the items that operationalize the 11 diagnostic criteria of the AUD were administered, which were coded with the values 1 (presence) and 0 (absence). A reliability value (estimated through Cronbach's alpha) of 0.93 was obtained for the study sample.

In addition, questions were included on sociodemographic variables related to gender, age, educational level, and employment.

2.3. Procedure

The instruments were administered to the community sample in an online format. Before administration, participants were asked to answer a series of questions to check that they could read and write correctly.

A trained psychologist administered the instruments to the sample of patients through individual interviews that took place in a room in the mental health center where they were being treated.

All participants (community sample and patients) were informed of the study objectives and the voluntary and anonymous nature of their participation and signed the informed consent form before completing the instruments. This study has been approved by the Bioethics Committee of Biomedical Research of Andalusia (Spain) (file number PI 040/18).

2.4. Data Analysis

The multivariate normality test revealed the absence of multivariate normality for skewness (Mardia = 60,874.19) and kurtosis (Mardia = 272.67). Therefore, the network was estimated using the GLASSO algorithm [27] in combination with the EBIC selection model (hyperparameter $\gamma = 0.5$) [28] applied to the nonparanormal transformation of the data set [29]. For the layout of the graph, the Fruchterman–Reingold algorithm was used [30]. The study's sample size ($n = 985$) was adequate to estimate the network according to the simulation study [31] (Supplementary Figure S1).

To detect community structures, the walktrap algorithm was employed [32]. The strength of centrality indices, one-step Expected Influence (EI1), and two-step Expected Influence

(EI2) were estimated [33]. Strength and EI provide information on the direct relationships between each node and the rest by summing the weights of the edges, considering the absolute values or the sign of the value (positive or negative), respectively. EI2 also sums the weights of indirectly related edges [33]. The stability of the centrality indices was quantified using a person-dropping bootstrap procedure that provides a correlation-stability coefficient (CS-coefficient). CS-coefficient values > 0.5 indicate strong stability and interpretability [31].

In addition, predictability (i.e., the proportion of variance of each node that is explained by its neighboring nodes) was estimated [34], along with the Participation Coefficient (PC), and Participation Ratio (PR) [35]. Higher PC values indicate that the edges of the nodes are distributed more equally among the network communities, while higher PR values indicate nodes with more numerous and stronger edges. The PC and PR values were transformed to a scale of 0 to 1 for ease of interpretation.

Regarding the bridge nodes, the bridge strength, bridge EI1, and bridge EI2 were estimated [36]. Bridge strength and bridge EI1 indicate the total connectivity of each node with nodes of other communities with which it is directly related, by summing the weights of the edges that connect the node with nodes of other communities considering absolute values (bridge strength) or the sign of the values (bridge EI1). Bridge EI2 also considers indirect relationships with nodes in other communities. A blind cut-off point at the 80th percentile of bridge strength was applied to identify bridge nodes [37].

Finally, network invariance for men (n = 495) and women (n = 490) was analyzed using the network comparison test [38] (5000 times repeated subsampling). In addition, the invariance of network structure and overall strength was analyzed. The M statistic indicates the differences in the connections between the edges of both networks, while the S statistic indicates the difference in global strength between the two networks. If the test for network-structure invariance is significant, the invariance of the individual edges will be examined [38].

All analyses were conducted in R 4.1.2 and R-Studio 2022.2.0.443. In addition, the packages mvn 5.9 [39], bootnet 1.5 [31], igraph 1.3.0 [40], network tools 1.4.0 [36], qgraph 1.9.2 [41], and Network-ComparisonTest 2.2.1 [38] were used.

3. Results

3.1. Network Structure with AMPD Personality Facets and AUD Criteria, and Invariance According to Gender

The estimated network is shown in Figure 1. The network consisted of 250 edges (out of a possible 630) that showed a partial correlation value different from zero. The weights of the edges ranged from −0.009 (Restricted Affectivity-Attention Seeking) to 0.431 (Depressivity-Anhedonia). The graphical analysis reveals an optimal 3-community solution (modularity index = 0.45), which organizes the nodes according to a structure that differentiates the facets most strongly linked to the internalizing spectrum (Anhedonia, Anxiousness, Depressivity, Distractibility, Eccentricity, Emotional Lability, Hostility, Intimacy Avoidance, Perceptual Dysregulation, Perseveration, Restricted Affectivity, Rigid Perfectionism, Separation Insecurity, Submissiveness, Suspiciousness, Unusual Beliefs and Experiences, and Withdrawal), to the externalizing spectrum (Attention Seeking, Callousness, Deceitfulness, Grandiosity, Impulsivity, Irresponsibility, Manipulativeness, and Risk Taking), and the AUD diagnostic criteria (Quit/Control, Time Spent, Activities Given Up, Tolerance, Withdrawal, Larger/Longer, Physical/Psychological Problems, Neglect Roles, Hazardous Use, Social/Interpersonal Problems, and Craving).

The standardized scores of the centrality indices, bridge-centrality indices, and the predictability of the nodes are displayed in Table 3. The nodes with the highest strength values were Anxiousness (1.94), Anhedonia (1.67), Perseveration (1.51), and Emotional lability (1.08). The highest EI1 values were for Perseveration (1.51), Anhedonia (1.48), Anxiousness (1.43), and Physical/ Psychological Problems (1.23). The highest EI2 values corresponded to Perseveration (1.57), Anhedonia (1.50), Eccentricity (1.24), and Anxiousness (1.20). The CS-coefficient (cor = 0.7) was 0.75 for Strength and 0.75 for EI (see Supplementary Figures S2 and S3, respectively), indicating strong stability and interpretability of the estimates. The nodes with the highest bridge strength, bridge EI1, and bridge EI2 values were Irresponsibility (bridge strength = 2.77; bridge EI1 = 2.91; bridge EI2 = 3.01), Impulsivity (2.49, 2.85, 2.84), Callousness (2.21, 1.34, 1.25), and Risk Taking (1.43, 1.47, 1.82). The predictability of each node is shown in Figure 1 and Table 3. The predictability values (R^2) ranged from 0.62 (Anhedonia) to 0.22 (Separation Insecurity), with an average value of 0.42. The symptoms with the least explained variance (i.e., the most independent) were Separation Insecurity (R^2 = 0.22), Quit/Control (R^2 = 0.24), Intimacy Avoidance (R^2 = 0.24), Larger/Longer (R^2 = 0.27), and Restricted Affectivity (R^2 = 0.27). In contrast, the symptoms with the greatest explained variance were Anhedonia (R^2 = 0.62), Depressivity (R^2 = 0.60), Anxiousness (R^2 = 0.57), and Perseveration (R^2 = 0.56). Table 3 also shows the PC and PR values. The highest PC values correspond to Hostility (PC = 0.53), Impulsivity (PC = 0.50), and Rigid Perfectionism (PC = 0.38), these being the nodes with edges that are distributed more equally among the communities. According to the PR values, the nodes with the strongest and most numerous edges were Irresponsibility (PR = 1), Perseveration (PR = 0.97), and Perceptual Dysregulation (PR = 0.90).

Concerning the invariance analysis, Table 4 shows the descriptive statistics (means and standard deviations) for the AMPD facets and AUD criteria in the total sample (n = 985), the male subsample (n = 495), and the female subsample (n = 490). It is observed that the mean difference between males and females has a small or null effect size for all AUD facets and criteria except for Emotional Lability, which yielded a medium effect size (d = 0.62).

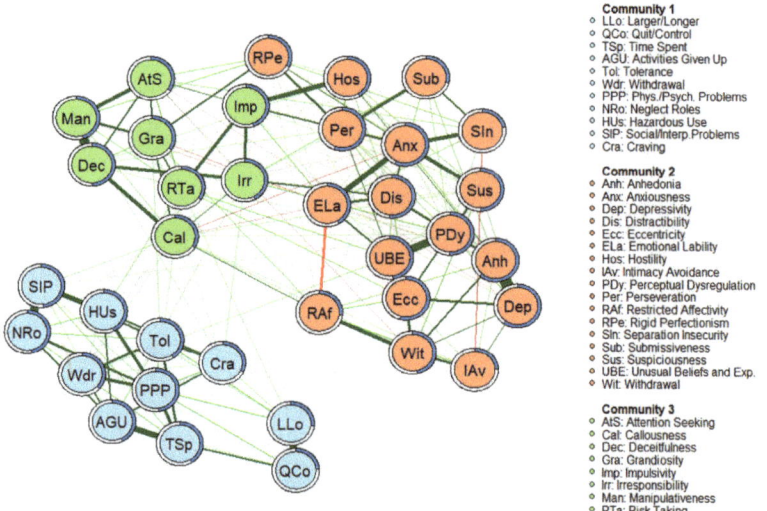

Figure 1. Empirical network model (network structure estimated from a walktrap modularity analysis) for the complete sample (n = 985). Note. Each node represents a symptom. The edges represent the relationships (partial correlations) between the symptoms. Positive relationships are represented in green, and negative relationships in red. The thickness of the edge reflects the strength of the association, so that the most strongly related symptoms are connected by thicker edges. The blue pie chart surrounding each node represents the predictability of each node (a higher proportion of blue indicates greater predictability). The membership of the nodes to the different communities is represented by different colors: the symptoms of Community 1 are shown in blue, the symptoms of Community 2 are shown in salmon, and the symptoms of Community 3 are shown in green. The arrangement of the nodes was established based on the Fruchterman-Reingold algorithm.

Table 3. Centrality indices and bridge-centrality indices of personality facets and alcohol-use disorder criteria.

Nodes	Strength	Expected Influence 1	Expected Influence 2	Bridge Strength	Bridge Expected Influence 1	Bridge Expected Influence 2	R^2	PC	PR
				Personality Facets of Alternative Model of Personality Disorder					
Anhedonia	1.67	1.48	1.50	−1.00	−1.14	−1.02	0.62	0.00	0.61
Anxiousness	1.94	1.43	1.20	−0.82	−1.33	−1.00	0.57	0.01	0.71
Attention Seeking	−0.21	−0.57	−0.64	0.32	−0.39	−0.14	0.34	0.11	0.45
Callousness	0.40	−0.24	−0.32	2.21	1.34	1.25	0.33	0.29	0.86
Deceitfulness	0.83	1.03	0.97	−0.33	−0.09	0.49	0.50	0.02	0.58
Depressivity	0.91	0.82	1.10	−0.89	−1.04	−1.00	0.60	0.00	0.59
Distractibility	0.35	0.61	0.75	−0.18	0.04	−0.12	0.51	0.15	0.64
Eccentricity	1.04	1.20	1.24	−0.46	−0.22	−0.08	0.54	0.05	0.67
Emotional Lability	1.08	−1.46	−1.19	0.20	−1.06	−1.25	0.41	0.09	0.86
Grandiosity	0.12	−0.10	−0.26	1.36	0.95	0.83	0.34	0.25	0.49
Hostility	−0.93	−0.46	−0.26	0.77	1.05	0.63	0.40	0.53	0.51
Impulsivity	0.16	0.47	0.41	2.49	2.85	2.84	0.44	0.50	0.37
Intimacy Avoidance	−1.75	−2.09	−2.01	−0.60	−0.37	−0.53	0.24	0.04	0.28
Irresponsibility	0.63	0.69	0.73	2.77	2.91	3.01	0.42	0.37	1
Manipulativeness	0.39	0.25	0.22	0.02	−0.27	−0.11	0.45	0.04	0.40
Perceptual Dysreg.	0.61	0.84	0.95	0.60	0.88	0.83	0.50	0.09	0.90
Perseveration	1.51	1.51	1.57	0.34	0.49	0.47	0.56	0.15	0.97
Restricted Affectivity	−0.49	−1.75	−1.72	0.29	0.43	0.15	0.27	0.18	0.35
Rigid Perfectionism	−0.75	−0.68	−0.70	0.96	0.75	0.60	0.33	0.38	0.48
Risk Taking	−0.17	−0.02	0.02	1.43	1.47	1.82	0.35	0.23	0.67
Separation Insecurity	−1.58	−2.15	−2.15	−0.53	−0.57	−0.72	0.22	0.05	0.20
Submissiveness	−1.84	−1.28	−1.28	−0.42	−0.28	−0.32	0.29	0.11	0.17
Suspiciousness	0.34	0.61	0.77	−0.40	−0.17	−0.15	0.50	0.04	0.85
Unusual Bel. and Exp.	−0.02	0.31	0.38	−0.05	0.21	0.30	0.48	0.05	0.48
Withdrawal	0.27	0.20	0.06	−0.56	−0.82	−0.74	0.46	0.03	0.39

Table 3. Cont.

Nodes	Strength	Expected Influence 1	Expected Influence 2	Bridge Strength	Bridge Expected Influence 1	Bridge Expected Influence 2	R^2	PC	PR
Alcohol-Use Disorders			Personality Facets of Alternative Model of Personality Disorder						
Larger/Longer	−1.54	−0.97	−1.23	−0.78	−0.55	−0.69	0.27	0.02	0.15
Quit/Control	−2.24	−1.59	−1.75	−1.14	−0.97	−1.07	0.24	0.00	0
Time spent	−0.36	0.03	0.01	−1.08	−0.88	−0.88	0.41	0.00	0.31
Activities given up	0.05	0.37	0.23	−0.74	−0.52	−0.53	0.43	0.02	0.36
Tolerance	0.12	0.36	0.22	−0.56	−0.44	−0.43	0.41	0.00	0.61
Withdrawal	−0.61	−0.35	−0.26	−0.15	−0.12	−0.21	0.37	0.03	0.56
Phys./Psych.Problems	1.07	1.23	0.99	−0.79	−0.57	−0.54	0.48	0.00	0.55
Neglect roles	0.06	0.19	0.28	−0.81	−0.85	−0.81	0.47	0.02	0.60
Hazardous use	−0.18	0.18	0.21	−0.56	−0.32	−0.35	0.43	0.02	0.27
Social/Interp.Prob.	0.18	0.48	0.50	−0.66	−0.43	−0.49	0.48	0.01	0.38
Craving	−1.07	−0.57	−0.54	−0.22	0.03	−0.04	0.32	0.04	0.44

Note. R^2 = Predictability; PC = Participation Coefficient; PR = Participation Ratio.

Table 4. Means, standard deviations, and Cohen's d of scores on the PID-5-SF subscales and alcohol-use disorder criteria.

	All Sample	Men	Women	Cohen's d
		PID-5 Subscales		
Anhedonia	6.78 (3.24)	6.18 (2.71)	7.38 (3.60)	0.38
Anxiousness	8.60 (3.38)	7.81 (3.17)	9.41 (3.39)	0.49
Attention Seeking	5.88 (2.50)	6.04 (2.55)	5.72 (2.44)	0.13
Callousness	4.75 (1.50)	4.90 (1.69)	4.59 (1.26)	0.34
Deceitfulness	5.24 (2.00)	5.40 (2.16)	5.08 (1.81)	0.16
Depressivity	5.88 (2.91)	5.39 (2.36)	6.38 (3.31)	0.34
Distractibility	7.97 (3.42)	7.40 (3.27)	8.54 (3.48)	0.34
Eccentricity	7.11 (3.39)	6.89 (3.28)	7.34 (3.48)	0.13
Emotional Lability	9.21 (3.14)	8.28 (2.85)	10.13 (3.15)	0.62
Grandiosity	5.50 (2.12)	5.74 (2.32)	5.25 (1.88)	0.23
Hostility	6.95 (2.85)	6.35 (2.69)	7.54 (2.88)	0.43
Impulsivity	6.47 (2.91)	6.10 (2.79)	6.85 (3.02)	0.26
Intimacy Avoidance	6.26 (3.26)	5.99 (2.76)	6.54 (3.66)	0.17
Irresponsibility	5.51 (1.91)	5.52 (2.01)	5.50 (1.80)	0.01
Manipulativeness	5.62 (2.13)	5.72 (2.18)	5.51 (2.08)	0.10
Perceptual Dysregulation	5.32 (2.20)	5.21 (2.13)	5.44 (2.25)	0.10
Perseveration	7.31 (2.96)	6.88 (2.79)	7.75 (3.07)	0.30
Restricted Affectivity	7.35 (2.66)	7.67 (2.68)	7.03 (2.59)	0.24
Rigid Perfectionism	8.06 (3.12)	7.84 (3.05)	8.27 (3.19)	0.14
Risk Taking	5.40 (2.23)	5.51 (2.30)	5.29 (2.14)	0.10
Separation Insecurity	7.90 (3.26)	7.78 (3.26)	8.03 (3.26)	0.08
Submissiveness	6.94 (2.82)	6.63 (2.56)	7.25 (3.02)	0.22
Suspiciousness	6.69 (2.57)	6.50 (2.51)	6.88 (2.63)	0.15
Unusual Beliefs and Exp.	5.92 (2.67)	5.63 (2.45)	6.21 (2.84)	0.22
Withdrawal	6.98 (2.93)	6.86 (2.86)	7.09 (3.00)	0.08
		Alcohol-Use Disorder criteria		
Larger/Longer	0.17 (0.17)	0.20 (0.40)	0.14 (0.35)	0.16
Quit/Control	0.19 (0.23)	0.25 (0.43)	0.13 (0.33)	0.31
Time spent	0.05 (0.20)	0.06 (0.24)	0.04 (0.20)	0.09
Activities given up	0.04 (0.38)	0.05 (0.22)	0.03 (0.17)	0.10
Tolerance	0.05 (0.39)	0.07 (0.25)	0.03 (0.18)	0.18
Withdrawal	0.05 (0.22)	0.06 (0.24)	0.04 (0.20)	0.09
Phys/Psych.Problems	0.08 (0.20)	0.09 (0.28)	0.06 (0.24)	0.12
Neglect roles	0.03 (0.22)	0.04 (0.21)	0.02 (0.13)	0.11
Hazardous use	0.06 (0.22)	0.08 (0.27)	0.03 (0.18)	0.21
Social/Interp.Problems	0.04 (0.26)	0.05 (0.22)	0.03 (0.18)	0.10
Craving	0.06 (0.24)	0.07 (0.26)	0.05 (0.22)	0.08

The above values are congruent with the invariance test conducted for men ($n = 495$) and women ($n = 490$), detecting no significant differences in terms of network structure (i.e., differences in the edge connections of the two networks, M = 0.22; $p = 0.838$) or global strength (i.e., difference in the sum of the absolute weights between the two networks, S = 0.34; $p = 0.494$). The overall strength of the network estimated for the male sample was 17.18, and for the female sample this was 16.84.

3.2. "Bridging Nodes" between AUD Criteria and Personality Facets

Figure 2 shows (in yellow) the facets that act as "bridge nodes" between the different network structures (i.e., the nodes more connected to nodes of other communities with which they are directly related), according to the highest values of bridge strength shown in Table 3. Through the edges, it is observed that most of the relationships between the AUD criteria and the personality facets occur through these "bridge nodes". Furthermore, it appears that most of the facets acting as "bridge nodes" correspond to the "antagonism" and "disinhibition" domains of the AMPD. Only the bridge node corresponding to the "hostility" facet falls within the "negative affectivity" domain of the AMPD.

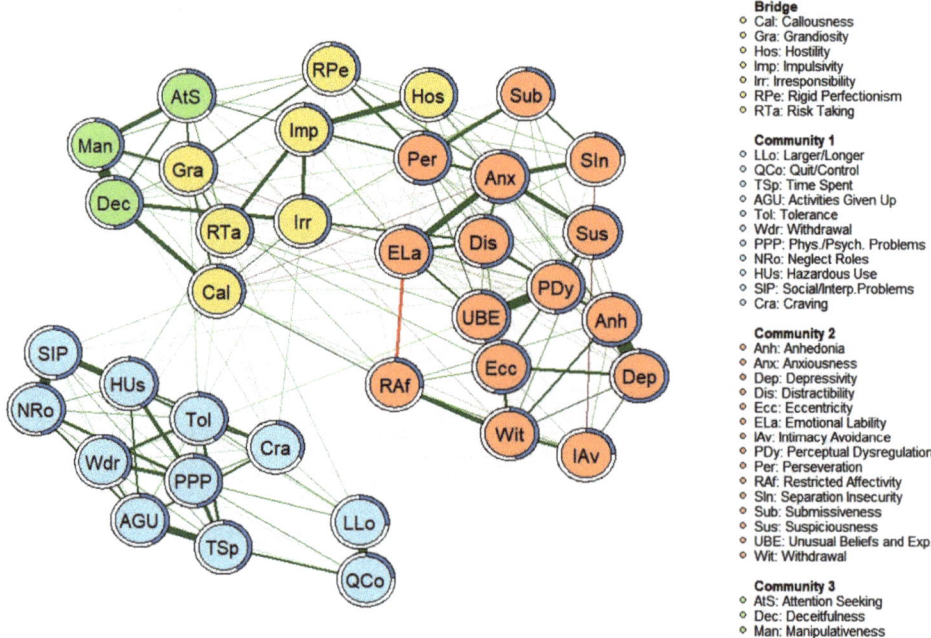

Figure 2. Empirical network model (network structure estimated from a walktrap modularity analysis) and bridge nodes for complete sample ($n = 985$). Note. Each node represents a symptom. The edges represent the relationships (partial correlations) between the symptoms. Positive relationships are represented in green. and negative relationships in red. The thickness of the edge reflects the strength of the association, so the most strongly related symptoms are connected by thicker edges. The blue pie chart surrounding each node represents the predictability of each node (a higher proportion of blue indicates greater predictability). The membership of the nodes to the different communities is represented by different colors: bridge symptoms are shown in yellow; the symptoms of Community 1 are shown in blue; the symptoms of Community 2 are shown in salmon; and the symptoms of Community 3 are shown in green. The arrangement of the nodes was established based on the Fruchterman-Reingold algorithm.

A detailed analysis of the relationships between the AUD criteria and the bridging nodes is displayed in Table 5, which shows the partial and Pearson correlations between the facets that constitute "bridging nodes" and the AUD diagnostic criteria. The bridge node "risk-taking" is the one that presents the most relationships with the AUD diagnostic criteria, followed by the facets of "irresponsibility" and "callousness." Concerning the AUD diagnostic criteria, it can be observed that the diagnostic criterion "withdrawal" shows the most associations with the bridging nodes, together with "neglect roles" and "craving".

Table 5. Partial and zero-order correlations between network symptoms on estimation sample.

	Scales	1	2	3	4	5	6	7	8	9	10	11	12	13	14	15	16	17	18
1.	Callousness	1	0.45	0.31	0.29	0.49	0.25	0.36	**0.14**	**0.13**	**0.25**	**0.27**	**0.31**	**0.32**	**0.26**	**0.31**	**0.29**	**0.33**	**0.31**
2.	Grandiosity	0.12	1	0.29	0.29	0.36	0.39	0.43	0.13	0.12	0.20	0.21	0.29	0.23	0.19	0.20	0.26	0.26	0.29
3.	Hostility	0.01	-	1	0.57	0.42	0.41	0.38	0.13	0.08	0.18	0.20	0.18	0.23	0.21	0.19	0.19	0.21	0.19
4.	Impulsivity	-	-	0.20	1	0.53	0.31	0.53	0.13	0.08	0.21	0.25	0.19	0.23	0.23	0.20	0.20	0.21	0.17
5.	Irresponsibility	0.12	-	0.00	0.16	1	0.23	0.43	**0.23**	**0.13**	**0.28**	**0.35**	**0.29**	**0.31**	**0.33**	**0.34**	**0.35**	**0.32**	**0.34**
6.	Rigid Perfectionism	-	0.12	0.04	0.13	−0.02	1	0.33	0.04	0.06	0.08	0.08	0.07	0.07	0.10	0.05	0.13	0.13	0.13
7.	Risk taking	0.03	0.12	-	0.18	-	-	1	**0.25**	**0.18**	**0.27**	**0.28**	**0.30**	**0.31**	**0.35**	**0.29**	**0.35**	**0.30**	**0.30**
8.	Larger/longer	-	-	-	-	-	-	0.05	1	0.48	0.35	0.28	0.39	0.30	0.42	0.34	0.36	0.34	0.34
9.	Quit/control	-	-	-	-	-	-	-	0.27	1	0.39	0.33	0.32	0.29	0.40	0.32	0.29	0.29	0.25
10.	Time Spent	-	-	-	-	-	-	0.01	0.19	0.23	1	0.58	0.52	0.48	0.55	0.48	0.46	0.50	0.40
11.	Activities given up	-	-	-	-	0.04	-	-	-	-	0.20	1	0.49	0.50	0.50	0.53	0.52	0.51	0.48
12.	Tolerance	-	-	-	-	-	-	0.02	0.04	-	0.22	0.09	1	0.51	0.52	0.51	0.44	0.53	0.48
13.	Withdrawal	0.03	-	0.01	-	0.02	-	0.04	0.08	-	0	0.10	0.19	1	0.55	0.49	0.45	0.46	0.41
14.	Phys./Psych.Problems	-	-	-	-	-	-	0.01	0.08	0.05	0.12	0.05	0.05	0.20	1	0.57	0.57	0.54	0.48
15.	Neglect roles	0.05	-	-	-	0.01	0.02	-	-	-	0.02	0.22	0.11	0.11	0.09	1	0.54	0.66	0.42
16.	Hazardous use	0.01	-	-	-	-	-	0.04	0.10	-	0.04	0.05	0.02	-	0.17	0.13	1	0.59	0.48
17.	Social/Interp.Problems	-	0.02	-	-	-	-	0.01	-	-	0.05	0.06	0.10	0.09	0.11	0.25	0.21	1	0.42
18.	Craving	0.03	0.02	-	-	0.05	-	-	0.10	0.05	-	-	0.27	0.08	0.11	0.01	0.06	0.04	1

Partial correlations are shown on the lower diagonal and zero-order correlations on the upper diagonal. The dashes represent correlation values = 0. The bold type reflects the relationships between the bridging nodes and the AUD criteria.

4. Discussion

The present study aimed to deepen our knowledge of the existing comorbidity between PDs and AUD. For this purpose, this study aimed to complement the existing evidence [10–12] with new evidence obtained through network analysis and use of the DSM-5 AMPD trait model. To our knowledge, no previous studies have used network analysis to examine the relationship between the DSM-5 AMPD traits and AUD criteria.

Analysis of the centrality indices of the AUD criteria has shown relatively low values, indicating their low capacity to influence the personality facets. This finding is also evident in the visualization of the network, in which the AMPD facets and the AUD criteria are organized into three independent communities—albeit empirically related and theoretically grounded. The alcohol diagnostic criteria maintain close relationships, leading them to be organized into an independent community, while the AMPD facets are organized into two interrelated communities, linked to the internalizing and externalizing spectrum. This organization of the AMPD facets is consistent with studies that have applied a hierarchical analysis of personality [42–44], and the independent organization of the AUD is congruent with the Hierarchical Taxonomy of Psychopathology (HiTOP) model [45] and previous network analysis studies [46–48]. Despite the relative independence of the three communities, the AUD diagnostic criteria show relationships with a set of personality facets that act as a bridge. These are mostly associated with the externalizing spectrum, highlighting the relationships with Callousness, Irresponsibility, and Risk Taking.

Our observation of these bridging facets is congruent with the relationships observed in previous studies analyzing FFM traits in alcohol consumers. The specialized literature supports an association between alcohol consumption and the FFM traits of conscientiousness and agreeableness [10,12], which are aligned with the disinhibition and antagonism domains of the AMPD [49]. This study has shown that these relationships could largely be due to the connection between the AUD criteria and the bridging facets within the disinhibition (risk taking, irresponsibility, impulsivity, and rigid perfectionism) and antagonism (callousness, grandiosity, and hostility) domains. Similarly, it is worth noting the connection between the AUD criterion "withdrawal" and the facet "hostility" framed in the negative affectivity domain of the AMPD (aligned with the neuroticism trait included in the FFM). This finding is congruent with the results of the meta-analysis conducted by Hakulinen et al. [12], which found that the domain "neuroticism" is associated primarily with people who engage in heavy alcohol consumption. It is also compatible with studies suggesting that people with AUD have biases toward recognizing and attributing hostile expressions and behaviors [50,51]. Thus, one hypothesis to explain this relationship could be that the occurrence of "withdrawal" exacerbates the "hostility" trait. Therefore, this association is observed mainly in heavy alcohol users and is weaker in those who consume alcohol in moderation.

On the other hand—and concerning PDs—some studies show that it is borderline and antisocial PDs that most frequently co-occur with AUD. According to the DSM-5 AMPD [52], antisocial PD is evaluated based on the presence of the facets "Callousness", "Irresponsibility", and "Risk Taking", among others, while Borderline PD includes the facets of "Risk Taking" and "Hostility" for its diagnosis. Thus, the bridging facets identified in this study are some of those required for the assessment of the two PDs mentioned above. Therefore, it is likely that the high comorbidity of AUD with these disorders is caused by the relationships between the diagnostic criteria of AUD and these bridging facets. This finding along with the results reported by other authors [53,54], could also help to explain why patients with antisocial and borderline PD have higher rates of relapse and treatment dropout. These authors found that patients who prematurely terminate treatment score higher on the facets of "Hostility", "Callousness", and "Risk-taking" than those who complete treatment. Thus, these bridging facets that are relevant to antisocial and borderline PD diagnoses, are also associated with premature patient dropout.

We consider the findings of this study to be useful for advancing our knowledge of the comorbidity of AUD with PDs. Nonetheless, it is also worth considering some aspects of the study sample that could have affected the results. As already indicated, the sample of patients shows the highest prevalence of emotional disorders (depressive and anxiety disorders). This may have maximized the relationships between the facets associated with the "negative affectivity" domain, which resulted in higher values of the centrality indices observed for these facets. However, aside from the centrality indices, the network structure is congruent with the hierarchical analysis reported in previous studies [42–44], and so the impact of this sample composition is more likely to be limited to the understanding of comorbidity between AUDs and PDs.

We would also like to point out that the partial correlations between the "bridging nodes" and the AUD criteria are low. It is possible that these weak relationships were found because this study did not include a specific sample of patients with AUDs, with the sample of the general population being more representative. Consequently, greater variability in the personality facets and AUD criteria are observed compared to the case in which AUD patients are specifically selected, which could negatively affect the values of the partial correlations. Despite this, the results have revealed the existence of "bridging nodes" congruent with evidence from previous meta-analysis [10–12]. Therefore, we consider that the results of this study provide novel insights that could help to improve our understanding of comorbidity between these disorders.

Finally, we consider it necessary to limit the generalizability of the relationships observed in this study to the cultural context in which it was carried out. In this sense, it should be noted that cultural studies analyzing the relationship between personality traits and alcohol consumption have shown differences in the relationships established between agreeableness, antisocial behavior, and alcohol-related consequences when comparing different countries [55]. Moreover, it should be considered that social norms about what constitutes, for example, "irresponsibility" or "risk taking" in the case of personality trait assessment, or "social/interpersonal problems" or "hazardous use" in the case of AUD assessment, may differ across cultures and even within a culture [56]. Therefore, we consider that the observed interrelationships be contextualized within the framework of Spanish culture as well as in other countries with equivalent social norms and legislation. Future cross-cultural studies should provide evidence on the stability of these relationships in other countries and cultures.

5. Conclusions

The present study has shown, through network analysis, connections between AUD diagnostic criteria and personality facets. It has been observed that the bridge nodes correspond to facets associated with the disinhibition and antagonism personality domains of the AMPD. This finding is congruent with the results of previous studies using the FFM model and applying other statistical techniques. This finding also helps to understand the comorbidities observed between AUD, borderline, and antisocial personality disorder. From a clinical perspective, the results indicate the importance of accurately assessing the risk-taking, callousness, and irresponsibility traits in patients with AUD, in order to differentiate between a possible primary personality disorder, or the existence of a syndrome induced by alcohol addiction. In addition, the observed connections may be useful to guide the development of interventions aimed at dual-pathology patients with AUD and PD.

Supplementary Materials: The following supporting information can be downloaded at: https://www.mdpi.com/article/10.3390/jcm11123468/s1, Figure S1: Simulation results using the estimated network adjusted to a real network structure for the complete sample (n = 985). From left to right this shows the correlation between the real network and the estimated network. The sensitivity (real positive rate). The specificity (real negative rate). And the correlation of the Strength and Expected Influence measures of centrality between the real network and the estimated network; Figure S2: Stability plot of the Strength of the network for the complete sample (n = 985). La línea representa la media de correlaciones entre un determinado porcentaje de la muestra y el total de la muestra y las sombras representan el área entre el 2.5% y el 97.5% de las correlaciones estimadas; Figure S3: Stability plot of the one-step Expected Influence of the network for the complete sample (n = 985). La línea representa la media de correlaciones entre un determinado porcentaje de la muestra y el total de la muestra y las sombras representan el área entre el 2.5% y el 97.5% de las correlaciones estimadas.

Author Contributions: Conceptualization: Ó.M.L.-R., M.N.-C., A.B.-M., D.D.-S.-S; Methodology: A.D.l.R.-C., Ó.M.L.-R., B.M.G.-P., C.M.-V., L.T.-R., N.R.-P.-P.; Formal analysis: A.D.l.R.-C., A.P.-G.; Writing original draft: all authors; Writing-review and editing: all authors. All authors have read and agreed to the published version of the manuscript.

Funding: This work was supported by the grant "Network-Psyco: Modelización a través de redes empíricas de las conexiones entre facetas y rasgos psicológicos", project UHU-1257470 on Programa Operativo FEDER Andalucía 2014–2020, provided by Fondo Europeo de Desarrollo Regional (EU) and Junta de Andalucía (Spain) and by Ministry of Universities of the Government of Spain (FPU2019/00144).

Institutional Review Board Statement: The study was conducted in accordance with the Declaration of Helsinki, and approved by the Bioethics Committee of Biomedical Research of Andalusia (Spain) (file number PI 040/18).

Informed Consent Statement: Informed consent was obtained from all subjects involved in the study.

Data Availability Statement: Database should be requested to the correspondence author.

Conflicts of Interest: The authors declare no conflict of interest.

References

1. World Health Organization. *Global Status Report on Alcohol and Health*; World Health Organization: Geneva, Switzerland, 2018.
2. Kapoor, M.; Wang, J.; Farris, S.; Liu, Y.; McClintick, J.; Gupta, I.; Goate, A. Analysis of whole genome-transcriptomic organization in brain to identify genes associated with alcoholism. *Transl. Psychiatry* **2019**, *9*, 89. [CrossRef] [PubMed]
3. Pearson, M.; Hustad, J. Personality and alcohol-related outcomes among mandated college students: Descriptive norms, injunctive norms, and college-related alcohol beliefs as mediatiors. *Addit. Behav.* **2014**, *39*, 879–884. [CrossRef] [PubMed]
4. Kwako, L.; Schawandt, M.; Ramchandani, V.; Diazgranados, N.; Koob, G.; Volkow, N.; Blanco, C.; Goldman, D. Neurofunctional domains derived from deep behavioral phenotyping in alcohol use disorder. *Am. J. Psychiatry* **2019**, *176*, 744–753. [CrossRef] [PubMed]
5. Cavicchioli, M.; Ramella, P.; Movalli, M.; Prudenziati, F.; Vassena, G.; Simone, G.; Maffei, C. DSM-5 maladaptive personality domains among treatment-seeking individuals with alcohol use disorder: The role of deshinibition and negative affectivity. *Subst. Use Misuse* **2020**, *55*, 1746–1758. [CrossRef] [PubMed]
6. Trull, T.J.; Jahng, S.; Tomko, R.L.; Wood, P.K.; Sher, K.J. Revised NESARC personality disorder diagnoses: Gender, prevalence, and comorbidity with substance dependence disorders. *J. Personal. Disord.* **2010**, *24*, 412–426. [CrossRef]
7. Grant, B.; Goldstein, R.B.; Saha, T.; Chou, P.; Jung, J.; Zhang, H.; Hasin, D. Epidemiology of DSM-5 Alcohol Use Disorder: Results from the National Epidemiologic Survey on Alcohol and Related Conditions III. *JAMA Psychiatry* **2015**, *72*, 757–766. [CrossRef]
8. Guy, K.; Newton-Howes, G.; Ford, H.; Williman, J.; Foulds, J. The prevalence of comorbid alcohol use disorder in the presence of personality disorder: Systematic review and explanatory modelling. *Personal. Ment. Health* **2018**, *12*, 216–228. [CrossRef]
9. Trull, T.J.; Solham, M.B.; Brown, W.C.; Tomko, R.L.; Schaefer, L.; Jahng, S. *Substance Use Disorders and Personality Disorders*; Sher, K., Ed.; Oxford Handbook of Substance Use Disorders; Oxford University Press: New York, NY, USA, 2016.
10. Malouf, J.M.; Thirsteinsson, E.; Rooke, S.; Chutte, N. Alcohol involvement and the Five-Factor Model of personality: A meta-analysis. *J. Drug Educ.* **2007**, *37*, 277–294. [CrossRef]
11. Kotov, R.; Gamez, W.; Schimidt, F.; Watson, D. Linking "Big" Personality traits to anxiety, depressive, and substance use disorders: A meta-analysis. *Psychol. Bull.* **2010**, *136*, 768–821. [CrossRef]
12. Hakulinen, C.; Elovainio, M.; Batty, G.D.; Virtanen, M.; Kivimäki, M.; Jokela, M. Personality and alcohol consumption: Pooled analysis of 72,949 adults from eight cohort studies. *Drug Alcohol Depend.* **2015**, *151*, 110–114. [CrossRef]
13. Moraleda, E.; Ramírez-lopez, J.; Fernández-Calderón, F.; Lozano, O.M.; Díaz-Batanero, C. Personality traits among the variuos profiles of substance use disorder patients: New evidence using the DSM-5 Section III Framework. *Eur. Addict. Res.* **2019**, *25*, 238–247. [CrossRef] [PubMed]
14. Ronningstam, E.; Keng, S.L.; Ridolfi, M.E.; Arbabi, M.; Grenyer, B. Cultural aspects in symptomatology, assessment and treatment of personality disorders. *Curr. Psychiatry Rep.* **2018**, *20*, 22. [CrossRef] [PubMed]
15. Contreras, A.; Nieto, I.; Valiente, C.; Espinosa, R.; Vazquez, C. The study of psychopathology from the network analysis perspective: A systematic review. *Psychother. Psychosom.* **2019**, *88*, 71–83. [CrossRef] [PubMed]
16. Borsboom, D. A network theory of mental disorders. *World Psychiatry* **2017**, *16*, 5–13. [CrossRef] [PubMed]
17. Borsboom, D.; Cramer, A.O.J. Network analysis: An integrative approach to the structure of psychopathology. *Annu. Rev. Clin. Psychol.* **2013**, *9*, 91–121. [CrossRef] [PubMed]
18. Boccaletti, S.; Latora, V.; Moreno, Y.; Chavez, M.; Hwang, D.U. Complex networks: Structure and dynamics. *Phys. Rep.* **2006**, *424*, 175–308. [CrossRef]
19. Kendler, K.S.; Zachar, P.; Craver, C. What kinds of things are psychiatric disorders? *Psychol. Med.* **2011**, *41*, 1143–1150. [CrossRef]
20. Anker, J.J.; Forbes, M.K.; Almquist, Z.W.; Menk, J.S.; Thuras, P.; Unruh, A.S.; Kushner, M.G. A network approach to modeling comorbid internalizing and alcohol use disorders. *J. Abnorm. Psychol.* **2017**, *126*, 325–339. [CrossRef]
21. Maples, J.L.; Carter, N.T.; Few, L.R.; Crego, C.; Gore, W.L.; Samuel, D.B.; Williamson, R.L.; Lynam, D.R.; Widiger, T.A.; Markon, K.E.; et al. Testing whether the DSM-5 personality disorder trait model can be measured with a reduced set of items: An item response theory investigation of the Personality Inventory for DSM-5. *Psychol. Assess.* **2015**, *27*, 1195–1210. [CrossRef]
22. Díaz-Batanero, C.; Ramírez-López, J.; Domínguez-Salas, S.; Fernández-Calderón, F.; Lozano, O.M. Personality inventory for DSM-5 Short Form (PID-5-SF): Reliability, factorial structure and relationship with functional impairment in dual diagnosis patients. *Assessment* **2019**, *26*, 853–866. [CrossRef]
23. American Educational Research Association; American Psychological Association; National Council on Measurement in Education. *Standards for Educational and Psychological Testing*; American Educational Research Association: Washington DC, USA, 2014.
24. Dacosta-Sánchez, D.; Fernández-Calderón, F.; González-Ponce, B.; Díaz-Batanero, C.; Lozano, O.M. Severity of substance use disorder: Utility as an outcome in clinical settings. *Alcohol. Clin. Exp. Res.* **2019**, *43*, 869–876. [CrossRef] [PubMed]
25. González-Sainz, F.; Lozano, O.M.; Vélez-Moreno, A.; Ramírez, J.L. *Manual de la Escala de Gravedad de la Dependencia de Sustancias*; Servicio de Publicaciones de la Universidad de Huelva: Huelva, Spain, 2014.
26. Miele, G.M.; Carpenter, K.M.; Cockerham, M.S.; Trautman, K.D.; Blaine, J.; Hasin, D.S. Substance Dependence Severity Scale (SDSS): Reliability and validity of a clinician-administered interview for DSM-IV substance use disorders. *Drug Alcohol Depend.* **2000**, *59*, 63–75. [CrossRef]
27. Friedman, J.; Hastie, T.; Tibshirani, R. Sparse inverse covariance estimation with the graphical lasso. *Biostatistics* **2008**, *9*, 432–441. [CrossRef] [PubMed]

28. Chen, J.; Chen, Z. Extended bayesian information criteria for model selection with large model spaces. *Biometrika* **2008**, *95*, 759–771. [CrossRef]
29. Liu, H.; Lafferty, J.; Wasserman, L. The nonparanormal: Semiparametric estimation of high dimensional undirected graphs. *J. Mach. Learn. Res.* **2009**, *10*, 2295–2328.
30. Fruchterman, T.M.J.; Reingold, E.M. Graph drawing by force-directed placement. *Softw. Pract. Exp.* **1991**, *21*, 1129–1164. [CrossRef]
31. Epskamp, S.; Borsboom, D.; Fried, E.I. Estimating psychological networks and their accuracy: A tutorial paper. *Behav. Res. Methods* **2018**, *50*, 195–212. [CrossRef]
32. Pons, P.; Latapy, M. Computing Communities in Large Networks Using Random Walks. In *Computer and Information Sciences—ISCIS*; Yolum, P., Güngör, T., Gürgen, F., Özturan, C., Eds.; Springer: Berlin/Heidelberg, Germany, 2005; pp. 284–293.
33. Robinaugh, D.J.; Millner, A.J.; McNally, R.J. Identifying highly influential nodes in the complicated grief network. *J. Abnorm. Psychol.* **2016**, *125*, 747–757. [CrossRef]
34. Haslbeck, J.M.B.; Waldorp, L.J. How well do network models predict observations? On the importance of predictability in network models. *Behav. Res. Methods* **2018**, *50*, 853–861. [CrossRef]
35. Letina, S.; Blanken, T.; Deserno, M.; Borsboom, D. Expanding network analysis tools in psychological networks: Minimal spanning trees, participation coefficients, and motif analysis applied to a network of 26 psychological attributes. *Complexity* **2019**, *2019*, 9424605. [CrossRef]
36. Jones, P. Networktools: Tools for Identifying Important Nodes in Networks. R Package Version 1.4.0. Available online: https://cran.r-project.org/package=networktools (accessed on 3 June 2022).
37. Jones, P.; Ma, R.; McNally, R.J. Bridge Centrality: A network approach to understanding comorbidity. *Multivar. Behav. Res.* **2019**, *56*, 353–367. [CrossRef] [PubMed]
38. van Borkulo, C.D.; Boschloo, L.; Kossakowski, J.J.; Tio, P.; Schoevers, R.A.; Borsboom, D.; Waldorp, L.J. Comparing network structures on three aspects: A permutation test. *Psychol. Methods* **2022**. [CrossRef] [PubMed]
39. Korkmaz, S.; Göksülük, D.; Zararsiz, G. MVN: An R package for assessing multivariate normality. *R J.* **2014**, *6*, 151–162. [CrossRef]
40. Csardi, G.; Nepusz, T. The Igraph Software Package for Complex Network Research. InterJournal Complex Systems 1695. 2006. Available online: http://igraph.org (accessed on 3 June 2022).
41. Epskamp, S.; Cramer, A.; Waldorp, L.; Schimittmann, V.; Borsboom, D. qgraph: Network visualizations of relationships in psychometric data. *J. Stat. Softw.* **2012**, *48*, 1–18. [CrossRef]
42. De Clercq, B.; Fruyt, F.; De Bolle, M.; Van Hiel, A.; Markon, K.E.; Krueger, R.F. The hierarchical structure and construct validity of the PID-5 trait measure in adolescence. *J. Personal.* **2014**, *82*, 158–169. [CrossRef]
43. Díaz-Batanero, C.; Aluja, A.; Sayans-Jiménez, -P.; Baillés, E.; Fernández-Calderón, F.; Peri, J.M.; Vall Lozano, O.M.; Gutiérrez, F. Alterntive DSM-5 Model for personality disorders through the lens of an empirical network model. *Assessment* **2021**, *28*, 773–787. [CrossRef]
44. Wright, A.G.; Thomas, K.M.; Hopwood, C.J.; Markon, K.E.; Pincus, A.L.; Krueger, R.F. The hierarchical structure of DSM-5 pathological personality traits. *J. Abnorm. Psychol.* **2012**, *121*, 951–957. [CrossRef]
45. Kotov, R.; Krueger, R.; Watson, D.; Achenbach, T.M.; Althoff, R.; Bagby, R.; Zimmerman, M. The Hierarchical Taxonomy of Psychopathology (HiTOP): A dimensional alternative to traditional nosologies. *J. Abnorm. Psychol.* **2017**, *126*, 454–477. [CrossRef]
46. Baggio, S.; Sapin, M.; Khazaal, Y.; Studer, J.; Wolff, H.; Gmel, G. Comorbidity of symptoms of alcohol and cannabis use disorders among a population-based sample of simultaneous users. Insight from a network perspective. *Int. J. Environ. Res. Public Health* **2018**, *15*, 2893. [CrossRef]
47. Rhemtulla, M.; Fried, E.I.; Aggen, S.H.; Tuerlinckx, F.; Kendler, K.S.; Borsboom, D. Network analysis of substance abuse and dependence symptoms. *Drug Alcohol Depend.* **2016**, *161*, 230–237. [CrossRef]
48. Sanchez-Garcia, M.; de la Rosa-Cáceres, A.; Díaz-Batanero, C.; Fernández-Calderón, F.; Lozano, O.M. Cocaine use disorder criteria in a clinical sample: An analysis using item response theory, factor and network analysis. *Am. J. Drug Alcohol Abus* **2021**. [CrossRef] [PubMed]
49. Widiger, T.A.; McCabe, G.A. The Alternative Model of Personality Disorders (AMPD) from the perspective of the Five-Factor Model. *Psychopathology* **2020**, *53*, 149–156. [CrossRef] [PubMed]
50. Freeman, C.; Wiers, C.; Sloan, M.; Zehra, A.; Ramirez, V.; Wang, G.; Volkow, N. Emotion recognition biases in alcohol use disorder. *Alcohol. Clin. Exp. Res.* **2018**, *42*, 1541–1547. [CrossRef] [PubMed]
51. Pabst, A.; Peyroux, E.; Rolland, B.; Timary, P.; Maurage, P. Hostile attributional bias in severe alcohol use disorder. *J. Psychiatr. Res.* **2020**, *129*, 176–180. [CrossRef]
52. American Psychiatric Association. *Diagnostic and Statistical Manual of Mental Disorders*, 5th ed.; American Psychiatric Publishing: Arlington, VA, USA, 2013.
53. Choate, A.; Gorey, C.; Rappaport, L.; Wiernik, B.; Bornovalova, M. Alternative model of personality disorders traits predict residential addictions treatment completion. *Drug Alcohol Depend.* **2021**, *228*, 109011. [CrossRef]
54. Gómez-Bujedo, J.; Lozano, O.M.; Pérez-Moreno, P.J.; Lorca-Marín, J.A.; Fernández-Calderón, F.; Díaz-Batanero, C.; Moraleda-Barreno, E. Personality traits and impulsivity task among substance use disorder patients: Their relations and links with retention in treatment. *Front. Psychiatry* **2020**, *11*, 566240. [CrossRef]

55. Mezquita, L.; Bravo, A.J.; Ortet, G.; Pilatti, A.; Rearson, M.R.; Ibañez, M.I. Cross-cultural examination of different personality pathways to alcohol use and misuse in emerging adulthood. *Drug Alcohol Depend.* **2018**, *19*, 193–200. [CrossRef]
56. Rhem, J.; Room, R. The cultural aspect: How to measure and interpret epidemiological data on alcohol-use disorders across cultures. *Nord. Stud. Alcohol Drugs* **2017**, *34*, 330–341. [CrossRef]

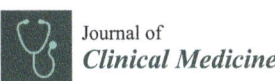

Article

Changes in the Care Activity in Addiction Centers with Dual Pathology Patients during the COVID-19 Pandemic

Cinta Mancheño-Velasco [1], Daniel Dacosta-Sánchez [1], Andrea Blanc-Molina [1], Marta Narvaez-Camargo [1] and Óscar Martín Lozano-Rojas [1,2,*]

[1] Department of Clinical and Experimental Psychology, University of Huelva, 21004 Huelva, Spain; cinta.mancheno@dpces.uhu.es (C.M.-V.); daniel.daco@dpces.uhu.es (D.D.-S.); andrea.blanc@dpces.uhu.es (A.B.-M.); marta.narvaez885@alu.uhu.es (M.N.-C.)
[2] Research Center on Natural Resources, Health and the Environment, University of Huelva, 21004 Huelva, Spain
* Correspondence: oscar.lozano@dpsi.uhu.es

Abstract: Background: Health care provision during the COVID-19 pandemic and confinement has led to significant changes in the activity of addiction centers. These changes in healthcare activity may have had a greater impact on patients with dual pathology. The aim of this study is to compare the treatment indicators of patients with dual pathology in addiction centers during the pre-confinement, confinement, and post-confinement periods. Methods: A retrospective observational study was conducted for the period between 1 February 2019 and 30 June 2021. A total of 2785 patients treated in specialized addiction services were divided into three periods according to their time of admission: pre-confinement, confinement, and post-confinement. Results: During the pre-pandemic period, the addiction centers attended to an average of 121.3 (SD = 23.58) patients, decreasing to 53 patients during confinement (SD = 19.47), and 80.69 during the post-confinement period (SD = 15.33). The number of appointments scheduled monthly for each patient decreased during the confinement period, although this number increased after confinement. There was a reduction in the number of toxicological tests carried out both during and after confinement (except for alcohol). Conclusions: The results show a reduction in the number of patients seen and the care activity delivered to dual diagnosis patients. These results, which were caused by the COVID-preventive measures, may affect the progress and recovery of dual patients. A greater investment is needed to bring the care activity up to the standards of the years prior to confinement.

Keywords: dual pathology; COVID-19; care activity; pandemic; drug addiction; mental health

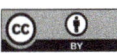

1. Introduction

The impact of the COVID-19 pandemic on mental health has been extensively documented [1–4]. Increased diagnoses of anxiety and depression have been described [5–8], as well as a rise in the number of suicides in the population [9]. In addition, several authors have pointed out that the consequences of the pandemic have been more negative for people who had previously been suffering from other mental disorders, including addictive disorders [10–12].

Some authors have reported that at the onset of confinement there was an increase in drug use, as reflected in indicators suggesting increased sales of alcohol [13,14] and cannabis [15]. Furthermore, higher rates of alcohol [16], cannabis, and other forms of drug abuse [17–21] have also been documented. For example, Chappuy et al. [19] reported a 29.2% increase in alcohol use, a 27.6% increase in cannabis use, a 36.2% increase in psychostimulant use, and a 25.9% increase in hypnosedative and opiate use. In addition, a 48.7% increase in behaviors associated with pathological gambling has also been detected. Other authors have reported increases in self-medication patterns in patients with opioid dependence [11] and a rise in overdose rates [22,23]. However, despite the above data, it should be borne in mind that consumption patterns may vary according to the country and the specific regulations in force during the pandemic [18,24].

In terms of health care provision, the pandemic, confinement, and the policy measures adopted by governments have led to significant changes in the care activities of specialized addiction centers. For example, Mark et al. [25] found a 28% decrease in admissions to treatment during the beginning of the pandemic compared to the previous year. In contrast, Aguilar et al. [26] noted an increase in care activity and higher relapse rates during the second half of confinement. In addition, other authors have reported changes in care patterns, with online appointments being prioritized and an increase in attendance at these appointments [27]. Likewise, it has been shown that confinement has led to an increase in the therapeutic needs of patients with addiction, with these patients also encountering more barriers to receiving therapeutic sessions and pharmacological treatments [11,28,29]. Some authors have also reported a slight increase in requests for pharmacological prescriptions by new patients, although an overall decrease in patients has also been noted [30]. On the other hand, Huskamp et al. [31] reported a decrease in the number of toxicological tests carried out in outpatient addiction centers.

These changes in healthcare activity may have had a greater impact on patients with dual pathology. Generally, these patients require more extensive follow-up due to the greater therapeutic complexity involved in comparison with patients without dual pathology [32,33]. In addition, the closure of some addiction centers [34] and the shift to virtual treatment have posed a major challenge to meeting the therapeutic needs of these patients. Therefore, some authors have warned of the worsening of comorbid mental disorders and disruptive behaviors both in confinement periods [35–37] and in the subsequent periods [38], in addition to a likely increase in relapses [39].

Although previous studies have suggested the potential impact of the pandemic on patients diagnosed with dual pathology, no studies have yet compared the treatment indicators of care activities implemented for patients with dual pathology in addiction centers across the pre-confinement, confinement, and post-confinement periods. Thus, the present study had the following objectives: (i) to examine the evolution of admissions to treatment for patients with dual pathology receiving coordinated care with mental health centers between February 2019 and June 2021; (ii) to analyze the sociodemographic profiles, consumption patterns, and psychopathological profiles of these patients; and (iii) to compare care indicators related to therapeutic appointments, toxicological tests, and treatment abandonment across the three specified time periods. As hypotheses based on those objectives, it is expected that:

(a) The evolution of admissions to treatment decreased during confinement;
(b) Patients with dual pathology who attend addiction care centers presented changes in their sociodemographic, consumption, and diagnosis profiles during the pandemic compared to the previous period;
(c) Care indicators related to therapeutic appointments, toxicological tests, and treatment abandonment changed during the pandemic compared to the previous period.

2. Material and Methods

2.1. Design

Retrospective observational study for the period between 1 February 2019 and 30 June 2021. Patients were divided into three periods according to their time of admission to the addiction centers: pre-confinement (1 February 2019 and 15 March 2020), confinement (16 March 2020–31 May 2020), and post-confinement (1 June 2020–30 June 2021).

2.2. Participants

For the current study, we included only patients admitted between 1 February 2019 to 30 June 2021 in specialized addiction services with dual pathology. Inclusion criteria were the following: (1) to be older than 18 years of age, (2) to have at least one diagnosis according to the International Classification of Diseases 10 (ICD-10) of an addictive disorder (cocaine, heroin, alcohol, cannabis, or pathological gambling) and another comorbid mental disorder, and (3) to have a clinical indication to receive coordinated care with mental health services.

The final sample consisted of 2785 patients diagnosed with an addictive disorder and another mental disorder according to ICD-10. In addition, all patients of the sample had therapeutic prescriptions to receive care in mental health services according to the Ries [40] classification. This is a dimensional model based on the severity of the addictive disorder and other mental disorders. Depending on the severity levels of these disorders, patients receive treatment exclusively in mental health (severe mental disorder and mild addictive disorder), in addiction centers (severe addictive disorder and mild mental disorder), or in both services in a coordinated manner (severe mental health and addictive disorder). All patients in this study received coordinated care between specialized addiction centers and mental health units in Andalusia [41]. These patients were admitted to treatment in one of the 121 outpatient centers of the Public Network for Addiction Care in Andalusia (Spain). Of the sample, 1576 (56.6%) were admitted during the year prior to confinement, 160 (5.7%) were admitted during confinement, and 1049 (37.7%) were admitted to treatment from the end of confinement until 06/30/2021.

Most patients were male (74.8%), with a mean age of 40.4 years (SD = 11.69) at the time of admission to treatment. Most patients had completed primary (37.6%) or secondary education (23.5%). Regarding employment status, 22.7% of the patients were employed, 44.9% were unemployed, 25% were retired, 3.7% were studying, and 3.7% were in an unknown employment situation.

According to ICD-10 criteria, 37.6% of the patients were diagnosed with alcohol dependence or harmful use, 33.6% with cocaine, 22.3% with cannabis, 16.3% with opiates, and 3.2 with hypnosedatives. In addition, 4.5% of the patients were admitted for pathological gambling. Excluding tobacco addiction, 13.9% of these patients were diagnosed with dependent or harmful use of more than one drug.

2.3. Procedure

The data used in the present study belong to the EHR of the Information System of the Andalusian Plan on Drugs (SiPASDA). The EHR begins by recording information corresponding to the variables of the Treatment Demand Indicator (TDI) Standard Protocol 3.0 of the European Monitoring Centre for Drugs and Drug Addiction [42]. The TDI provides basic information on sociodemographic variables, drug use history, previous treatments, and infectious diseases at the start of treatment. In addition, clinical data collected during the periodic appointments that patients attend (with physicians, psychologists, nurses, and social workers) are incorporated into the clinical history of each patient. In these appointments, each team member (physicians, psychologists, nurses, and social workers) inputs the relevant patient information into the EHR. This information includes the diagnosis of the patients according to ICD-10 criteria, prescribed pharmacological treatments, psychological evaluation and treatments, results of toxicological tests, social status of the patient, and evolution of treatment. All this information is stored in a centralized database, and therapists can access the information at any time. Previous research conducted with this same data set has shown good reliability values [43].

Due to the pandemic, most of the Andalusian centers used telephones as the main channel for treatment admissions and follow-up. Critically ill patients received face-to-face care from professionals, while telephone services have been maintained for patient follow-up after the confinement period. The requests are recorded by health professionals in the Electronic Health Record (EHR).

2.4. Ethics and Approvals

This research has been approved by the Research Ethics Committee of the Andalusian Ministry of Health, who certified compliance with the requirements for the ethical handling of the information.

To access the EHRs, the researchers made a request to the General Secretary of Social Services of the Department of Equality and Social Policies of the Regional Government of Andalusia (Spain). Patients gave their authorization so the information could be registered in the system. The database is fully anonymized for both patients and professionals, so it is not possible to inform the participants about the study. The storage and encoding of this data comply with the General Health Law of 25 April 1986 (Spain) and Law 41/2002 of 14 November on patient autonomy, rights, and obligations regarding clinical information and documentation. It also complies with the Organic Law 3/2018 of 5 December 2018, regarding the protection of personal data and the assurance of digital rights, adapted to European regulations.

2.5. Statistical Analysis

The three groups were compared using nonparametric analyses, given the differences in sample size between the confinement group and the pre- and post-confinement groups.

The differences between qualitative variables were analyzed using Pearson's chi-square test, and Cramer's V statistic was used to calculate effect sizes. Quantitative variables were analyzed with the Kruskal–Wallis test, using the epsilon-squared test to calculate effect sizes.

Analyses were conducted using IBM SPSS Statistics software version 27 (Chicago, IL, USA).

3. Results

3.1. Evolution of Treatment Admissions between 1 February 2019 and 30 June 2021

Figure 1 shows the monthly evolution of the number of treatment admissions for each month analyzed, with respect to the patients receiving coordinated care with mental health services. This shows the downward trend in admissions of these patients. Thus, during the pre-pandemic period, the addiction centers attended to an average of 121.3 (SD = 23.58) patients with dual pathology per month, decreasing to 53 patients during confinement (SD = 19.47), and 80.69 (SD = 15.33) patients during the post-confinement period.

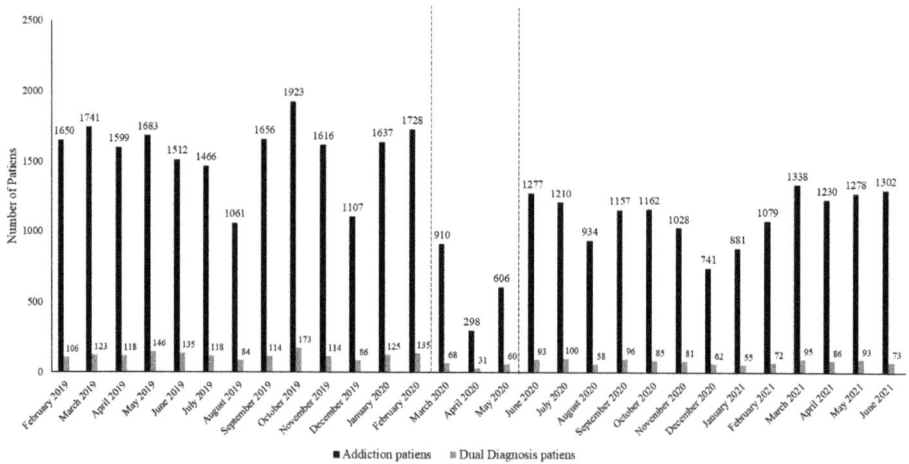

Figure 1. Evolution of patient admissions for treatment in the addiction centers.

In percentage terms, the number of patients with dual pathology seen during the year prior to confinement was 7.2%, with this number increasing slightly during confinement (8.1%) and then falling to 6.7% in the year after confinement, and these differences were statistically significant ($\chi^2 = 6.646$; $d.f. = 4$; $p = 0.036$; $V = 0.013$). As shown in Table 1, the variations observed in these periods run parallel to the readmissions to treatment (patients requesting treatment who had previously been in treatment), with the highest percentage of readmissions to treatment occurring during confinement.

Table 1. Sociodemographic characteristics, consumption profile, and diagnosis of patients with dual pathology.

	Admission Period			Statistics (d.f.)	p	Effect Size
	19 February–20 February	March–20 May	20 June–21 June			
No. of patients	1577 (56.6%)	159 (5.7%)	1049 (37.7%)			
% Patients (out of total patients)	7.2	8.1	6.7	$\chi^2 (4) = 6.646$	0.036 *	V = 0.013
Readmissions	67.4%	74.8%	63.2%	$\chi^2 (4) = 10.549$	0.005 **	V = 0.062
Sociodemographic variables						
Admission age (Mean, SD)	40.36 (11.536)	39.25 (11.698)	40.58 (11.920)	H (2) = 1.482	0.477	$\varepsilon^2 = 0.001$
Gender (%)						
Male	75.8	72.5	73.8	$\chi^2 (2) = 1.796$	0.407	V = 0.025
Female	24.2	27.5	26.2			
Educational level (%)						
No education	17.0	14.1	14.6			
Primary	39.1	37.8	35.3			
Secondary	22.3	22.4	25.6	$\chi^2 (8) = 13.402$	0.099	V = 0.049
Baccalaureate/Degree	14.9	20.5	17.8			
Higher	6.7	5.1	6.8			
Employment status (%)						
Employed	22.7	18.5	23.3			
Unemployed	44.9	45.9	44.8			
Retired	24.7	26.1	25.1	$\chi^2 (8) = 6.830$	0.555	V = 0.035
Student	3.5	6.4	3.6			
Others	4.2	3.2	3.1			
Main referral source (%)						
Legal Services	3.1	4.4	2.5			
Own initiative	41.9	48.1	42.2			
Family members	13.2	8.9	12.8	$\chi^2 (10) = 7.263$	0.700	V = 0.036
Health Services	14.4	13.9	15.7			
Social Services	23.3	22.2	22.7			
Others	4.1	2.5				
Variables related to consumption						
Age of onset of consumption (Mean, SD)	19.64 (10.91)	20.81 (14.28)	19.74 (11.29)	H (2) = 0.739	0.691	$\varepsilon^2 = 0.000$
Admission drug (%)						
Alcohol	36.4	34.4	39.3	2.930	0.231	V = 0.032
Cocaine	34.1	30.6	33.4	0.819	0.664	V = 0.017
Cannabis	23.4	20.2		4.447	0.108	V = 0.040
Opioids	18.3	21.3	12.5	18.840	0.000 **	V = 0.082
Hypnosedatives	2.9	4.4	3.5	1.455	0.483	V = 0.023
Pathological gambling	4.7	1.9	4.7	2.759	0.252	V = 0.031
Other drugs used prior to admission (%)						
Alcohol	55.6	55.0	58.0	$\chi^2 (2) = 1.522$	0.467	V = 0.023
Cocaine	36.8	35.0	39.4	$\chi^2 (2) = 2.284$	0.319	V = 0.029
Cannabis	39.9	40.6	37.4	$\chi^2 (2) = 1.901$	0.387	V = 0.026
Opioids	18.6	22.5	13.7	$\chi^2 (2) = 14.231$	0.001 **	V = 0.071
Hypnosedatives	8.1	6.3	7.9	$\chi^2 (2) = 0.653$	0.721	V = 0.015

Table 1. Cont.

	Admission Period			Statistics (d.f.)	p	Effect Size
	19 February–20 February	March–20 May	20 June–21 June			
Frequency of consumption in the 30 days prior to admission (%)						
Every day	44.1	45.2	42.4			
4–6 days/week	7.4	5.1	9.1			
2–3 days/week	13.9	12.7	14.1	$\chi^2 (10) = 12.011$	0.284	V = 0.048
1 day/week	5.5	10.8	5.9			
Less 1 day/week	7.8	6.4	8.2			
Did not consume	21.3	19.7	20.4			
Variables related to the diagnosis of comorbid mental disorders						
F 20. Schizophrenia, schizotypal disorders, and delusional disorders	16.2	16.4	16.2	0.004	0.998	V = 0.001
F 30–39. Mood disorders	17.4	13.8	16.9	1.297	0.523	V = 0.022
F 40–49. Neurotic, secondary to stressful situations, and somatoform disorders	31.9	34.0	32.6	0.362	0.834	V = 0.011
F 41. Mixed Anxiety-Depressive Disorder	16.8	20.1	17.6	1.241	0.538	V = 0.021
F 90. Hyperkinetic disorders	4.6	3.8	3.3	2.480	0.289	V = 0.030
Mental retardation	1.3	1.9	1.5	0.409	0.815	V = 0.012
Adult personality and behavioral disorders (%)						
Any personality disorder (F 60–F 60.9)	24.4	24.5	20.2	6.421	0.040 *	V = 0.048
F 60.0 and 60.1. Paranoid or schizoid personality disorder	2.0	2.5	1.3	2.220	0.330	V = 0.028
F 60.2–60.4. Antisocial, borderline, histrionic or narcissistic disorder	12.6	8.8	10.9	3.268	0.195	V = 0.034
F 60.5–60.7. Avoidance, dependence, or obsessive-compulsive disorder.	1.2	1.3	1.0	0.394	0.821	V = 0.012
F 60.9. Unspecified Personality disorder	8.8	11.9	7.2	4.688	0.096	V = 0.041
Patients without specified ICD-10 diagnosis	13.1	10.7	16.4	7.441	0.024 *	V = 0.052

Abbreviations: d.f.—degrees of freedom; SD—Standard Deviation; H—Kruskal–Wallis; V— Cramer's V; * p-value ≤ 0.05; ** p-value < 0.01

3.2. Sociodemographic Characteristics, Consumption Patterns, and Comorbid Diagnoses

Table 1 compares the three time periods according to sociodemographic variables, consumption patterns, and psychopathological diagnoses. There were no statistically significant differences in the sociodemographic profiles of the patients, although there was an increase in the number of women who were admitted to treatment during confinement. With respect to consumption patterns, it should be noted that treatment admissions for opiate use increased during confinement (and although the number of admissions subsequently decreased, the differences were statistically significant). Concerning admissions for patients with alcohol abuse/dependence, a slight decrease was observed during confinement, after which an increase of almost 5% was observed after confinement. However, admissions for cannabis dependence/abuse decreased after confinement. Finally, admissions for pathological gambling decreased during confinement, subsequently returning to pre-confinement levels.

Concerning the diagnoses of comorbid mental disorders, in general terms, no statistically significant differences were observed between the three periods, except for personality disorders. However, an increase in diagnoses of anxiety spectrum disorders was observed during confinement, mainly due to mixed anxiety-depressive disorders. On the other hand, a reduction in personality disorders diagnosed after confinement was observed. However, it should be borne in mind that after confinement, there was an increase in the number of patients with clinical indications for coordinated care with mental health services, although the diagnosis provided in the clinical history was generic (severe mental disorder-SMD-together with an addictive disorder of difficult clinical management).

3.3. Care Provision Indicators

Table 2 shows the care indicators for the three periods analyzed. With respect to the therapeutic sessions planned by the clinicians, the number of monthly appointments scheduled for each patient decreased during the confinement period, although this number increased after confinement. Regarding the care activity of the patients, it was observed that they attended a greater percentage of scheduled appointments during the confinement period, with no difference between pre-and post-confinement.

Table 2. Care indicators for patients with dual pathology.

		Admission Period			Statistics (d.f.)	p	Effect Size
		19 February–20 February	March–20 May	20 June–21 June			
			Appointments (mean, SD)				
Scheduled monthly		1.12 (2.22)	0.64 (0.74)	1.28 (2.32)	H (2) = 62.655	0.000 **	ε^2 = 0.023
Percentage attendance		0.76 (0.23)	0.88 (0.25)	0.77 (0.25)	H (2) = 92.348	0.000 **	ε^2 = 0.033
			Toxicological controls (mean, SD)				
Alcohol	% Patients tested	7.7	0	10.4	χ^2 (2) = 7.701	0.021 **	V = 0.086
	Average per patient	4.91 (4.88)	0	5.72 (14.82)	H (2) = 0.631	0.427	ε^2 = 0.000
	Positive ratio	0.14 (8.75)	0	0.19 (0.35)	H (2) = 3.565	0.168	ε^2 = 0.001
Cocaine	% Patients tested	53.6	24.5	45.4	χ^2 (2) = 18.174	0.000 **	V = 0.139
	Average per patient	6.51 (12.75)	0.8 (1.14)	5.20 (5.83)	H (2) = 17.721	0.000 **	ε^2 = 0.006
	Positive ratio	0.38 (0.40)	0.50 (0.58)	0.37 (0.41)	H (2) = 0.287	0.866	ε^2 = 0.000
Cannabis	% Patients tested	52.3	20.0	40.1	χ^2 (2) = 19.761	0.000 **	V = 0.178
	Average per patient	5.16 (6.16)	1.87 (0.64)	4.86 (4.59)	H (2) = 6.142	0.046 **	ε^2 = 0.002
	Positive ratio	0.64 (0.42)	0.63 (0.52)	0.53 (0.45)	H (2) = 3.437	0.179	ε^2 = 0.001
Opioids	% Patients tested	45.7	14.7	37.4	χ^2 (2) = 13.031	0.001 **	V = 0.169
	Average per patient	4.75 (6.69)	1.60 (0.89)	5.04 (6.55)	H (2) = 2.825	0.243	ε^2 = 0.001
	Positive ratio	0.30 (0.41)	0.75 (0.50)	0.75 (0.29)	H (2) = 28.033	0.000 **	ε^2 = 0.010
Benzodiazepines	% Patients tested	21.7	14.3	13.5	χ^2 (2) = 1.013	0.603	V = 0.106
	Average per patient	2.10 (2.18)	0	2.20 (1.30)	H (2) = 2.827	0.243	ε^2 = 0.001
	Positive ratio	0.69 (0.46)	0	0.40 (0.55)	H (2) = 1.296	0.255	ε^2 = 0.001
% Patients that dropped out of treatment		40.1	34.4	13.3	215.46	0.000	V = 0.280

Abbreviations: d.f.—degrees of freedom; SD—Standard Deviation; H—Kruskal–Wallis; V—Cramer's V; ** p-value ≤ 0.05.

There was a reduction in the number of toxicological tests carried out both during and after confinement (except for alcohol). In the case of patients with alcohol-related problems, a greater number of tests were carried out after confinement. For the remaining substances, there was a significant reduction in the percentage of patients who underwent toxicological tests. It should be noted that of the five substances analyzed, a statistically significant increase in positive test results was only observed for opiates.

Concerning treatment retention, a significant reduction in the percentage of patients abandoning treatment was observed across the three periods.

4. Discussion

Various studies have shown how the pandemic has resulted in changes in the treatment demands placed on addiction centers and the healthcare provision patterns of clinicians [25–27,44], along with the associated impact on patients [35–38]. Unlike previous studies, this study focused exclusively on patients with dual pathology and analyzed the evolution of treatment admissions, profiles, and care indicators corresponding to the periods before, during, and after confinement, when various anti-COVID-19 measures were implemented in addiction and mental health services.

Concerning the first hypothesis, the present study has clearly shown a change in the evolution of treatment admissions of patients with dual pathology. Specifically, we have observed an increase in admissions during confinement followed by a drop in such admissions post-confinement. The increase in the number of patients admitted during confinement might be explained by treatment readmissions (patients who had previously been in treatment). This finding is similar to that of Di Lorenzo et al. [45]. Although these authors did not exclusively analyze patients with substance use disorders, they observed a reduction in urgent psychiatric consultations during confinement while this number increased in people who were already being treated. Therefore, the observed increase could be due to the fact that patients with pre-existing mental disorders experienced a marked deterioration of symptoms during this period. Concerning the decline in admissions post-confinement, other authors have reported a similar observation, and this may pattern be due to infection-control measures associated with COVID-19 [25,46].

With regard to our second hypothesis, we expected to find differences in the profiles of patients admitted across the three-time periods analyzed, a prediction that was not supported by our results. However, there was a notable percentage increase in women admitted to treatment during confinement. This may be due to the characteristic symptomatology of anxious-depressive disorder experienced during this stage since the percentage of women with this diagnosis increased from 24.9% before confinement to 41.4% during confinement. Other authors have also found that these emotional stress symptoms are more frequent in women [35,38]. Therefore, the symptomatology associated with this disorder is likely to be the factor that explains the percentage increase observed in this gender.

We also observed a significant increase in the number of patients admitted for opiate dependence. The reduced availability of opiates in the illegal market has possibly prompted patients dependent on this substance to come to addiction centers demanding pharmacological treatment [30]. However, barriers to obtaining epidemiological data on illicit drug use during the pandemic in Spain, especially for drugs such as opiates [47], make it difficult to test this hypothesis.

Concerning diagnoses of mental disorders, the results of the present study agree with those reported by other authors, indicating an increase in symptoms characteristic of mixed anxiety-depressive disorders during confinement [48]. However, we found no increase in the number of admissions to treatment in patients with personality disorders, which might be expected based on other studies [49]. In fact, quite the opposite trend was found—the number of admissions to treatment for these patients decreased after confinement. However, this decrease may be due to methodological problems associated with the data recording techniques since, as described above, there was a significant increase in patients without a specific ICD-10 diagnosis after confinement.

The analysis of our third hypothesis revealed that patients with dual pathology received less care during confinement, although some post-confinement indicators were similar to those observed pre-pandemic. Other authors have also reported this lower attendance to psychiatric services [50]. These observations may be due to the implementation of care protocols designed to protect these patients against COVID-19. However, despite this reduction in scheduled appointments, it was found that patients in treatment attended more appointments and showed a reduction in treatment dropout, in congruence with other studies conducted in addiction centers [44]. Thus, patients showed greater treatment adherence during confinement, although subsequently, care indicators showed activity equivalent to that of pre-confinement levels, with a notable reduction in treatment dropout. In addition, fewer toxicological tests were carried out during confinement, as reported by other authors [31], with no recovery of pre-confinement levels. It is likely that the risk of contagion associated with the collection of biological samples has influenced this reduction in care activity, with priority given to self-report measures of drug use.

We should consider some limitations to correctly interpret these findings and compare the results. One of the main aspects to consider is that patients receive treatment coordinated with mental health services. In this study, while the activity of addiction services has been analyzed, the activity of these patients in mental health services has not. Thus, we are observing only a part of the care provided to these patients without knowing the care indicators of these patients in mental health services. Previous studies conducted in patients with dual pathology under this care modality have shown that sometimes patients leave one of the care networks and remain in the other, depending on the addiction profile and psychopathological disorder of the patients [51,52]. Moreover, the present study was based on data obtained from the EHR registry. Although clinicians have been using EHRs in a standardized manner since 2015, the pressure of care experienced in the months studied herein could have produced slight errors in the completion of EHRs. This could explain, for example, the increase in patients without a specific ICD-10 diagnosis observed in the data. On the other hand, it is necessary to keep in mind that the study included patients with high severities of their respective addictive disorders and other mental disorders, and not only patients with other comorbid disorders. Consequently, it is likely that the prevalence of dual pathology observed in this study is lower than that observed in other studies of dual pathology conducted in addiction centers.

Despite these limitations, the present study provides useful information for understanding the changes produced by the COVID-19 pandemic. In particular, our results provide relevant knowledge about a large sample of patients with dual diagnosis and the health care provided in several addiction centers. As this is a coordinated treatment modality, we have observed only the care that has occurred in addiction centers and not the care that these patients have received in mental health centers. Bearing this in mind, the data have shown a reduction in the healthcare received by these patients. Moreover, it is striking that after confinement, the number of patients with dual pathology has decreased. Therefore, it is likely that there is a group of patients with dual pathology who are presently either only receiving care in mental health centers or are not attending health services. Thus, we suggest that the coordinated treatment modality followed by these patients with dual pathology has proven to be insufficient for providing adequate clinical care during the pandemic period. Therefore, we believe that it is now more necessary than ever to integrate mental health and addiction services for the coordinated treatment of these patients with dual pathology.

Future studies should continue to provide information on care activity and confirm the results found with these patients, so that these data can be used to inform the development of effective and efficient treatments for patients with dual pathology. In addition, future analyses could identify factors that may mediate and prevent some of the major risks in similar situations.

5. Conclusions

We can conclude that: (1) the period of confinement resulting from the coronavirus pandemic has triggered a reduction in the number of patients seen and the care activity delivered to dual diagnosis patients, including treatment admissions. At the end of the isolation period, the care activity of the addiction centers increased again. (2) There has been an increase in the number of patients admitted for opiate dependence and in reported symptoms characteristic of mixed anxiety-depressive disorders during confinement. (3) These results—due to the COVID-19 preventive measures—may impact the progress and recovery of dual patients. (4) A greater investment is needed to raise the current level of care up to the standards of the pre-pandemic period. (5) A precise evaluation of the impact of the pandemic on patients with dual pathology and care activity will require more time to analyze the full extent of its effects.

Author Contributions: Conceptualization, C.M.-V., D.D.-S. and Ó.M.L.-R.; Formal analysis, C.M.-V., A.B.-M., M.N.-C. and Ó.M.L.-R.; Methodology, D.D.-S.; Writing—original draft, C.M.-V., D.D.-S.,

A.B.-M., M.N.-C. and Ó.M.L.-R.; Writing—review & editing, C.M.-V. and Ó.M.L.-R. All authors have read and agreed to the published version of the manuscript.

Funding: This work was supported by the grant "COMPARA: Psychiatric Comorbidity in Addictions and Outcomes in Andalusia. Modelización a través de Big Data", project P20-00735 of the Andalusian Research, Development, and Innovation Plan, provided by Fondo Europeo de Desarrollo Regional (EU) and Junta de Andalucía (Spain).

Institutional Review Board Statement: This research has been approved by the Research Ethics Committee of the Andalusian Ministry of Health, who certified compliance with the requirements for the ethical handling of the information.

Informed Consent Statement: Not applicable.

Data Availability Statement: Database should be request to the correspondence author.

Acknowledgments: This study has been carried out thanks to the transfer of data by the Department of Equality, Social Policies, and Conciliation of the Junta de Andalucía.

Conflicts of Interest: The authors declare no conflict of interest.

References

1. Chiappini, S.; Guirguis, A.; John, A.; Corkery, J.M.; Schifano, F. COVID-19: The Hidden Impact on Mental Health and Drug Addiction. *Front. Psychiatry* **2020**, *11*, 767. [CrossRef]
2. Da, B.L.; Im, G.Y.; Schiano, T.D. COVID-19 Hangover: A Rising Tide of Alcohol Use Disorder and Alcohol-Associated Liver Disease. *Hepatology* **2020**, *72*, 1102–1108. [CrossRef] [PubMed]
3. Ornell, F.; Moura, H.F.; Scherer, J.N.; Pechansky, F.; Kessler, F.H.P.; von Diemen, L. The COVID-19 Pandemic and Its Impact on Substance Use: Implications for Prevention and Treatment. *Psychiatry Res.* **2020**, *289*, 113096. [CrossRef] [PubMed]
4. García-Rivera, B.R.; García-Alcaraz, J.L.; Mendoza-Martínez, I.A.; Olguin-Tiznado, J.E.; García-Alcaráz, P.; Aranibar, M.F.; Camargo-Wilson, C. Influence of COVID-19 Pandemic Uncertainty in Negative Emotional States and Resilience as Mediators against Suicide Ideation, Drug Addiction and Alcoholism. *Int. J. Environ. Res. Public Health* **2021**, *18*, 12891. [CrossRef] [PubMed]
5. Ahmed, M.Z.; Ahmed, O.; Aibao, Z.; Hanbin, S.; Siyu, L.; Ahmad, A. Epidemic of COVID-19 in China and Associated Psychological Problems. *Asian J. Psychiatry* **2020**, *51*, 102092. [CrossRef]
6. Erquicia, J.; Valls, L.; Barja, A.; Gil, S.; Miquel, J.; Leal-Blanquet, J.; Schmidt, C.; Checa, J.; Vega, D. Emotional Impact of the COVID-19 Pandemic on Healthcare Workers in One of the Most Important Infection Outbreaks in Europe. *Clin. Med.* **2020**, *155*, 434–440. [CrossRef] [PubMed]
7. Liu, S.; Yang, L.; Zhang, C.; Xiang, Y.-T.; Liu, Z.; Hu, S.; Zhang, B. Online Mental Health Services in China during the COVID-19 Outbreak. *Lancet Psychiatry* **2020**, *7*, e17–e18. [CrossRef]
8. Nicolini, H. Depresión y Ansiedad En Los Tiempos de La Pandemia de COVID-19. *Cirugía Cirujanos* **2020**, *88*, 542–547. [CrossRef] [PubMed]
9. Griffiths, M.D.; Mamun, M.A. COVID-19 Suicidal Behavior among Couples and Suicide Pacts: Case Study Evidence from Press Reports. *Psychiatry Res.* **2020**, *289*, 113105. [CrossRef]
10. Allen, B.; El Shahawy, O.; Rogers, E.S.; Hochman, S.; Khan, M.R.; Krawczyk, N. Association of Substance Use Disorders and Drug Overdose with Adverse COVID-19 Outcomes in New York City: January–October 2020. *J. Public Health* **2020**, *43*, 462–465. [CrossRef]
11. Dubey, M.J.; Ghosh, R.; Chatterjee, S.; Biswas, P.; Chatterjee, S.; Dubey, S. COVID-19 and Addiction. *Diabetes Metab. Syndr. Clin. Res. Rev.* **2020**, *14*, 817–823. [CrossRef] [PubMed]
12. Wildberger, J.; Wenzel, K.; Fishman, M. Assessing Clinical Impacts and Attitudes Related to COVID-19 among Residential Substance Use Disorder Patients. *Subst. Abus.* **2022**, *43*, 756–762. [CrossRef] [PubMed]
13. Finlay, I.; Gilmore, I. COVID-19 and Alcohol—A Dangerous Cocktail. *BMJ* **2020**, *369*, m1987. [CrossRef] [PubMed]
14. The Nielsen Company. Rebalancing the "COVID-19 Effect" on Alcohol Sales. Available online: https://nielseniq.com/global/en/insights/analysis/2020/rebalancing-the-covid-19-effect-on-alcohol-sales/ (accessed on 3 May 2021).
15. MacKillop, J.; Cooper, A.; Costello, J. National Retail Sales of Alcohol and Cannabis during the COVID-19 Pandemic in Canada. *JAMA Netw. Open* **2021**, *4*, e2133076. [CrossRef]
16. Pollard, M.S.; Tucker, J.S.; Green, H.D. Changes in Adult Alcohol Use and Consequences during the COVID-19 Pandemic in the US. *JAMA Netw. Open* **2020**, *3*, e2022942. [CrossRef]
17. Rolland, B.; Haesebaert, F.; Zante, E.; Benyamina, A.; Haesebaert, J.; Franck, N. Global Changes and Factors of Increase in Caloric/Salty Food, Screen, and Substance Use, during the Early COVID-19 Containment Phase in France: A General Population Online Survey. *JMIR Public Health Surveill.* **2020**, *6*, e19630. [CrossRef]
18. Been, F.; Emke, E.; Matias, J.; Baz-Lomba, J.A.; Boogaerts, T.; Castiglioni, S.; Campos-Mañas, M.; Celma, A.; Covaci, A.; de Voogt, P.; et al. Changes in Drug Use in European Cities during Early COVID-19 Lockdowns—A Snapshot from Wastewater Analysis. *Environ. Int.* **2021**, *153*, 106540. [CrossRef]

19. Chappuy, M.; Peyrat, M.; Lejeune, O.; Duvernay, N.; David, B.; Joubert, P.; Lack, P. Drug Consumption during Prolonged Lockdown due to COVID-19 as Observed in French Addiction Center. *Therapies* **2021**, *76*, 379–382. [CrossRef]
20. Gili, A.; Bacci, M.; Aroni, K.; Nicoletti, A.; Gambelunghe, A.; Mercurio, I.; Gambelunghe, C. Changes in Drug Use Patterns during the COVID-19 Pandemic in Italy: Monitoring a Vulnerable Group by Hair Analysis. *Int. J. Environ. Res. Public Health* **2021**, *18*, 1967. [CrossRef]
21. Schmidt, R.A.; Genois, R.; Jin, J.; Vigo, D.; Rehm, J.; Rush, B. The Early Impact of COVID-19 on the Incidence, Prevalence, and Severity of Alcohol Use and Other Drugs: A Systematic Review. *Drug Alcohol Depend.* **2021**, *228*, 109065. [CrossRef]
22. Slavova, S.; Rock, P.; Bush, H.M.; Quesinberry, D.; Walsh, S.L. Signal of Increased Opioid Overdose during COVID-19 from Emergency Medical Services Data. *Drug Alcohol Depend.* **2020**, *214*, 108176. [CrossRef] [PubMed]
23. Imtiaz, S.; Nafeh, F.; Russell, C.; Ali, F.; Elton-Marshall, T.; Rehm, J. The Impact of the Novel Coronavirus Disease (COVID-19) Pandemic on Drug Overdose-Related Deaths in the United States and Canada: A Systematic Review of Observational Studies and Analysis of Public Health Surveillance Data. *Subst. Abus. Treat. Prev. Policy* **2021**, *16*, 1–14. [CrossRef]
24. Kilian, C.; Rehm, J.; Allebeck, P.; Braddick, F.; Gual, A.; Barták, M.; Bloomfield, K.; Gil, A.; Neufeld, M.; O'Donnell, A.; et al. Alcohol Consumption during the COVID-19 Pandemic in Europe: A Large-Scale Cross-Sectional Study in 21 Countries. *Addiction* **2021**, *116*, 3369–3380. [CrossRef]
25. Mark, T.L.; Gibbons, B.; Barnosky, A.; Padwa, H.; Joshi, V. Changes in Admissions to Specialty Addiction Treatment Facilities in California During the COVID-19 Pandemic. *JAMA Netw. Open* **2021**, *4*, e2117029. [CrossRef] [PubMed]
26. Aguilar, L.; Vicente-Hernández, B.; Remón-Gallo, D.; García-Ullán, L.; Valriberas-Herrero, I.; Maciá-Casas, A.; Pérez-Madruga, A.; Garzón, M.Á.; Álvarez-Navares, A.; Roncero, C. A Real-World Ten-Week Follow-up of the COVID Outbreak in an Outpatient Drug Clinic in Salamanca (Spain). *J. Subst. Abus. Treat.* **2021**, *125*, 108303. [CrossRef] [PubMed]
27. Milani, R.M.; Keller, A.; Roush, S. Dual Diagnosis Anonymous (DDA) and the Transition to Online Support During COVID-19. *J. Concurr. Disord.* **2021**. [CrossRef]
28. Arya, S.; Gupta, R. COVID-19 outbreak: Challenges for Addiction services in India. *Asian J. Psychiatry* **2020**, *51*, 102086. [CrossRef]
29. Green, T.C.; Bratberg, J.; Finnell, D.S. Opioid use disorder and the COVID 19 pandemic: A call to sustain regulatory easements and further expand access to treatment. *Subst. Abus.* **2020**, *41*, 147–149. [CrossRef]
30. Cance, J.D.; Doyle, E. Changes in Outpatient Buprenorphine Dispensing During the COVID-19 Pandemic. *JAMA* **2020**, *324*, 2442–2444. [CrossRef]
31. Huskamp, H.A.; Busch, A.B.; Uscher-Pines, L.; Barnett, M.L.; Riedel, L.; Mehrotra, A. Treatment of Opioid Use Disorder Among Commercially Insured Patients in the Context of the COVID-19 Pandemic. *JAMA* **2020**, *324*, 2440–2442. [CrossRef]
32. Torrens-Mèlich, M. Dual pathology: Current situation and future challenges. *Adicciones* **2008**, *20*, 315–320. [CrossRef] [PubMed]
33. Tirado-Muñoz, J.; Farré, A.; Mestre-Pintó, J.; Szerman, N.; Torrens, M. Dual pathology in depression: Recommendations in treatment. *Adicciones* **2017**, *30*, 66–76. [CrossRef]
34. Sivertsen, K.; Sørly, R.; Mydland, T.; Ekberg, J.I. Perspectives on Challenges and Opportunities in Norwegian Peer Recovery Services for People Living with Dual Diagnosis During a Pandemic. *J. Patient Exp.* **2021**, *8*, 237437352199695. [CrossRef] [PubMed]
35. Daigre, C.; Grau-López, L.; Palma-Álvarez, R.F.; Perea-Ortueta, M.; Sorribes-Puertas, M.; Serrano-Pérez, P.; Quesada, M.; Segura, L.; Coronado, M.; Ramos-Quiroga, J.A.; et al. A Multicenter Study on the Impact of Gender, Age, and Dual Diagnosis on Substance Consumption and Mental Health Status in Outpatients Treated for Substance Use Disorders during COVID-19 Lockdown. *J. Dual Diagn.* **2022**, *18*, 71–80. [CrossRef] [PubMed]
36. Grau-López, L.; Daigre, C.; Palma-Álvarez, R.F.; Sorribes-Puertas, M.; Serrano-Pérez, P.; Quesada-Franco, M.; Segura, L.; Coronado, M.; Ramos-Quiroga, J.A.; Colom, J. COVID-19 Lockdown and Consumption Patterns among Substance Use Disorder Outpatients: A Multicentre Study. *Eur. Addict. Res.* **2022**, *28*, 243–254. [CrossRef]
37. Sher, L. Dual disorders and suicide during and following the COVID-19 pandemic. *Acta Neuropsychiatr.* **2021**, *33*, 49–50. [CrossRef]
38. Rao, R.; Mueller, C.; Broadbent, M. Dual diagnosis in older drinkers during the COVID-19 pandemic. *Adv. Dual Diagn.* **2021**, *14*, 70–79. [CrossRef]
39. Gastón-Guerrero, A. Dual pathology: Drug dependence and depression. *Apunt. Psicol.* **2021**, *38*, 13–22.
40. Ries, R.K. Serial, parallel and integrated models of dual diagnosis treatment. *J. Health Care Poor Underserved* **1992**, *3*, 173–180. [CrossRef]
41. Arenas, F.; Ariza, M.J. *Protocolo de Actuación Conjunta Entre Unidades de Salud Mental Comunitaria y Centros de Tratamiento Ambulatorio de Drogodependencias*; Servicio Andaluz de Salud: Seville, Spain, 2012.
42. European Monitoring Centre for Drugs and Drug Addiction. *Treatment Demand Indicator (TDI) Standard Protocol 3.0: Guidelines for Reporting Data on People Entering Drug Treatment in European Countries*; EMCDDA: Lisbon, Portugal, 2012.
43. Dacosta-Sánchez, D.; Díaz-Batanero, C.; Fernández-Calderón, F.; Lozano, O.M. Impact of cluster B personality disorders in drugs therapeutic community treatment outcomes: A study based on Real World Data. *J. Clin. Med.* **2021**, *10*, 2572. [CrossRef]
44. Roncero, C.; Vicente-Hernández, B.; Casado-Espada, N.M.; Aguilar, L.; Gamonal-Limcaoco, S.; Garzón, M.A.; Martínez-González, F.; Llanes-Álvarez, C.; Martínez, R.; Franco-Martín, M.; et al. The Impact of COVID-19 Pandemic on the Castile and Leon Addiction Treatment Network: A Real-Word Experience. *Front. Psychiatry* **2020**, *11*, 575755. [CrossRef] [PubMed]
45. di Lorenzo, R.; Frattini, N.; Dragone, D.; Farina, R.; Luisi, F.; Ferrari, S.; Bandiera, G.; Rovesti, S.; Ferri, P. Psychiatric Emergencies During the COVID-19 Pandemic: A 6-Month Observational Study. *Neuropsychiatr. Dis. Treat.* **2021**, *17*, 1763–1778. [CrossRef] [PubMed]

46. Harris, M.T.H.; Peterkin, A.; Bach, P.; Englander, H.; Lapidus, E.; Rolley, T.; Weimer, M.B.; Weinstein, Z.M. Adapting inpatient addiction medicine addiction consult services during the COVID-19 pandemic. *Addict. Sci. Clin. Pract.* **2021**, *16*, 1–6. [CrossRef] [PubMed]
47. Manthey, J.; Kilian, C.; Carr, S.; Bartak, M.; Bloomfield, K.; Braddick, F.; Rehm, J. Use of alcohol, tobacco, cannabis, and other substances during the first wave of the SARS-CoV-2 pandemic in Europe: A survey on 36,000 European substance users. *Subst. Abus. Treat. Prev. Policy* **2021**, *16*, 1–11. [CrossRef]
48. Bonati, M.; Campi, R.; Segre, G. Psychological impact of the quarantine during the COVID-19 pandemic on the general European adult population: A systematic review of the evidence. *Epidemiol. Psychiatr. Sci.* **2022**, *31*, e27. [CrossRef]
49. Preti, E.; di Pierro, R.; Fanti, E.; Madeddu, F.; Calati, R. Personality disorders in time of pandemic. *Curr. Psychiatry Rep.* **2020**, *22*, 1–9. [CrossRef]
50. Patel, R.; Irving, J.; Brinn, A.; Broadbent, M.; Shetty, H.; McGuire, P. Impact of the COVID-19 pandemic on remote mental healthcare and prescribing in psychiatry: An electronic health record study. *BMJ Open* **2021**, *11*, e046365. [CrossRef]
51. Mancheño-Barba, J.J.; Navas-León, S.; Gutiérrez-López, M.L.; Rosa-Cáceres, A.D.L.; Cáceres-Pachón, P. Analysis of the profiles of patients with dual pathology attending addiction centers, mental health centers, and a coordinated service. *Ann. Psychol.* **2019**, *35*, 233–241. [CrossRef]
52. Mancheño-Barba, J.J.; Navas-León, S.; Fernández-Calderón, F.; Gutiérrez, M.; Sánchez-García, M.; Díaz-Batanero, C.; Lozano, O.M. Coordinated treatment between addiction and mental health centers vs uncoordinated treatment for patients with dual pathology: Greater dropout, but less deterioration of functional disability. *Actas Españolas Psiquiatr.* **2021**, *49*, 71–80.

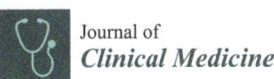

Journal of
Clinical Medicine

Article

Machine Learning Prediction of Comorbid Substance Use Disorders among People with Bipolar Disorder

Vincenzo Oliva [1,2,†], Michele De Prisco [1,3,†], Maria Teresa Pons-Cabrera [4], Pablo Guzmán [4], Gerard Anmella [1], Diego Hidalgo-Mazzei [1], Iria Grande [1], Giuseppe Fanelli [2,5], Chiara Fabbri [2,6], Alessandro Serretti [2], Michele Fornaro [3], Felice Iasevoli [3], Andrea de Bartolomeis [3], Andrea Murru [1], Eduard Vieta [1,*] and Giovanna Fico [1]

[1] Bipolar and Depressive Disorders Unit, Institute of Neurosciences, Hospital Clinic, University of Barcelona, IDIBAPS, CIBERSAM, 170 Villarroel St., 12-0, 08036 Barcelona, Catalonia, Spain; voliva@clinic.cat (V.O.); mdeprisco@clinic.cat (M.D.P.); anmella@clinic.cat (G.A.); dahidalg@clinic.cat (D.H.-M.); igrande@clinic.cat (I.G.); amurru@clinic.cat (A.M.); gfico@clinic.cat (G.F.)
[2] Department of Biomedical and Neuromotor Sciences, University of Bologna, 40123 Bologna, Italy; giuseppe.fanelli5@unibo.it (G.F.); chiara.fabbri@yahoo.it (C.F.); alessandro.serretti@unibo.it (A.S.)
[3] Section of Psychiatry, Department of Neuroscience, Reproductive Science and Odontostomatology, Federico II University of Naples, 80131 Naples, Italy; dott.fornaro@gmail.com (M.F.); felice.iasevoli@unina.it (F.I.); adebarto@unina.it (A.d.B.)
[4] Addictions Unit, Department of Psychiatry and Psychology, Institute of Neuroscience, Hospital Clinic, University of Barcelona, IDIBAPS, CIBERSAM, 170 Villarroel St., 12-0, 08036 Barcelona, Catalonia, Spain; mtpons@clinic.cat (M.T.P.-C.); prguzman@clinic.cat (P.G.)
[5] Department of Human Genetics, Radboud University Medical Center, Donders Institute for Brain, Cognition and Behavior, 6525 GD Nijmegen, The Netherlands
[6] Social, Genetic & Developmental Psychiatry Centre, Institute of Psychiatry, Psychology & Neuroscience, King's College London, London SE5 9NU, UK
* Correspondence: evieta@clinic.cat
† These authors contributed equally to this work.

Abstract: Substance use disorder (SUD) is a common comorbidity in individuals with bipolar disorder (BD), and it is associated with a severe course of illness, making early identification of the risk factors for SUD in BD warranted. We aimed to identify, through machine-learning models, the factors associated with different types of SUD in BD. We recruited 508 individuals with BD from a specialized unit. Lifetime SUDs were defined according to the DSM criteria. Random forest (RF) models were trained to identify the presence of (i) any (SUD) in the total sample, (ii) alcohol use disorder (AUD) in the total sample, (iii) AUD co-occurrence with at least another SUD in the total sample (AUD+SUD), and (iv) any other SUD among BD patients with AUD. Relevant variables selected by the RFs were considered as independent variables in multiple logistic regressions to predict SUDs, adjusting for relevant covariates. AUD+SUD could be predicted in BD at an individual level with a sensitivity of 75% and a specificity of 75%. The presence of AUD+SUD was positively associated with having hypomania as the first affective episode (OR = 4.34 95% CI = 1.42–13.31), and the presence of hetero-aggressive behavior (OR = 3.15 95% CI = 1.48–6.74). Machine-learning models might be useful instruments to predict the risk of SUD in BD, but their efficacy is limited when considering socio-demographic or clinical factors alone.

Keywords: bipolar disorder; substance use disorder; cannabis use disorder; alcohol use disorder; machine learning

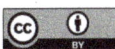

1. Introduction

Substance use disorder (SUD) frequently occurs among people with bipolar disorder (BD), worsening their clinical trajectories [1,2]. A comorbid diagnosis of BD and SUD occurs in up to 30–60% of people with SUD, depending on the substance used, including alcohol [3], cannabis [4], tobacco [5], or others [3,6,7], with men having higher lifetime risks of SUD than women [8]. The presence of SUD accounts for a higher number of lifetime mood episodes and hospitalizations [9]; lifetime medical comorbidities [10]; reduced cognitive and psychosocial functioning [11]; and an increased risk for suicide [12], impulsive and aggressive behavior [13], or mortality [14]. Substance use may also attenuate the efficacy or compliance to psychopharmacological treatments, further worsening BD course [15,16].

The strongest comorbid associations of SUD among individuals with BD are found with alcohol use disorder (AUD), followed by cannabis and other illicit drugs [8]. Interestingly, the most current report by the National Epidemiological Survey on alcohol and related conditions [17] suggests that the presence of both alcohol use and having a psychiatric diagnosis, including BD, are associated with higher utilization rates of lifetime poly-substance abuse [18] compared with individuals without these clinical characteristics. Patients with BD with multiple SUDs have even more severe outcomes, including the risk of overdose, criminal conviction, low adherence to treatments, and reduced global functioning [10,19,20].

Despite its burden, the relationship between SUDs and BD has been minimally studied. Indeed, a few longitudinal studies have examined the predictors of SUD onset in BD, reporting that alcohol use disorder (AUD) might be predicted by psychotic symptoms [21], while cannabis use disorder might be predicted by younger age, lower education, and previous substance use [22]. In addition, the generalizability of much-published research on this issue is problematic, given that individuals who exclusively meet the criteria for a single SUD do not represent the naturalistic population in clinical settings [19]. This more significant symptomatic burden of comorbid SUDs in adults with BD points out the necessity of identifying the risk factors of co-occurrence in order to implement appropriate preventative strategies.

Evidence has suggested the feasibility of developing predictive models in psychiatry through machine-learning algorithms [23,24]. Several studies have used data mining and machine learning techniques to predict patient outcomes, including SUD [25]. However, to the best of our knowledge, no study has applied machine-learning techniques to date to predict the presence of comorbid SUD in individuals with BD. In addition, no studies on the topic have analyzed to what extent BD phenotypes differ according to the type of SUD.

The current study aims at identifying the most meaningful variables associated with SUD, AUD, and AUD in comorbidity with any other SUD in a large sample of patients with BD through the use of a random forest (RF) model. These variables will then be used in a regression model to provide further information on the associations between BD and specific types of SUD.

2. Materials and Methods

2.1. Participants

The present study included all the patients enrolled in the systematic prospective follow-up of the Bipolar Disorders Unit of the Hospital Clinic, University of Barcelona, Catalunia, Spain, from October 1998 to November 2021. Barcelona's Bipolar and Depressive Disorders Unit provides both tertiary- and secondary-level care. The unit enrolls difficult-to-treat BD patients BD derived from all over Spain, and patients from a catchment area of approximately 170,000 inhabitants in Barcelona in particular [26]. Trained psychiatrists regularly treat more than 700 patients according to a local protocol based on international clinical guidelines [27,28]. The inclusion criteria were as follows: (i) older than 18 years of age, and (ii) diagnosis of BD type I (BDI) or type II (BDII) according to the Diagnostic and Statistical Manual of Mental Disorders (DSM) IV [29], DSM-IV-TR [30], or DSM-5 criteria [31]. In addition, the exclusion criteria were the presence of severe organic diseases requiring urgent treatment at baseline assessment or severe cognitive, motor, or visual impairment. All participants provided written informed consent for this ethical committee-approved study (approval code: HCB/2017/0432).

2.2. Clinical Variables Assessment

Patients were assessed using the Structured Clinical Interview for DSM Disorders [32]. The main sociodemographic and clinical characteristics were collected through an ad hoc schedule. If specific information was not collected during the baseline assessment, the electronic clinical records of each patient were inquired. Collected variables included age, education, working and living status, duration of illness, current pharmacological treatment (if maintained for at least six months), the number of hospitalizations and affective episodes, and lifetime aggressive behavior, among other variables of interest (see Table 1). Predominant polarity was defined according to the standard definition created in our unit and repeatedly validated [33]. A family history of psychiatric disorder was defined as having a first-degree relative diagnosed with and/or treated for any mood disorder, including major depression, cyclothymia, and dysthymia. The term "suicide attempt" refers to intentional self-inflicted poisoning, injury, or self-harm with a deadly intent without death. The presence of lifetime SUD was assessed according to DSM-IV [29], DSM-IV-TR [30], or DSM-5 criteria [31], including drug-specific diagnoses for ten substances: alcohol, cannabis, cocaine, heroin, hallucinogens, inhalants, prescription opioids, sedatives/tranquilizers, stimulants, and other drugs (e.g., ecstasy or ketamine). Each DSM-5 SUD diagnosis required positive responses to 2 or more of the 11 criteria for each drug-specific SUD.

2.3. Statistical Analyses

All of the analyses were conducted with RStudio, R version 4.1.2 [34]. The Kolmogorov–Smirnov test was used to assess whether continuous variables displayed a normal distribution. The parametric comparative analyses for the demographic and clinical characteristics of the groups (SUD vs. non-SUD) were done with unpaired t-test with Bonferroni post hoc correction for continuous variables; for non-parametric distributions, a Mann–Whitney *U* Test or Kruskal–Wallis Test was used, where appropriate. Categorical data were analyzed by Chi-square analysis.

2.3.1. Missing Data

We inspected missing data using the R package "skimr" [35], and these were assumed to be missing at random. Therefore, we included only the variables presenting at least 75% of the available data in the model. For those contributing less than 25% of missing data, missing data were imputed using the R package "missRanger" [36], which is based on the algorithm of "missForest" (Stekhoven and Bühlmann 2012) and uses a random forest (RF) approach. The parameter "num.trees" was set at 5000, and the out-of-bag (OOB) errors were calculated for each variable in order to measure the accuracy according to the method outlined in previous evidence [37]. OOB errors ranged from 0 (better performance) to 1 (worse performance).

2.3.2. Random Forest

We performed RFs using the R packages "RandomForest" [38] and "caret" [39] to tune the algorithm. A series of RFs were primarily used to select the most important features, which predicted different outcomes. To select the most critical variables, the "mean decrease of Gini coefficient" was adopted to observe which variables substantially contributed to the homogeneity of the nodes and leaves in the resulting RF.

We conducted a first RF considering the presence of lifetime SUD as the predicted condition in the entire sample. Next, among people with SUD, as the first step, we selected only people with a lifetime diagnosis of AUD who consumed alcohol alone or combined with other substances (i.e., cocaine, cannabis, hallucinogens, or MDMA). Then, we conducted a second and third RF considering the presence of AUD mono-use or comorbid with another SUD as the predicted conditions, compared with non-abusing controls; finally, we performed a fourth RF to differentiate people with AUD mono-use from people with AUD+SUD. RF is a classification algorithm that combines multiple decision trees made by randomly selected bootstrap samples, mainly affected by unbalanced data. We used the R package "ROSE" [40] to under sample the predicted class that presented the most observations in order to obtain a balanced dataset. As a secondary step, to exploratory assess the accuracy of the prediction model, a "train" and a "test" dataset were prepared, containing 80% and 20% of the original observations, respectively. We initially used a repeated cross-validated RF (10-folds, ten repeats) on the "train" dataset and then tuned some hyperparameters (i.e., number of trees, number of features randomly selected at each node, and size of the node) during the learning phase, to obtain the best accuracy value. Then, we applied the trained model to the "test" dataset, and calculated measures such as accuracy, sensitivity, specificity, the OOB estimate, and the F-score (F1), which alternatively are tests of the model's accuracy. To graphically present our results, we produced a confusion matrix.

Table 1. Socio-demographic and clinical characteristics of the sample classified according to the presence of substance use disorder(s).

	SUD (n = 262; 51.57%)	Non-SUD (n = 246; 48.4%)	$t/Z/\chi^2$	p
Gender (n; %)				
- Female	109; 41.6%	167; 67.9%	35.32	<0.001
Living status (n; %)				
- Parents	45; 18.8%	83; 33.2%		
- Family	141; 59%	114; 45.6%	14.27	0.003
- Alone	33; 18.8%	36; 14.4%		
- Other (community)	20; 8.4%	17; 6.8%		
Relationship status (n; %)				
- Not in a relationship	72; 29.8%	125; 48.4%		
- Married	117; 48.3%	84; 32.6%	27.8	<0.001
- Divorced	40; 16.5%	47; 18.2%		
- Widow	13; 5.4%	2; 0.8%		
Working status (n; %)				
- Full-time or part-time job	127; 53.8%	131; 52.8%		
- Unemployed	27; 11.4%	23; 9.3%	14.78	0.011
- Retired	33; 14%	45; 18.1%		
- Not able to work	34; 14.4%	17; 6.9%		
Diagnosis (n; %)				
- BDI	190; 72.5%	155; 63%	5.26	0.014
- BDII	72; 27.5%	91; 37%		
Age and illness duration (mean ± SD)				
Age at assessment	48.6 ± 15.08	43.77 ± 26.46	26.397	<0.001
Age at onset	29.3 ± 13.19	26.4 ± 10.63	28.307	<0.001
Duration of illness	19.27 ± 12.1	17.32 ± 12.06	29.959	0.048
Number of affective episodes, lifetime (mean ± SD)				
- Depressive	8.39 ± 11.87	7.13 ± 9.17	28.285	0.084
- Manic	2.25 ± 4.1	2.52 ± 3.69	35.186	0.066
- Hypomanic	5.51 ± 10.2	4.04 ± 7.76	28.288	<0.001
- Mixed	0.63 ± 1.89	0.65 ± 1.77	32.958	0.54
- Total	16.84 ± 22.61	14.34 ± 16.66	30.338	0.25
Polarity of the first affective episode (n; %)				
- Depressive	168; 70.9%	66; 26.2%		
- Manic	52; 21.9%	22; 8.7%	7.94	0.09
- Hypomanic	9; 3.8%	155; 61.5%		
- Mixed	6; 2.5%	5; 2%		

Table 1. Cont.

	SUD (n = 262; 51.57%)	Non-SUD (n = 246; 48.4%)	t/Z/χ²	p
Number of Psychiatric admissions, lifetime (mean ± SD)	1.59 ± 2.14	1.61 ± 2.01	30.023	0.61
Clinical course variables, lifetime (n; %)				
- Suicide attempts	73; 51.4%	172; 47%	0.702	0.23
- Aggressive behaviours				
- Self-directed	52; 21%	52; 19.8%	0.130	0.4
- Hetero-directed	26; 10.6%	54; 20.6%	9.64	0.001
- Psychotic symptoms	119; 49.2%	132; 51.2%	0.198	0.36
- Rapid cycling	60; 22.9%	68; 27.6%	1.51	0.130
- Seasonality	63; 25.6%	53; 20.2%	2.08	0.09
- Family history of Mood Disorder	143; 62.2%	153; 61.4%	0.027	0.47
- Comorbidity with Personality Disorder				
- Cluster A	4; 1.7%	7; 2.9%	7.31	0.063
- Cluster B	20; 8.7%	34; 13.9%		
- Cluster C	11; 4.8%	4; 1.6%		

BD = bipolar disorder; SUD = substance use disorder; n = number of cases; p = statistical significance; SD = standard deviation; χ² = Chi-square test; t = Independent Samples t-test; Z = Mann–Whitney U test.

2.3.3. Multiple Logistic Regression

The variables selected by the RFs that mostly decreased the homogeneity of the nodes and leaves of the model were considered as independent variables in multiple logistic regressions, adjusting for sex, duration of illness, and age at BD onset, as these are known factors associated with SUD in previous studies [6,20,41]. The dependent variables were the same ones considered in the corresponding RFs. Odds ratios (ORs) and their 95% confidence intervals (CIs) were estimated to assess the significance of each result. The variance explained was calculated as Nagelkerke's pseudo R^2 with the R package "fmsb" [42]. These regression models were useful to provide further information on the association between the relevant variables identified by the RFs and the various SUD comorbidities of interest.

3. Results

3.1. Characteristics of the Sample

A total of 508 patients were included, of which 276 were female (54.3%). The mean age of the total sample was 46.11 (standard deviation—SD = 14.47) years old. Our sample consisted of 345 (67.9%) patients with BD-I and 163 (32.1%) patients with BD-II. Of all of the patients, 262 (51.57%) fulfilled the DSM criteria for lifetime SUD of any type. The most used substance was alcohol (42.1%), followed by cannabis (22.6%), cocaine (12%), amphetamine (4.7%), MDMA (4.7%), and hallucinogens (2.1%). A total of 106 patients (20.8%) had AUD with at least another SUD (AUD+SUD). The sample characteristics are presented in Table 1.

3.2. Missing Data

Among the variables presenting missing data, 22 of them presented less than 25% of missing values. Of these, 17 presented fewer than 10% of missing values. Errors estimated during the imputation of missing data were less than 20%, except for the number of lifetime hospitalization (OOB = 0.29).

3.3. Patients with SUD vs. without SUD

The RF model performance outputs are reported in Table 2. The variables presenting higher values of mean decrease of gini were "number of total affective episodes", "number of total depressive episodes", "number of total hypomanic episodes", "number of total manic episodes", "number of lifetime hospitalization", "being in a relationship", "diagnosis of cluster B personality disorder", "number of attempted suicides", "number of mixed episodes", and "treatment with benzodiazepines".

These variables were tested in a multiple logistic regression adjusted for relevant covariates (see Methods). The presence of SUD was positively associated with a diagnosis of cluster B personality disorder (OR = 2.31 [95% CI = 1.26–4.23]; p = 0.006), and negatively associated with being in a relationship (OR = 0.6 [95% CI = 0.39–0.91]; p = 0.015) (Figure 1). The model explained 16.9% of the total variance in the sample of BD with SUD vs. non-SUD.

3.4. Patients with AUD vs. without SUD

RF model performance outputs are reported in Table 2. The variables presenting higher values of mean decrease of gini were "number of total affective episodes", "number of total depressive episodes", "number of total hypomanic episodes", "number of total manic episodes", "number of mixed episodes", "number of lifetime hospitalization", "number of attempted suicides", "being in a relationship", "diagnosis of cluster B personality disorder, any", "treatment with mood stabilizers other than lithium".

In a multiple logistic regression model adjusted for relevant covariates (see Methods), none of these variables was significantly associated with the presence of AUD (Figure 1). The model explained 14.2% of the total variance.

Table 2. Random forest model performance outputs.

Data Set	Number of Trees	Number of Features	Node Size	Accuracy%	95% CI	p	Sensitivity	Specificity	F1-Score
SUD VS. NO-SUD	800	9	6	65.3%	54.8–74.7	0.004	69.6%	61.2%	0.66
AUD VS. NO-SUD	350	3	43	53.8%	39.5–67.8	0.44	44%	63%	0.48
AUD+SUD VS. NO-SUD	500	26	47	75%	56.6–88.5	0.003	75%	75%	0.75
AUD+SUD VS. AUD	800	2	14	62.5%	43.6–78.9	0.107	43.8%	81.2%	0.54

Substance use disorder: SUD; alcohol use disorder (AUD); confidence interval (CI).

3.5. Patients with AUD+SUD vs. without SUD or AUD

RF model performance outputs are reported in Table 2. The variables presenting higher values of mean decrease of gini were "number of total hypomanic episodes", "presence of hetero-directed aggressivity", "number of total affective episodes", "number of total depressive episodes", "violent suicide attempt", "number of total manic episodes", "being in a relationship", "number of lifetime hospitalization", "first episode as hypomanic", "presence of melancholia".

In a multiple logistic regression adjusted for relevant covariates, hypomania as the first affective episode (OR = 4.34 [95% CI = 1.42–13.31]; p = 0.01) and hetero-directed aggressivity (OR = 3.15 [95% CI = 1.48–6.74]; p = 0.003) were associated with AUD+SUD (Figure 1). The model explained 31.5% of the total variance in AUD+SUD.

3.6. Patients with AUD+SUD vs. with AUD

RF model performance outputs are reported in Table 2. The variables presenting higher values of mean decrease of gini were "number of total affective episodes", "number of total manic episodes", "number of total depressive episodes", "number of total hypomanic episodes", "mood disorders familiarity", "number of lifetime hospitalization", "number of total mixed episodes", "first episode as depressive", "presence of rapid-cycling", and "atypical depression".

These variables were considered in an adjusted multiple logistic regression. The presence of another SUD in the context of AUD was negatively associated with having depression as the first affective episode (OR = 0.41 [95% CI = 0.21–0.81]; p = 0.011) (Figure 1). The model explained 30.5% of the total variance.

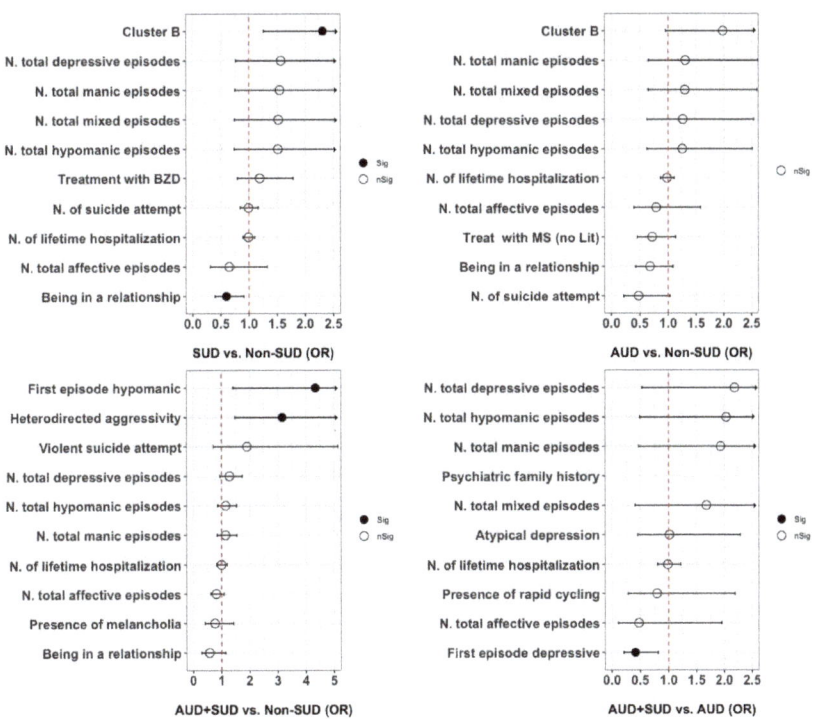

Figure 1. Logistic regression plots of odds ratio (OR) and 95% confidence intervals (CI). Independent variables were selected among the top ten features derived from the random forest (RF) models. The four models predicted (from left to right): any substance use disorder (SUD) in the total sample, alcohol use disorder (AUD) in the total sample, AUD co-occurrence with at least another SUD in the total sample, and AUD co-occurrence with at least another SUD among BD patients with AUD.

4. Discussion

To the best of our knowledge, this is the first study attempting to examine the value of socio-demographic and clinical factors for the prediction of SUD in a large, naturalistic sample of adults with BD using a machine-learning approach.

Using a random forest classifier, we developed models to predict the presence of SUD, AUD, or the co-occurrence of AUD and other SUDs in BD. Although the specificities of the models were acceptable, their accuracies were low to moderate. The comparison of the performance of our models with previously developed models is limited by the scarce evidence on the topic [20].

The model with the highest accuracy was the one predicting the co-occurrence of another SUD among individuals with AUD and compared with those without SUD, correctly classifying up to 75% of the sample. The top features were similar among the four random forest models and included clinical factors associated with a severe course of illness in BD, such as the lifetime number of affective episodes and the respective episode polarity [43], type of index episode [44], the presence of comorbid cluster B personality disorder [45], and suicide or aggressive behavior [46]. It should be remarked that the top features extracted might be highly correlated with other relevant variables associated with poor BD outcomes (e.g., presence of psychotic symptoms, and low socioeconomic status) [47,48], thus hindering their effect on SUD prediction. However, the effect of other variables could be considered minimal compared with that of the selected top features [49]. While we found similarities among the top features identified by the RF models, their association with SUD comorbidities varied among the logistic regression models.

A lifetime comorbid diagnosis of cluster B personality disorder and not being in a relationship predicted the presence of SUD vs. no-SUD. This result is not surprising as SUD, cluster B personality disorders, and BD are characterized by impulsivity and poor behavioral control [50–52]. The complex phenotypic overlap between BD and cluster B personality disorders is a clinical challenge [53], with problematic clinical and genetic boundaries [54], frequently leading to a misdiagnosis of BD in people with personality disorders, such as borderline personality disorder (BPD) [55,56]. The risk of substance use and abuse in individuals with BD and comorbid BPD is two to three times higher than in individuals with BD alone [57]. This could be possibly justified by an even higher tendency toward risky behaviors, mood instability, impulsivity, affective reactivity, and context-specific increased sensitivity to rewards in patients with comorbid BD and BPD, ultimately leading to substance misuse [58]. Another variable associated with SUD risk is the lack of a stable relationship, which is in line with previous evidence [59]. Similarly, socio-economic functioning is substantially decreased in patients with BD, with lower odds of being in a stable relationship compared with the general population (Sletved et al., 2021 [60]), while social or family support improves patients' global functioning [61].

Given the extremely high prevalence of AUD in BD and their strong interplay, we analyzed predictors of AUD alone or comorbid with another SUD. The relationship between AUD and BD is complex and comprises shared biological pathways [62], as well as clinical and psychological characteristics [63]. However, previous observational studies on AUD in BD were mainly conducted on individuals with a co-occurrence of other SUDs [3,21,64], without clinical phenotyping, based on a distinct pattern of use. After controlling for sex, age of onset, and duration of illness, no other factors were associated with AUD without other SUDs in our sample. However, AUD comorbid with another SUD was positively associated with a history of a hypomanic episode at BD onset and hetero-aggressive behavior compared with non-use, and negatively associated with a history of a depressive episode at BD onset when compared with non-use. The polarity of the first episode has a relevant influence on the course of BD, with the depressive one being the most common and being related to suicide attempts [65], with (hypo)manic being related to alcohol or other substance misuses [44]. Given that polarity at onset might predict subsequent predominant polarity in BD [44,66], its evaluation may guide long-term therapeutic planning [67]. The link between first-episode polarity or predominant polarity, SUDs, and BD requires further analysis in prospective longitudinal studies, as affective episodes may be triggered by substance use, thus influencing lifetime affective episodes of a specific polarity [68]. Aggressive behavior is considered a trait and a state factor associated with BD, often driven/worsened by substance use [52]. Proneness to impulsivity may lead to greater involvement in substance use and an increased risk for criminal, violent, or aggressive acts. However, these premises and the existence of putative common biological underpinnings of aggressive behavior and BD suggest that this undesirable outcome might result from environmental–gene interactions [69].

Individuals that reported substance misuse before the onset of BD are sometimes considered to have a "milder" BD phenotype [70]. In addition, sub-threshold mood symptoms or mood instability might be the result of substance use and might lead to BD misdiagnosis [71]. Therefore, the direction of the association between SUD and BD is relevant, as it might depict two different subpopulations of individuals according to the onset of SUD (i.e., before or after BD onset) with distinct clinical needs. However, our study lacked information about the differences between these subpopulations and the direction of the association. Several other limitations in this study should be considered. The cross-sectional design of the study, as well as the use of clinical variables, collected retrospectively from electronic clinical records, may have affected the accuracy and reliability of our data, particularly regarding previous affective episodes, hypomanic onsets—for which retrospective diagnosis is a clinical challenge—or mixed episodes—for which the DSM definition varied across the years. Obviously, a longitudinal study would be a better design to test our models [72]. In addition, we only included data on current psychopharmacological treatment, but not on psychosocial, psychoeducational, or other psychological interventions that are highly recommended for comorbid SUD management in major guidelines [73] because they improve adherence to pharmacological treatment, leading to a more stable BD course [74]. Secondly, SUD might have been underdiagnosed because of internalized stigma [75]. Given that patients were recruited from a specialized unit, a potential selection bias should also be taken into account, as we could assessed the most severe cases that were ultimately forwarded to a tertiary clinic or, conversely, the less severe ones. Furthermore, when considering lifetime SUD, we might have excluded people with current SUD, thus inflating the risk for Berkson's bias, and ultimately reducing the overall generalizability of the results. Finally, RFs are a "black box", making any local interpretation of a specific prediction quite impractical.

Despite its possible limitations, the present study is the first one to develop algorithms to identify SUD in patients with BD and to describe potential sociodemographic and clinical predictors of comorbidity. Furthermore, our data come from a highly specialized unit, in which patients are regularly followed-up by trained psychiatrists.

5. Conclusions

Bipolar disorder that occurs in comorbidity with substance use disorder represents a severe clinical phenotype of bipolar illness. Alcohol use disorder is the most frequent comorbid substance use disorder in individuals with bipolar disorder, and it frequently presents in co-occurrence with other substance use. Machine-learning models might be used to predict the risk of having a comorbid substance use disorder in bipolar disorder, but their accuracy is limited when they include socio-demographical or clinical factors alone, as done in this study. Complex models integrating biological and clinical predictors represent a promising alternative to improve the performance of prediction.

Author Contributions: Data curation, V.O., G.F. (Giuseppe Fanelli) and G.F. (Giovanna Fico); Formal analysis, V.O., M.D.P. and G.F. (Giovanna Fico); Methodology, C.F., A.S. and G.F. (Giovanna Fico); Supervision, E.V.; Writing—original draft, G.F. (Giovanna Fico); Writing—review & editing, M.T.P.-C., P.G., G.A., D.H.-M., I.G., M.F., F.I., A.d.B., A.M. and G.F. (Giovanna Fico). All authors have read and agreed to the published version of the manuscript.

Funding: This research received no external funding.

Institutional Review Board Statement: The study was conducted in accordance with the Declaration of Helsinki, and was approved by the Ethics Committee (Drug Research Ethics Committee (CEIm); Approval Code: HCB/2017/0432; Approval Date: 7 June 2017).

Informed Consent Statement: Informed consent was obtained from all of the subjects involved in the study.

Data Availability Statement: Data are available upon request.

Acknowledgments: G.A.'s research is supported by a Rio Hortega 2021 grant (CM21/00017) financed by the Instituto de Salud Carlos III (ISCIII) and cofinanced by the Fondo Social Europeo Plus (FSE+). I.G. thanks the support of the Spanish Ministry of Science and Innovation (MCIN) (PI19/00954) integrated into the Plan Nacional de I+D+I and cofinanced by the ISCIII-Subdirección General de Evaluación y el Fondos Europeos de la Unión Europea (FEDER, FSE, Next Generation EU/Plan de Recuperación Transformación y Resiliencia_PRTR); the Instituto de Salud Carlos III; the CIBER of Mental Health (CIBERSAM); and the the Secretaria d'Universitats i Recerca del Departament d'Economia i Coneixement (2017 SGR 1365), CERCA Programme /Generalitat de Catalunya. E.V. thanks the support of the Spanish Ministry of Science and Innovation (PI15/00283, PI18/00805) integrated into the Plan Nacional de I+D+I and co-financed by the ISCIII-Subdirección General de Evaluación and the Fondo Europeo de Desarrollo Regional (FEDER); the Instituto de Salud Carlos III; the CIBER of Mental Health (CIBERSAM); the Secretaria d'Universitats i Recerca del Departament d'Economia i Coneixement (2017 SGR 1365), the CERCA Programme, and the Departament de Salut de la Generalitat de Catalunya for the PERIS grant SLT006/17/00357. A.M. has received a grant

(PI19/00672) from the Instituto de Salud Carlos III Subdirección General de Evaluación y Fomento de la investigación, Plan Nacional 2019–2022. The project that gave rise to these results received the support of a fellowship from "La Caixa" Foundation (ID 100010434). G.F. (Giovanna Fico) fellowship code is LCF/BQ/DR21/11880019.

Conflicts of Interest: I.G. has received grants and served as consultant, advisor, or CME speaker for the following identities: Angelini, Casen Recordati, Ferrer, Janssen Cilag, and Lundbeck, Lundbeck-Otsuka, Luye, SEI Healthcare outside the submitted work. C.F. was a speaker for Janssen. A.S. is or has been a consultant/speaker for Abbott, Abbvie, Angelini, AstraZeneca, Clinical Data, Boehringer, Bristol-Myers Squibb, Eli Lilly, GlaxoSmithKline, Innovapharma, Italfarmaco, Janssen, Lundbeck, Naurex, Pfizer, Polifarma, Sanofi, and Servier. G.A. has received CME-related honoraria, or consulting fees from Janssen-Cilag, Lundbeck, Lundbeck/Otsuka, and Angelini, with no financial or other relationship relevant to the subject of this article. A.M. has received funding unrelated to the present work for research projects and/or honoraria as a consultant or speaker from the following entities: Angelini, Janssen, Lundbeck, Otsuka, Sanofi-Aventis and Spanish Ministry of Science and Innovation-Instituto de Salud Carlos III. E.V. has received grants and served as consultant, advisor, or CME speaker unrelated to the present work for the following entities: AB-Biotics, Abbott, Abbvie, Adamed, Angelini, Biogen, Dainippon Sumitomo Pharma, Ferrer, Gedeon Richter, Janssen, Lundbeck, Otsuka, Rovi, Sage, Sanofi-Aventis, Sunovion, Takeda, and Viatris. G.F. (Giovanna Fico) has received CME-related honoraria, or consulting fees from Angelini, Janssen-Cilag and Lundbeck. M.F. has none to disclose in conjunction with the present piece of work. A.d.B. has received unrestricted research support from Janssen, Lundbeck, and Otsuka and lecture honoraria for educational meeting from Chiesi, Lundbeck, Roche, Sunovion, Vitria, Recordati, Angelini and Takeda; he has served on advisory boards for Eli Lilly, Jansen, Lundbeck, Otsuka, Roche, and Takeda, Chiesi, Recordati, Angelini, Vitria.

References

1. Ostacher, M.J.; Perlis, R.H.; Nierenberg, A.A.; Calabrese, J.; Stange, J.P.; Salloum, I.; Weiss, R.D.; Sachs, G.S. Impact of Substance Use Disorders on Recovery From Episodes of Depression in Bipolar Disorder Patients: Prospective Data From the Systematic Treatment Enhancement Program for Bipolar Disorder (STEP-BD). *Am. J. Psychiatry* **2010**, *167*, 289. [CrossRef] [PubMed]
2. Menculini, G.; Steardo, L.; Verdolini, N.; Cirimbilli, F.; Moretti, P.; Tortorella, A. Substance Use Disorders in Bipolar Disorders: Clinical Correlates and Treatment Response to Mood Stabilizers. *J. Affect. Disord.* **2022**, *300*, 326–333. [CrossRef] [PubMed]
3. Simhandl, C.; Radua, J.; König, B.; Amann, B.L. Prevalence and Impact of Comorbid Alcohol Use Disorder in Bipolar Disorder: A Prospective Follow-up Study. *Aust. N. Z. J. Psychiatry* **2016**, *50*, 345–351. [CrossRef] [PubMed]
4. Pinto, J.V.; Medeiros, L.S.; Santana da Rosa, G.; Santana de Oliveira, C.E.; de Souza Crippa, J.A.; Passos, I.C.; Kauer-Sant'Anna, M. The Prevalence and Clinical Correlates of Cannabis Use and Cannabis Use Disorder among Patients with Bipolar Disorder: A Systematic Review with Meta-Analysis and Meta-Regression. *Neurosci. Biobehav. Rev.* **2019**, *101*, 78–84. [CrossRef]
5. Fornaro, M.; Carvalho, A.F.; de Prisco, M.; Mondin, A.M.; Billeci, M.; Selby, P.; Iasevoli, F.; Berk, M.; Castle, D.J.; de Bartolomeis, A. The Prevalence, Odds, Predictors, and Management of Tobacco Use Disorder or Nicotine Dependence among People with Severe Mental Illness: Systematic Review and Meta-Analysis. *Neurosci. Biobehav. Rev.* **2022**, *132*, 289–303. [CrossRef]
6. Cerullo, M.A.; Strakowski, S.M. The Prevalence and Significance of Substance Use Disorders in Bipolar Type I and II Disorder. *Subst. Abus. Treat. Prev. Policy* **2007**, *2*, 1–9. [CrossRef]
7. Grant, B.F.; Stinson, F.S.; Hasin, D.S.; Dawson, D.A.; Chou, S.P.; Ruan, W.J.; Huang, B. Prevalence, Correlates, and Comorbidity of Bipolar I Disorder and Axis I and II Disorders: Results from the National Epidemiologic Survey on Alcohol and Related Conditions. *J. Clin. Psychiatry* **2005**, *66*, 1205–1215. [CrossRef]
8. Hunt, G.E.; Malhi, G.S.; Cleary, M.; Lai, H.M.X.; Sitharthan, T. Prevalence of Comorbid Bipolar and Substance Use Disorders in Clinical Settings, 1990–2015: Systematic Review and Meta-Analysis. *J. Affect. Disord.* **2016**, *206*, 331–349. [CrossRef]
9. Lagerberg, T.V.; Icick, R.; Aminoff, S.R.; Nerhus, M.; Barrett, E.A.; Bjella, T.D.; Olsen, S.H.; Høegh, M.C.; Melle, I. Substance Misuse Trajectories and Risk of Relapse in the Early Course of Bipolar Disorder. *Front. Psychiatry* **2021**, *12*, 656962. [CrossRef]
10. McIntyre, R.S.; Nguyen, H.T.; Soczynska, J.K.; Lourenco, M.T.C.; Woldeyohannes, H.O.; Konarski, J.Z. Medical and Substance-Related Comorbidity in Bipolar Disorder: Translational Research and Treatment Opportunities. *Dialog. Clin. Neurosci.* **2022**, *10*, 203–213. [CrossRef]
11. Xu, N.; Huggon, B.; Saunders, K.E.A. Cognitive Impairment in Patients with Bipolar Disorder: Impact of Pharmacological Treatment. *CNS Drugs* **2020**, *34*, 29–46. [CrossRef] [PubMed]
12. Dalton, E.J.; Cate-Carter, T.D.; Mundo, E.; Parikh, S.V.; Kennedy, J.L. Suicide Risk in Bipolar Patients: The Role of Co-Morbid Substance Use Disorders. *Bipolar Disord.* **2003**, *5*, 58–61. [CrossRef]
13. Grunebaum, M.F.; Galfalvy, H.C.; Nichols, C.M.; Caldeira, N.A.; Sher, L.; Dervic, K.; Burke, A.K.; Mann, J.J.; Oquendo, M.A. Aggression and Substance Abuse in Bipolar Disorder. *Bipolar Disord.* **2006**, *8*, 496–502. [CrossRef] [PubMed]

14. Hjorthøj, C.; Østergaard, M.L.D.; Benros, M.E.; Toftdahl, N.G.; Erlangsen, A.; Andersen, J.T.; Nordentoft, M. Association between Alcohol and Substance Use Disorders and All-Cause and Cause-Specific Mortality in Schizophrenia, Bipolar Disorder, and Unipolar Depression: A Nationwide, Prospective, Register-Based Study. *Lancet Psychiatry* **2015**, *2*, 801–808. [CrossRef]
15. Mazza, M.; Mandelli, L.; di Nicola, M.; Harnic, D.; Catalano, V.; Tedeschi, D.; Martinotti, G.; Colombo, R.; Bria, P.; Serretti, A.; et al. Clinical Features, Response to Treatment and Functional Outcome of Bipolar Disorder Patients with and without Co-Occurring Substance Use Disorder: 1-Year Follow-Up. *J. Affect. Disord.* **2009**, *115*, 27–35. [CrossRef] [PubMed]
16. Swartz, M.S.; Wagner, H.R.; Swanson, J.W.; Stroup, T.S.; McEvoy, J.P.; Reimherr, F.; Miller, D.D.; McGee, M.; Khan, A.; Canive, J.M.; et al. The Effectiveness of Antipsychotic Medications in Patients Who Use or Avoid Illicit Substances: Results from the CATIE Study. *Schizophr. Res.* **2008**, *100*, 39–52. [CrossRef] [PubMed]
17. Grant, B.F.; Goldstein, R.B.; Saha, T.D.; Patricia Chou, S.; Jung, J.; Zhang, H.; Pickering, R.P.; June Ruan, W.; Smith, S.M.; Huang, B.; et al. Epidemiology of DSM-5 Alcohol Use Disorder: Results From the National Epidemiologic Survey on Alcohol and Related Conditions III. *JAMA Psychiatry* **2015**, *72*, 757–766. [CrossRef]
18. Blanco, C.; Flórez-Salamanca, L.; Secades-Villa, R.; Wang, S.; Hasin, D.S. Predictors of Initiation of Nicotine, Alcohol, Cannabis, and Cocaine Use: Results of the National Epidemiologic Survey on Alcohol and Related Conditions (NESARC). *Am. J. Addict.* **2018**, *27*, 477–484. [CrossRef]
19. John, W.S.; Zhu, H.; Mannelli, P.; Schwartz, R.P.; Subramaniam, G.A.; Wu, L.T. Prevalence, Patterns, and Correlates of Multiple Substance Use Disorders among Adult Primary Care Patients. *Drug Alcohol Depend.* **2018**, *187*, 79–87. [CrossRef]
20. Cassidy, F.; Ahearn, E.P.; Carroll, B.J. Substance Abuse in Bipolar Disorder. *Bipolar Disord.* **2001**, *3*, 181–188. [CrossRef]
21. Strakowski, S.M.; DelBello, M.P.; Fleck, D.E.; Adler, C.M.; Anthenelli, R.M.; Keck, P.E.; Arnold, L.M.; Amicone, J. Effects of Co-Occurring Alcohol Abuse on the Course of Bipolar Disorder Following a First Hospitalization for Mania. *Arch. Gen. Psychiatry* **2005**, *62*, 851–858. [CrossRef] [PubMed]
22. Strakowski, S.M.; DelBello, M.P.; Fleck, D.E.; Adler, C.M.; Anthenelli, R.M.; Keck, P.E.; Arnold, L.M.; Amicone, J. Effects of Co-Occurring Cannabis Use Disorders on the Course of Bipolar Disorder after a First Hospitalization for Mania. *Arch. Gen. Psychiatry* **2007**, *64*, 57–64. [CrossRef] [PubMed]
23. Bzdok, D.; Meyer-Lindenberg, A. Machine Learning for Precision Psychiatry: Opportunities and Challenges. *Biol. Psychiatry Cogn. Neurosci. Neuroimag.* **2018**, *3*, 223–230. [CrossRef] [PubMed]
24. Radua, J.; Carvalho, A.F. Route Map for Machine Learning in Psychiatry: Absence of Bias, Reproducibility, and Utility. *Eur. Neuropsychopharmacol.* **2021**, *50*, 115–117. [CrossRef]
25. Hasan, M.M.; Young, G.J.; Patel, M.R.; Modestino, A.S.; Sanchez, L.D.; Noor-E-Alam, M. A Machine Learning Framework to Predict the Risk of Opioid Use Disorder. *Mach. Learn. Appl.* **2021**, *6*, 100144. [CrossRef]
26. Vieta, E. Terciarismo En Psiquiatría: El Programa de Trastornos Bipolares Del Clínic de Barcelona. *J. Psychiatry Ment. Health* **2011**, *4*, 1–4. [CrossRef]
27. Goodwin, G.M.; Haddad, P.M.; Ferrier, I.N.; Aronson, J.K.; Barnes, T.; Cipriani, A.; Coghill, D.R.; Fazel, S.; Geddes, J.R.; Grunze, H.; et al. Evidence-Based Guidelines for Treating Bipolar Disorder: Revised Third Edition Recommendations from the British Association for Psychopharmacology. *J. Psychopharmacol.* **2016**, *30*, 495–553. [CrossRef]
28. Verdolini, N.; Hidalgo-Mazzei, D.; del Matto, L.; Muscas, M.; Pacchiarotti, I.; Murru, A.; Samalin, L.; Aedo, A.; Tohen, M.; Grunze, H.; et al. Long-Term Treatment of Bipolar Disorder Type I: A Systematic and Critical Review of Clinical Guidelines with Derived Practice Algorithms. *Bipolar Disord.* **2020**, *23*, 324–340. [CrossRef]
29. APA. *Diagnostic and Statistical Manual of Mental Disorders*, 4th ed.; American Psychiatric Association: Arlington, VA, USA, 1994.
30. APA. *Diagnostic and Statistical Manual of Mental Disorders*, 4th ed.; Text Rev.; American Psychiatric Association: Arlington, VA, USA, 2000.
31. APA. *Diagnostic and Statistical Manual of Mental Disorders: DSM-5*; American Psychiatric Association (APA): Arlington, VA, USA, 2013; ISBN 089042554X.
32. First, M.B.; Williams, J.B.; Karg, R.S.; Spitzer, R.L. *Structured Clinical Interview for DSM-5—Research Version (SCID-5 for DSM-5, Research Version SCID-5-RV)*; American Psychiatric Association: Arlington, VA, USA, 2017; pp. 1–94.
33. Colom, F.; Vieta, E.; Daban, C.; Pacchiarotti, I.; Sanchez-Moreno, J. Clinical and Therapeutic Implications of Predominant Polarity in Bipolar Disorder. *J. Affect. Disord.* **2006**, *93*, 13–17. [CrossRef]
34. R Foundation for Statistical Computing; R Core Team. *R: A Language and Environment for Statistical Computing*; R Core Team: Vienna, Austria, 2021.
35. Waring, E.; Quinn, M.; McNamara, A.; de la Rubia, E.A.; Zhu, H.; Lowndes, J.; Ellis, S.; McLeod, H.; Wickham, H.; Müller, K.; et al. Skimr: Compact and Flexible Summaries of Data, R Package, Version 1.0.7. 2019. Available online: https://CRAN.R-project.org/package=skimr (accessed on 8 June 2022).
36. Wright MN, Z.A. Ranger: A Fast Implementation of Random Forests for High Dimensional Data in C++ and R. *J. Stat. Softw.* **2017**, *77*, 1–17. [CrossRef]
37. Breiman, L. Random Forests. *Mach. Learn.* **2001**, *45*, 5–32. [CrossRef]
38. Liaw, A.; Wiener, M. Classification and Regression by RandomForest. *R News* **2002**, *2*, 18–22.
39. Kuhn, M. Caret: Classification and Regression Training, R Package Version 6.0-71. 2016. Available online: https://CRAN.R-project.org/package=caret (accessed on 8 June 2022).
40. Lunardon, N.; Menardi, G.; Torelli, N. ROSE: A Package for Binary Imbalanced Learning. *R J.* **2014**, *6*, 82–92.

41. Baethge, C.; Baldessarini, R.J.; Khalsa, H.M.K.; Hennen, J.; Salvatore, P.; Tohen, M. Substance Abuse in First-Episode Bipolar I Disorder: Indications for Early Intervention. *Am. J. Psychiatry* **2005**, *162*, 1008–1010. [CrossRef]
42. Minato Nakazawa, M. Package "fmsb" Title Functions for Medical Statistics Book with Some Demographic Data Depends R (>= 2.2.0). 2022. Available online: https://cran.r-project.org/web/packages/fmsb/fmsb.pdf (accessed on 8 June 2022).
43. Fico, G.; Anmella, G.; Sagué-Villavella, M.; Gomez-Ramiro, M.; Hidalgo-Mazzei, D.; Vieta, E.; Murru, A. Undetermined Predominant Polarity in a Cohort of Bipolar Disorder Patients: Prevalent, Severe, and Overlooked. *J. Affect. Disord.* **2022**, *303*, 223–229. [CrossRef]
44. Daban, C.; Colom, F.; Sanchez-Moreno, J.; García-Amador, M.; Vieta, E. Clinical Correlates of First-Episode Polarity in Bipolar Disorder. *Compr. Psychiatry* **2006**, *47*, 433–437. [CrossRef]
45. Bezerra-Filho, S.; Galvao-de Almeida, A.; Studart, P.; Rocha, M.; Lopes, F.L.; Miranda-Scippa, A. Personality Disorders in Euthymic Bipolar Patients: A Systematic Review. *Rev. Bras. Psiquiatr.* **2015**, *37*, 162–167. [CrossRef]
46. Verdolini, N.; Perugi, G.; Samalin, L.; Murru, A.; Angst, J.; Azorin, J.-M.; Bowden, C.L.; Mosolov, S.; Young, A.H.; Barbuti, M.; et al. Aggressiveness in Depression: A Neglected Symptom Possibly Associated with Bipolarity and Mixed Features. *Acta Psychiatr. Scand.* **2017**, *136*, 362–372. [CrossRef]
47. Altamura, A.C.; Buoli, M.; Caldiroli, A.; Caron, L.; Cumerlato Melter, C.; Dobrea, C.; Cigliobianco, M.; Zanelli Quarantini, F. Misdiagnosis, Duration of Untreated Illness (DUI) and Outcome in Bipolar Patients with Psychotic Symptoms: A Naturalistic Study. *J. Affect. Disord.* **2015**, *182*, 70–75. [CrossRef]
48. Salvatore, P.; Baldessarini, R.J.; Khalsa, H.M.K.; Vázquez, G.; Perez, J.; Faedda, G.L.; Amore, M.; Maggini, C.; Tohen, M. Antecedents of Manic versus Other First-Psychotic Episodes in 263 Bipolar-I Disorder Patients. *Acta. Psychiatr. Scand.* **2014**, *129*, 275. [CrossRef]
49. Uher, R.; Pallaskorpi, S.; Suominen, K.; Mantere, O.; Pavlova, B.; Isometsä, E. Clinical Course Predicts Long-Term Outcomes in Bipolar Disorder. *Psychol. Med.* **2019**, *49*, 1109–1117. [CrossRef] [PubMed]
50. Najt, P.; Perez, J.; Sanches, M.; Peluso, M.A.M.; Glahn, D.; Soares, J.C. Impulsivity and Bipolar Disorder. *Eur. Neuropsychopharmacol.* **2007**, *17*, 313–320. [CrossRef] [PubMed]
51. Dervic, K.; Garcia-Amador, M.; Sudol, K.; Freed, P.; Brent, D.A.; Mann, J.J.; Harkavy-Friedman, J.M.; Oquendo, M.A. Bipolar I and II versus Unipolar Depression: Clinical Differences and Impulsivity/Aggression Traits. *Eur. Psychiatry* **2015**, *30*, 106–113. [CrossRef]
52. Swann, A.C.; Dougherty, D.M.; Pazzaglia, P.J.; Pham, M.; Moeller, F.G. Impulsivity: A Link between Bipolar Disorder and Substance Abuse. *Bipolar Disord.* **2004**, *6*, 204–212. [CrossRef] [PubMed]
53. Zimmerman, M.; Morgan, T.A. The Relationship between Borderline Personality Disorder and Bipolar Disorder. *Dialogues Clin. Neurosci.* **2013**, *15*, 155. [CrossRef] [PubMed]
54. Witt, S.H.; Streit, F.; Jungkunz, M.; Frank, J.; Awasthi, S.; Reinbold, C.S.; Treutlein, J.; Degenhardt, F.; Forstner, A.J.; Heilmann-Heimbach, S.; et al. Genome-Wide Association Study of Borderline Personality Disorder Reveals Genetic Overlap with Bipolar Disorder, Major Depression and Schizophrenia. *Transl. Psychiatry* **2017**, *7*, e1155. [CrossRef] [PubMed]
55. Ruggero, C.J.; Zimmerman, M.; Chelminski, I.; Young, D. Borderline Personality Disorder and the Misdiagnosis of Bipolar Disorder. *J. Psychiatr. Res.* **2010**, *44*, 405–408. [CrossRef]
56. Post, R.M.; Leverich, G.S.; McElroy, S.L.; Kupka, R.; Suppes, T.; Altshuler, L.L.; Nolen, W.A.; Frye, M.A.; Keck, P.E.; Grunze, H.; et al. Are Personality Disorders in Bipolar Patients More Frequent in the US than Europe? *Eur. Neuropsychopharmacol.* **2022**, *58*, 47–54. [CrossRef]
57. Hidalgo-Mazzei, D.; Walsh, E.; Rosenstein, L.; Zimmerman, M. Comorbid Bipolar Disorder and Borderline Personality Disorder and Substance Use Disorder. *J. Nerv. Ment. Dis.* **2015**, *203*, 54–57. [CrossRef]
58. Bodkyn, C.N.; Holroyd, C.B. Neural Mechanisms of Affective Instability and Cognitive Control in Substance Use. *Int. J. Psychophysiol.* **2019**, *146*, 1–19. [CrossRef]
59. Heinz, A.J.; Wu, J.; Witkiewitz, K.; Epstein, D.H.; Preston, K.L. Marriage and Relationship Closeness as Predictors of Cocaine and Heroin Use. *Addict. Behav.* **2009**, *34*, 258. [CrossRef] [PubMed]
60. Sletved, K.S.O.; Ziersen, S.C.; Andersen, P.K.; Vinberg, M.; Kessing, L.V. Socio-Economic Functioning in Patients with Bipolar Disorder and Their Unaffected Siblings—Results from a Nation-Wide Population-Based Longitudinal Study. *Psychol. Med.* **2021**, *2021*, 1–8. [CrossRef] [PubMed]
61. Verdolini, N.; Amoretti, S.; Mezquida, G.; Cuesta, M.J.; Pina-Camacho, L.; García-Rizo, C.; Lobo, A.; González-Pinto, A.; Merchán-Naranjo, J.; Corripio, I.; et al. The Effect of Family Environment and Psychiatric Family History on Psychosocial Functioning in First-Episode Psychosis at Baseline and after 2 Years. *Eur. Neuropsychopharmacol.* **2021**, *49*, 54–68. [CrossRef]
62. Wiström, E.D.; O'Connell, K.S.; Karadag, N.; Bahrami, S.; Hindley, G.F.L.; Lin, A.; Cheng, W.; Steen, N.E.; Shadrin, A.; Frei, O.; et al. Genome-Wide Analysis Reveals Genetic Overlap between Alcohol Use Behaviours, Schizophrenia and Bipolar Disorder and Identifies Novel Shared Risk Loci. *Addiction* **2022**, *117*, 600–610. [CrossRef] [PubMed]
63. Janiri, D.; di Nicola, M.; Martinotti, G.; Janiri, L. Who's the Leader, Mania or Depression? Predominant Polarity and Alcohol/Polysubstance Use in Bipolar Disorders. *Curr. Neuropharmacol.* **2017**, *15*, 409–416. [CrossRef] [PubMed]
64. Lagerberg, T.V.; Aminoff, S.R.; Aas, M.; Bjella, T.; Henry, C.; Leboyer, M.; Pedersen, G.; Bellivier, F.; Icick, R.; Andreassen, O.A.; et al. Alcohol Use Disorders Are Associated with Increased Affective Lability in Bipolar Disorder. *J. Affect. Disord.* **2017**, *208*, 316–324. [CrossRef] [PubMed]

65. Cremaschi, L.; Dell'Osso, B.; Vismara, M.; Dobrea, C.; Buoli, M.; Ketter, T.A.; Altamura, A.C. Onset Polarity in Bipolar Disorder: A Strong Association between First Depressive Episode and Suicide Attempts. *J. Affect. Disord.* **2017**, *209*, 182–187. [CrossRef]
66. Baldessarini, R.J.; Tondo, L.; Visioli, C.; Baldessarini, R.J.; Research Center, M. First-Episode Types in Bipolar Disorder: Predictive Associations with Later Illness. *Acta Psychiatr. Scand.* **2014**, *129*, 383–392. [CrossRef]
67. Pallaskorpi, S.; Suominen, K.; Rosenstrom, T.; Mantere, O.; Arvilommi, P.; Valtonen, H.; Leppamaki, S.; Garcia-Estela, A.; Grande, I.; Colom, F.; et al. Predominant Polarity in Bipolar I and II Disorders: A Five-Year Follow-up Study. *J. Affect. Disord.* **2019**, *246*, 806–813. [CrossRef]
68. Li, D.J.; Lin, C.H.; Wu, H.C. Factors Predicting Re-Hospitalization for Inpatients with Bipolar Mania—A Naturalistic Cohort. *Psychiatry Res.* **2018**, *270*, 749–754. [CrossRef]
69. Fico, G.; Anmella, G.; Pacchiarotti, I.; Verdolini, N.; Sagué-Vilavella, M.; Corponi, F.; Manchia, M.; Vieta, E.; Murru, A. The Biology of Aggressive Behavior in Bipolar Disorder: A Systematic Review. *Neurosci. Biobehav. Rev.* **2020**, *119*, 9–20. [CrossRef] [PubMed]
70. Pacchiarotti, I.; di Marzo, S.; Colom, F.; Sánchez-Moreno, J.; Vieta, E. Bipolar Disorder Preceded by Substance Abuse: A Different Phenotype with Not so Poor Outcome? *World J. Biol. Psychiatry* **2009**, *10*, 209–216. [CrossRef]
71. Stewart, C.; El-mallakh, R.S. Is Bipolar Disorder Overdiagnosed among Patients with Substance Abuse? *Bipolar Disord.* **2007**, *9*, 646–648. [CrossRef] [PubMed]
72. Vieta, E.; Angst, J. Bipolar Disorder Cohort Studies: Crucial, but Underfunded. *Eur. Neuropsychopharmacol.* **2021**, *47*, 31–33. [CrossRef] [PubMed]
73. González-Pinto, A.; Goikolea, J.M.; Zorrilla, I.; Bernardo, M.; Arrojo, M.; Cunill, R.; Castell, X.; Becoña, E.; López, A.; Torrens, M.; et al. Guía de Práctica Clínica Para El Tratamiento Farmacológico y Psicológico de Los Pacientes Adultos Con Trastorno Bipolar y Un Diagnóstico Comórbido de Trastorno Por Uso de Sustancias. *Adicciones* **2021**, *34*, 142–156. [CrossRef] [PubMed]
74. Grunze, H.; Schaefer, M.; Scherk, H.; Born, C.; Preuss, U.W. Comorbid Bipolar and Alcohol Use Disorder—A Therapeutic Challenge. *Front. Psychiatry* **2021**, *12*, 660432. [CrossRef]
75. Hansen, S.S.; Munk-Jørgensen, P.; Guldbæk, B.; Solgård, T.; Lauszus, K.S.; Albrechtsen, N.; Borg, L.; Egander, A.; Faurholdt, K.; Gilberg, A.; et al. Psychoactive Substance Use Diagnoses among Psychiatric In-Patients. *Acta Psychiatr. Scand.* **2000**, *102*, 432–438. [CrossRef]

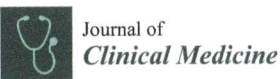

Article

Circadian Characteristics in Patients under Treatment for Substance Use Disorders and Severe Mental Illness (Schizophrenia, Major Depression and Bipolar Disorder)

Ana Belén Serrano-Serrano [1,†], Julia E. Marquez-Arrico [1,†], José Francisco Navarro [2], Antonio Martinez-Nicolas [3,4,5] and Ana Adan [1,6,*]

1. Department of Clinical Psychology and Psychobiology, School of Psychology, University of Barcelona, Passeig de la Vall d'Hebrón 171, 08035 Barcelona, Spain; anik_83@hotmail.com (A.B.S.-S.); jmarquez@ub.edu (J.E.M.-A.)
2. Department of Psychobiology, Campus de Teatinos s/n, School of Psychology, University of Málaga, 29071 Málaga, Spain; navahuma@uma.es
3. Chronobiology Lab, Department of Physiology, Mare Nostrum Campus, IMIB-Arrixaca, IUIE, College of Biology, University of Murcia, 30100 Murcia, Spain; antilas@um.es
4. Human Physiology Area, Faculty of Sport Sciences, University of Murcia, Santiago de la Ribera-San Javier, 30720 Murcia, Spain
5. Ciber Fragilidad y Envejecimiento Saludable (CIBERFES), 28029 Madrid, Spain
6. Institute of Neurosciences, University of Barcelona, 08035 Barcelona, Spain
* Correspondence: aadan@ub.edu; Tel.: +34-933125060
† Equal contribution.

Abstract: Dual disorders (substance use and mental illness comorbidity) are a condition that has been strongly associated with severe symptomatology and clinical complications. The study of circadian characteristics in patients with Severe Mental Illness or Substance Use Disorder (SUD) has shown that such variables are related with mood symptoms and worse recovery. In absence of studies about circadian characteristics in patients with dual disorders we examined a sample of 114 male participants with SUD and comorbid Schizophrenia (SZ+; $n = 38$), Bipolar Disorder (BD+; $n = 36$) and Major Depressive Disorder (MDD+; $n = 40$). The possible differences in the sample of patients according to their psychiatric diagnosis, circadian functioning with recordings of distal skin temperature during 48 h (Thermochron iButton®), circadian typology and sleep-wake schedules were explored. MDD+ patients were more morning-type, while SZ+ and BD+ had an intermediate-type; the morning-type was more frequent among participants under inpatient SUD treatment. SZ+ patients had the highest amount of sleeping hours, lowest arousal and highest drowsiness followed by BD+ and MDD+, respectively. These observed differences suggest that treatment for patients with dual disorders could include chronobiological strategies to help them synchronize patterns with the day-light cycle, since morning-type is associated with better outcomes and recovery.

Keywords: circadian rhythm; dual disorders; chronobiology; substance use disorders; schizophrenia; major depressive disorder; bipolar disorder; distal skin temperature

Citation: Serrano-Serrano, A.B.; Marquez-Arrico, J.E.; Navarro, J.F.; Martinez-Nicolas, A.; Adan, A. Circadian Characteristics in Patients under Treatment for Substance Use Disorders and Severe Mental Illness (Schizophrenia, Major Depression and Bipolar Disorder). *J. Clin. Med.* **2021**, *10*, 4388. https://doi.org/10.3390/jcm10194388

Academic Editor: Nuri B. Farber

Received: 30 July 2021
Accepted: 23 September 2021
Published: 25 September 2021

Publisher's Note: MDPI stays neutral with regard to jurisdictional claims in published maps and institutional affiliations.

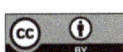

Copyright: © 2021 by the authors. Licensee MDPI, Basel, Switzerland. This article is an open access article distributed under the terms and conditions of the Creative Commons Attribution (CC BY) license (https://creativecommons.org/licenses/by/4.0/).

1. Introduction

As defined by the Word Health Organization in its lexicon of alcohol and drug terms, Dual Disorders are defined as the comorbidity of at least one Substance Use Disorder (SUD) and one Severe Mental Illness (SMI) in the same person [1], being the most frequent psychotic, bipolar and depressive spectrum disorders [2,3]. Given the heterogeneous nature, high prevalence and clinical and functional implications of dual disorders, in recent years interest in its study has increased with the aim of improving both the detection and the therapeutic approach [2–4].

Different studies have shown that addictive behavior has negative effects on circadian rhythmic expression [5,6] which can persist weeks or months after starting substance withdrawal [7,8] and they do not always respond to treatment with medication [9,10] Rhythmic alterations commonly observed in patients with SUD are amplitude reduction and phase delay, which in severe cases can lead to chronodisruption or disappearance of rhythmicity [8]. This affectation is related both to the type of substance used and to the person's metabolism and tolerance (i.e., sensitivity to reward) [11].

The relationship between circadian rhythms and SUD is bidirectional, with evening-type as a precipitating factor for drug use and with drug use generating chronodisruption [8,9]. Moreover, sleep disturbances have been associated with a higher risk of drug use and relapses [12,13], while the magnitude of the phase delay with the degree of dependence [14]. Thus, the exploration of the affectation and recovery of circadian rhythmicity seems to be of special relevance in patients under treatment for SUD [7,15]. In relation to the circadian typology, there seem to be rhythmic differences depending on the chronotype. The evening typology has been identified as a probable risk factor for the development of SUD, while the morning typology has been identified as a protective factor [16,17]. The reinforcing effect of the substances, mediated by clock genes, is greater in evening typology, especially during adolescence and early youth [16,18].

Studies in patients with SUD who have completed a detoxification phase indicated they have a higher prevalence of the morning and intermediate typologies, compared with those who have not initiated treatment, which seems to be a positive characteristic linked to better adherence to treatment [7,15]. Likewise, these patients exhibited a more robust circadian pattern of distal skin temperature (DST) than healthy controls, which is associated with longer abstinence periods and related to some of the treatment strategies used in therapeutic communities (e.g., strong daytime activity and morning habits). Furthermore, poorer sleep quality in patients with SUD is linked to their age and to a greater fragility of the circadian rhythm and chronodisruption [15].

There is a great lack of knowledge about the circadian characteristics in patients with SUD and comorbid SMI. Thus, to date no study has been conducted in dual patients with the diagnoses of schizophrenia (SZ+), bipolar disorder (BD+) and major depressive disorder (MDD+). In this sense, the available evidence on circadian rhythmicity in psychiatric conditions without SUD is limited and heterogeneous, indicating disruptions in prodromal phases in patients without medication [19,20] and in those with remission symptoms or in a sustained withdrawal phase [15,21–23]. All of this evidence suggests that circadian alterations could not only be symptoms but a significant clinical characteristic that affects the appearance and development of SMI [24,25].

Patients with schizophrenia show phase delays, free-running rhythms of 48 h or less than 24 h in the sleep-wake cycle or in melatonin secretion, flat amplitude and fragmentation of the activity-rest pattern [26–29]. All these alterations could be related to poor endogenous control and/or inadequate exposure to external synchronizers [28]. On the other hand, disruptions in the sleep-wake rhythm in schizophrenia have been associated with both clinical and functional prognosis. Deficits in sleep quality have been related with the predominance of positive symptoms [28,30,31] and a lower amplitude and inter-daily stability in the activity-rest rhythm, with poorer neurocognitive performance [27]. Some authors have observed an evening typology predominance in these patients compared to healthy controls [32,33], while in other work no differences have been appreciated [34]. None of these studies found a relationship between circadian typology and the age of the patient, as observed in healthy control subjects. Overall, no previous work has evaluated the circadian rhythm of DST in patients with schizophrenia.

Regarding patients with bipolar disorder, the findings indicate a reduced amplitude activity-rest rhythm, with phase delays (for example, melatonin secretion), greater rhythm fragmentation and more prevalent evening-type [35,36]. Furthermore, although depressive and maniac mood episodes change the rest and activity patterns, circadian alterations persist in euthymic phases [22], which seems to be relevant for the differential diagnosis and for non-psychiatric groups at risk of bipolar disorder [37,38].

Stabilized bipolar patients do not differ in nocturnal activation but they do show less intradaily variability compared to control participants, which may be due to depressive symptoms dependent on variable mood [23,39]. Two systematic reviews that examined activation and energy patterns found that both the euthymic and depressed bipolar groups differ from the controls by a lower mean activity mediated by mood, also concluding that it may be a consequence of bipolar disorder itself [21,40]. It is remarkable that the results that point out a delayed circadian phase in these patients are associated with a younger age, a shorter duration of bipolar disorder and more frequent depressive episodes [41], while those patients who show an advanced phase presented manic episodes and more suicide attempts [42].

Finally, in relation to circadian characteristics in MDD+ patients, only one published study [15] compared these dual patients with SUD ones and explored the possible influence of outpatient vs. residential treatment in therapeutic community. Such work described that the SUD group in therapeutic community presented a better adjustment to the light-dark cycle and a better DST pattern (greater amplitude, relative amplitude and percentage of rhythm and lower minimum temperature average) compared with MDD+ and with patients under outpatient treatment. Furthermore, the therapeutic community patients had the highest prevalence of morning-type regardless of their psychiatric diagnosis. These observations contrast with studies that have described an association of the evening typology with SUD [6,14] and with depression [43,44], although in none of these studies the participants were under residential treatment.

Even though the circadian rhythmic alteration or even its chronodisruption are not precipitating factors for mental disorders, they are related to a greater clinical symptomatology, more difficulties for remission, worse clinical prognosis, lesser healthy habits and worse quality of life [6,45]. All of this can be applicable to both SUD and the three comorbid diagnoses (SZ+, BD+ and MDD+) that have focused our attention on this study.

Therefore, the main goal of this work is to explore the possible differences in circadian rhythmicity in a sample of under treatment patients with SUD taking into account their comorbid SMI. Additionally, we aim to elucidate the possible relationship among circadian rhythmicity with epidemiological and clinical characteristics. This research could provide data of interest and applicability at the therapeutic level, especially when it comes to improve treatment adherence and recovery of dual patients with different SMI.

2. Materials and Methods

2.1. Study Design and Participants

The present study has a cross-sectional multicenter design, with a sample of 114 male patients with a diagnosis of dual disorder undergoing treatment for SUD (outpatient or residential) in different public and private specialized services located in the province of Barcelona. All patients with SUD were divided into three groups according to the comorbid psychiatric diagnosis: SZ+ ($n = 38$), BD+ ($n = 36$) and MDD+ ($n = 40$).

The inclusion criteria for the study were: (a) men between 20 and 50 years of age; (b) diagnosis of SUD (dependence) in initial remission phase according to Diagnostic and Statistical Manual of Mental Disorders (DSM-5) criteria [46] (c) comorbid psychiatric diagnosis of Schizophrenia, Bipolar Disorder or Major Depressive Disorder, not induced by substances or due to medical condition and (d) a minimum abstinence period of three months up to one year. The consideration of including only men patients in our sample is based on the higher prevalence of SUD in this gender and due to significant greater proportion of men in treatment facilities [2]. Moreover, only males were included to avoid possible biases in the circadian characteristics generated by the differential consumption patterns observed in men vs. women [2]. On the other hand, the exclusion criteria were: (a) patients with unstable or uncontrolled psychiatric symptoms or (b) inability (intellectual, cognitive, developmental or physical) to complete the assessment. Disorders related to caffeine and nicotine consumption were not considered as SUD, although data related to the consumption of both substances were recorded.

For the comparison of temperature data, a group of 40 male healthy control (HC) volunteers (mean age 36.50 yrs.; SD = 8.83; age range 21–51 yrs. old) recruited and assessed at the University of Murcia was also included. Regarding these participants 62.5% were married/with a stable partner, 25% were single and 12.5% were separated/divorced; the majority of them were active (working 88%), and very few were unemployed (10%) or with a disability pension (2%). None of the participants in the HC group had a medical or psychiatric diagnosis, nor any past or present SUD, and they were not under any kind of pharmacological treatment.

This study was approved by the Ethics Committee of the University of Barcelona (registration number: IRB00003099) and complied with the ethical principles of the Declaration of Helsinki. Participation in the study was voluntary and the patients did not receive any compensation except for individualized verbal feedback of their results.

2.2. Sociodemographic and Clinical Assessment Instruments

Sociodemographic and clinical data were collected through the Structured Clinical Interview for Axis I Disorders of the DSM-IV (SCID-I) [47], together with a structured interview specifically designed for our study. All collected data were corroborated by the psychologist/psychiatrist in charge of patient's treatment, as well as checked in the clinical records of each treatment center.

The Positive and Negative Syndrome Scale (PANSS) [48] in its Spanish version was used [49] for the assessment of psychiatric symptoms in the SZ+ group. The PANSS scale yields scores in four areas related to different symptomatology: positive syndrome, negative syndrome, composite scale and general psychopathology. In the BD+ group, we used the Young Mania Rating Scale (YMRS) [50] to measure the severity of maniac symptoms as well as the Hamilton Depression Rating Scale (HDRS) [51]. The YMRS in its Spanish version [52] gives a total score from 0 to 60 understood as it follows: 0–6 euthymic, 7–20 mixed episode and >20 possible maniac episode. On the other hand, the HDRS was used to assess depressive symptoms for the BD+ and MDD+ groups, with its 17-item Spanish version [53] and cut-off points being: 0–7, no current depression; 8–13, low; 14–18, mild; 19–22, severe; and >23, very severe depressive symptoms.

2.3. Circadian Assessment Instruments

To evaluate the circadian typology, the Spanish version of the Composite Morning Scale (CSM) [54] was used, consisting of 13 items and a total score from 0 to 55. Its interpretation considers the following cut-off points: 13–25 as an evening typology, 26–36 as an intermediate typology and 37–55 as a morning typology. The sleep-wake schedules were recorded using the structured interview designed for our study.

DST was recorded using the Thermochron iButton® DS1921H (Maxim Integrated Products, San Jose, CA, USA), previously programmed to take measurements every 2 min for 48 consecutive hours with an accuracy of ±0.125 °C. The sensor, which is attached to a strap similar to that of a wristwatch, was placed on the wrist of the non-dominant hand over the temporal artery [55].

2.4. Statistical Analysis

For the sociodemographic, clinical and SUD data, descriptive statistics were calculated for the three groups of patients (mean, standard deviation, frequencies and percentages) and subsequent contrasts were performed with ANOVA and Chi-square, depending on the data were parametric or non-parametric.

For the analysis of the DST data, the CircadianwareTM software version 7.1.1 [56] was used. The parametric analyses of cosinor (maximum and minimum temperature, mesor, amplitude, acrophase and percentage of variance explained by the cosine wave), and the analysis of the Rayleigh vector and the Fourier analysis with the first 12 harmonics were made to characterize the circadian rhythm of the DST. The circadianity index was calculated as detailed in previous publications [57]. Non-parametric analyses were performed [55,58] to obtain the values of interdaily stability (IS), intradaily variability (IV), relative amplitude (RA), maximum mean temperature in 5 consecutive hours (M5), temperature minimum average in 2 and 10 consecutive hours (L2 and L10).

DST values, both parametric and non-parametric, and sleep schedules (after transformation to the centesimal system) were evaluated using MANCOVA, while IS and CSM scores were analyzed with ANCOVA. In all cases, age was considered as a covariate, the analyses were performed with the diagnostic group as a factor (SZ+, BD+ and MDD+) and they were repeated considering treatment modality (outpatient/residential). Furthermore, in the parametric analyses for the DST the HC group was also incorporated together with the three clinical groups. Correlational analyses were also performed among DST and clinical variables. Subsequently, a linear regression analysis was carried out with significant correlations at the level of $p = 0.01$. The effect size was calculated as an estimate of the risk of committing type I error with the partial square index of Eta (ηp^2), assuming values of 0.01 as low, 0.06 as moderate and 0.14 as high [59]. Bonferroni test was applied in all the post-hoc contrasts. The data of the present study have been analyzed using the Statistical Package for the Social Sciences program (IBM SPSS Statistics 25.0, Armonk, New York, United States). Two-sided statistical significance was established with a predefined type I error of 5% ($p < 0.05$).

3. Results

3.1. Sociodemographic and Clinical Characteristics

The groups showed significant differences (see Table 1) in the sociodemographic variables studied such as age ($p = 0.009$), marital status ($p = 0.011$), number of children ($p = 0.002$), family situation ($p = 0.001$), employment status ($p = 0.001$) and years of study ($p = 0.026$). The mean age of the total sample of patients was 37.72 yrs. old (SD = 7.68), observing a higher mean age in SZ+ with respect to MDD+ ($p = 0.005$). The comparison among the three groups and HC subjects did not show differences for age ($F_{(3,153)} = 3.176$; $p = 0.167$) while they did for marital status ($\chi^2_{(3)} = 39.771$; $p < 0.001$), economic situation ($\chi^2_{(3)} = 125.086$; $p < 0.001$) and years of schooling ($F_{(3,153)} = 8.903$; $p < 0.001$).

Table 1. Sociodemographic data for the three groups of patients. Means, standard deviation, percentages and statistical contrasts (ANOVA and Chi Square test).

Sociodemographic Data	SZ+ (n = 38)	BD+ (n = 37)	MDD+ (n = 39)	Contrasts
Age (years)	35.13 ± 8.20	37.58 ± 8.19	40.41 ± 5.67	$F_{(2,111)} = 4.87$ **
Marital status				$\chi^2_{(3)} = 16.55$ *
Single	86.8%	55.6%	47.5%	
Married/stable partner	2.6%	8.3%	10.0%	
Separated/divorced	10.5%	33.3%	42.5%	
Widower	0%	2.8%	0%	
Family situation				$\chi^2_{(1)} = 11.78$ **
Without children	86.8%	61.1%	50.5%	
With children	13.2%	38.9%	50.0%	
Living arrangements				$\chi^2_{(3)} = 21.88$ ***
Alone	7.9%	16.7%	5.0%	
Sharing	65.8%	61.1%	45.0%	
Therapeutic community	15.8%	22.2%	50.0%	
Supported accommodation	10.5%	0%	0%	
Economic situation				$\chi^2_{(3)} = 26.64$ ***
Working	13.2%	11.1%	12.5%	
Unemployed	21.1%	22.52%	55.0%	
Under sick leave	7.9%	5.6%	20.0%	
Disability pension	57.9%	61.1%	12.5%	
Years of schooling	10.00 ± 2.36	11.54 ± 3.07	10.64 ± 2.57	$F_{(2,111)} = 3.77$ *

SZ+: Substance use disorder with comorbid schizophrenia; BD+: Substance use disorder with comorbid bipolar disorder; MDD+: Substance use disorder with comorbid major depressive disorder; * $p < 0.05$; ** $p < 0.01$; *** $p < 0.001$.

The analysis of the clinical variables (see Table 2) confirmed that a high percentage of patients with MDD+ were under a residential treatment in therapeutic community, in contrast with the SZ+ ($\chi^2_{(1)} = 19.90$; $p = 0.001$) and BD+ groups ($\chi^2_{(1)} = 8.85$; $p = 0.003$) who were receiving an outpatient follow-up. The SMI age of onset was later in the MDD+ group compared with SZ+ ($p = 0.001$) and to BD+ ($p = 0.019$). In contrast, no differences were found among the groups for medical disease comorbidities, family history and years of duration of the SMI, and global functioning (not showed in table). Regarding pharmacological treatment, the SZ+ group took a greater amount of psychotropic daily drugs than the MDD+ group ($p = 0.026$), while the BD+ group was in an intermediate position. In all groups the percentage of smoking patients was >80%, with no differences in the active smoking years (>17 years; not showed in table). The mean score of the Fagerström questionnaire for nicotine dependence was higher in the SZ+ group compared to MDD+ ($p = 0.008$). Instead, the caffeine daily intake did not exhibit differences among the groups (not showed in table). Scores on the PANSS, Hamilton and YMRS clinical scales indicated that all groups were clinically stable, although the MDD+ group (11.23 ± 5.14) had a higher HDRS score than the BD+ group (6.86 ± 5.17) ($F_{(1,74)} = 5.44$; $p = 0.024$).

Table 2. Clinical data for the three groups of patients regarding psychiatric diagnosis and substance use disorders. Means, standard deviation, percentages and statistical contrasts (ANOVA and Chi Square test).

Clinical Data	SZ+ (n = 38)	BD+ (n = 37)	MDD+ (n = 39)	Contrasts
Treament modality				$\chi^2_{(1)} = 20.93$ ***
Outpatient	78.9%	62.2%	28.2%	
Residential	21.1%	37.8%	71.8%	
SMI age of onset (years)	23.53 ± 7.50	26.26 ± 9.75	31.74 ± 8.14	$F_{(2,109)} = 9.37$ ***
Suicide attempts	1.08 ± 1.86	1.38 ± 3.14	0.77 ± 0.98	$F_{(2,111)} = 0.74$
Pharmacological treatment (N/day)	3.35 ± 1.54	3.14 ± 1.82	2.32 ± 1.64	$F_{(2,109)} = 3.98$ *
Typical antipsychotic	26.3%	8.1%	2.6%	$\chi^2_{(1)} = 11.17$ **
Atypical antipsychotic	94.7%	64.9%	12.8%	$\chi^2_{(1)} = 55.55$ ***
Mood stabilizers	36.8%	70.3%	15.4%	$\chi^2_{(1)} = 23.22$ ***
Anxiolytics	42.1%	35.1%	43.6%	$\chi^2_{(1)} = 0.82$
Antidepressants	34.2%	43.2%	71.8%	$\chi^2_{(1)} = 12.44$ **
Anticholinergic	26.3%	2.7%	0%	$\chi^2_{(1)} = 18.36$ ***
Alcohol-aversive-agent	26.3%	21.6%	28.2%	$\chi^2_{(1)} = 0.56$
Other psychotropics	13.2%	13.5%	17.9%	$\chi^2_{(1)} = 0.47$
Chlorpromazine equivalent dose (mg)	406.08 ± 34.73	145.95 ± 35.71	32.44 ± 34.27	$F_{(2,108)} = 30.65$ *
Daily cigarettes per day	21.95 ± 11.54	18.84 ± 8.76	13.23 ± 6.87	$F_{(2,111)} = 8.80$ ***
Fagerström total score	6.11 ± 2.60	5.03 ± 2.75	4.28 ± 2.40	$F_{(2,111)} = 4.82$ **
SUD age of onset (years)	17.24 ± 5.16	20.81 ± 10.10	18.59 ± 7.01	$F_{(2,110)} = 2.04$
Duration of the SUD (years)	17.63 ± 1.42	17.02 ± 1.45	21.82 ± 1.10	$F_{(2,110)} = 3.39$ *
Quantity substances used	3.74 ± 1.44	2.54 ± 1.19	2.95 ± 1.41	$F_{(2,111)} = 7.55$ ***
Type of substance [a]				
Cocaine	94.7%	64.9%	87.2%	$\chi^2_{(1)} = 12.47$ **
Alcohol	76.3%	89.2%	89.7%	$\chi^2_{(1)} = 3.46$
Cannabis	78.9%	48.6%	53.8%	$\chi^2_{(1)} = 8.31$ *
Ectasis	18.4%	10.8%	5.1%	$\chi^2_{(1)} = 3.25$
Hallucinogens	39.5%	16.2%	20.5%	$\chi^2_{(1)} = 6.10$ *
Opioids	28.9%	13.5%	25.6%	$\chi^2_{(1)} = 2.87$
Anxiolytics/hypnotics	28.9%	10.8%	12.8%	$\chi^2_{(1)} = 5.17$
DAST-20 total score	12.68 ± 3.18	12.74 ± 9.47	13.74 ± 3.94	$F_{(2,111)} = 0.30$
Severity of addiction				$\chi^2_{(3)} = 17.58$ *
Low	2.6%	10.8%	2.6%	
Mild	13.2%	16.2%	12.8%	
High	42.1%	13.5%	35.9%	
Severe	7.9%	10.8%	28.2%	
Months of abstinence	10.88 ± 1.15	8.44 ± 1.18	7.33 ± 1.14	$F_{(2,111)} = 2.48$
Quantity of relapses	1.05 ± 1.57	0.75 ± 1.30	0.87 ± 1.23	$F_{(2,111)} = 0.44$

SZ+: Substance use disorder with comorbid schizophrenia; BD+: Substance use disorder with comorbid bipolar disorder; MDD+: Substance use disorder with comorbid major depressive disorder; SMI: Severe mental illness; N: Number; SUD: Substance use disorder; DAST-20: Drug abuse screening test. [a] Percentages will not equal 100 as each patient may have taken more than one substance. * $p < 0.05$; ** $p < 0.01$; *** $p < 0.001$.

The results in the clinical variables related to SUD did not indicate any differences among groups for the SUD age of onset, but they did in its duration, being higher in MDD+ patients compared to SZ+ ($p = 0.05$). The SZ+ group consumed more amounts of substances compared to BD+ ($p = 0.001$) and MDD+ ($p = 0.037$), although we obtained a majority pattern of polydrug use in the entire sample (>80% in each group; not showed in table), regardless of the SMI diagnosis. The most commonly used substances in all groups were cocaine, alcohol and cannabis. The DAST-20 revealed a higher proportion of MDD+ patients with high and severe dependence compared to BD+ ($\chi^2_{(3)} = 7.83; p = 0.035$). The groups did not contribute differences in the abstinence period, or in the number of relapses prior to the start of treatment. The presence of family, work and legal related problems did not exhibit differences either (not showed in table).

3.2. Circadian Typology and Sleep-Wake Data

The ANCOVA analysis (see Table 3) showed a mean score for the CSM questionnaire in the morningness range for the MDD+ group ($p = 0.026$; $\eta p^2 = 0.064$), in contrast with for patients with SZ+ ($p = 0.008$) and BD+ ($p = 0.002$), who were placed in the intermediate range. The percentage of patients in the morning typology was also higher in the MDD+ group compared to the SZ+ ($\chi^2_{(2)} = 9.60; p = 0.008$) and BD+ ($\chi^2_{(2)} = 7.81; p = 0.02$) groups. In both SZ+ and BD+ the predominating typology was the intermediate one. Regarding sleep-wake schedules, a greater total sleep duration was observed for SZ+ patients compared to MDD+ ($p = 0.001$); without differences from the BD+ group, which showed an intermediate position. Furthermore, the MDD+ group got up earlier than SZ+ ($p = 0.009$) and BD+ ($p = 0.015$).

Table 3. Circadian typology and sleep-wake data for the three groups of patients. Means, percentages and differences according to the type of treatment.

	SZ+ (n = 38)	BP+ (n = 37)	MDD+ (n = 39)	Contrasts	Outpatient (n = 63)	Residential (n = 51)	Contrasts
CSM total	34.04 ± 1.11	33.56 ± 1.10	37.55 ± 1.10	$F_{(2,111)} = 3.77$ * $\chi^2_{(2)} = 12.66$ *	34.14 ± 0.86	36.29 ± 0.97	$F_{(2,112)} = 2.70$ $\chi^2_{(2)} = 10.96$ **
Circadian typology							
Morning-type	28.9%	32.4%	64.1%		29.7%	58%	
Intermediate-type	57.9%	48.6%	28.02%		57.8%	28%	
Evening-type	13.12%	18.9%	7.7%		12.5%	14%	
Total sleeping (h)	9.44 ± 0.25	8.75 ± 0.24	8.03 ± 0.24	$F_{(2,112)} = 7.84$ ***	9.03 ± 0.18	7.09 ± 0.20	$F_{(2,112)} = 24.89$ ***
Bedtime	23:07 ± 0.20	23:26 ± 0.20	23:05 ± 0.20	$F_{(2,112)} = 0.93$	23:29 ± 0.15	22:51 ± 0.17	$F_{(2,112)} = 7.72$ **
Getting up time	08:01 ± 0.22	07:93 ± 0.22	07:02 ± 0.22	$F_{(2,112)} = 5.78$ **	08:36 ± 0.15	06:73 ± 0.17	$F_{(2,112)} = 50.97$ ***
Nap (yes)	34.2%	24.3%	20.5%	$\chi^2_{(1)} = 1.97$	39.1%	10.0%	$\chi^2_{(1)} = 12.22$ ***
Nap total time (min)	24.93 ± 5.55	13.77 ± 5.03	10.03 ± 5.41	$F_{(2,112)} = 1.90$	25.21 ± 3.96.03	04.22 ± 4.48	$F_{(2,112)} = 12.99$ ***

SZ+: Substance use disorder with comorbid schizophrenia; BD+: Substance use disorder with comorbid bipolar disorder; MDD+: Substance use disorder with comorbid major depressive disorder; * $p < 0.05$; ** $p < 0.01$; *** $p < 0.001$.

On the other hand, the mean score on the CSM scale according to the type of treatment (outpatient vs. residential) provided a similar score for both modalities. However, the percentage of morning typology patients was higher in the residential treatment modality than in the outpatient one ($p = 0.004$). Being under an outpatient treatment program was associated to the intermediate circadian typology. The proportion of people with evening chronotype was also the minority for both treatment modalities. The influence of the type of treatment on sleep-wake schedules showed that outpatients slept for more hours ($p = 0.001$), went to bed and got up later ($p = 0.006$ and $p = 0.001$, respectively). Furthermore, the percentage of patients who took naps and its duration was also higher in the outpatient treatment group ($p = 0.001$).

3.3. Distal Skin Temperature

Table 4 shows the results of the DST analyses for the three groups of patients and the data for the HC group. The MANCOVA carried out, both for the parametric and non-parametric indexes, showed significant differences depending on the comorbid SMI diagnoses (see Figure 1). The SZ+ group presented the highest minimum and mesor compared to the MDD+ group ($p = 0.021$), without differences from the BD+ group, which was in an intermediate position. We also found a higher M5 value for BD+ patients compared with MDD+ ($p = 0.025$).

Table 4. Distal skin temperature for the three groups of patients and the healthy controls group. Means, standard error and MANCOVA analyses.

	SZ+ (n = 38)	BP+ (n = 37)	MDD+ (n = 39)	MANCOVA $F_{(2,111)}$	ηp^2	HC Group (n = 40)	MANCOVA $F_{(3,150)}$	ηp^2
Maximum	36.08 ± 0.09	36.12 ± 0.90	35.98 ± 0.09	0.64	0.01	36.17 ± 0.09	0.98	0.02
Minimum	31.65 ± 0.28	31.16 ± 0.28	30.58 ± 0.28	3.78 *	0.07	30.40 ± 0.21	5.15 **	0.10
Mesor	34.01 ± 0.15	33.83 ± 0.15	33.45 ± 0.15	3.23 *	0.06	33.60 ± 0.09	3.23 *	0.06
Amplitude	0.82 ± 0.13	1.00 ± 0.13	1.10 ± 0.13	1.11	0.02	0.88 ± 0.06	1.08	0.02
Acrophase [a]	01:30 ± 0.74	00:36 ± 0.74	23:59 ± 0.74	0.97	0.02	02:19 ± 0.43	0.42	0.01
Rayleigh	0.88 ± 0.03	0.88 ± 0.03	0.94 ± 0.03	0.88	0.02	0.80 ± 0.02	2.71 *	0.05
P1	0.56 ± 0.19	0.95 ± 0.19	0.65 ± 0.19	1.15	0.02	0.48 ± 0.07	1.53	0.03
P12	1.01 ± 0.31	1.59 ± 0.32	1.88 ± 0.31	1.83	0.03	0.81 ± 0.11	3.18 *	0.06
CI	0.39 ± 0.03	0.43 ± 0.03	0.34 ± 0.03	1.50	0.03	0.55 ± 0.02	7.47 ***	0.14
IS	0.66 ± 0.02	0.72 ± 0.02	0.72 ± 0.02	1.14	0.02	0.44 ± 0.02	26.45	0.00
IV	0.02 ± 0.00	0.02 ± 0.00	0.02 ± 0.00	0.83	0.02	0.19 ± 0.01	107.56 ***	0.70
RA_10	0.25 ± 0.03	0.32 ± 0.03	0.30 ± 0.03	1.30	0.02	0.26 ± 0.01	1.35	0.03
M5	35.01 ± 0.10	35.12 ± 0.10	34.71 ± 0.10	3.78 *	0.07	34.68 ± 0.07	5.07 **	0.10
TM5 [a]	01:48 ± 0.72	01:12 ± 0.72	02:03 ± 0.72	0.36	0.01	03:20 ± 0.44	1.81	0.04
L10	33.30 ± 0.22	32.96 ± 0.22	32.66 ± 0.22	1.97	0.04	32.93 ± 0.12	1.80	0.04
TL10 [a]	16:50 ± 1.03	18:35 ± 1.04	15:16 ± 1.03	2.55	0.05	15:98 ± 0.94	2.06	0.04

SZ+: Substance use disorder with comorbid schizophrenia; BD+: Substance use disorder with comorbid bipolar disorder; MDD+: Substance use disorder with comorbid major depressive disorder; HC: healthy control group; ηp^2: Partial square index of eta (effect size); P1: first armonic power; P12: Cumulative power of the twelfth harmonic; CI: Circadianity index; IS: Interdaily stability; IV: Intradaily variability; RA_10: Relative amplitude multiplied by 10; M5: Mean value of the five consecutive hours of maximum temperature values; TM5: M5 time location; L10: Mean value of the 10 consecutive hours of minimum temperature values; TL10: L10 time location. [a] Data expressed in hours and minutes (mean and standard error). * $p < 0.05$; ** $p < 0.01$; *** $p < 0.001$.

The comparison of the DST parameters between the dual groups and the HC group showed a higher minimum value ($p = 0.002$) and mesor ($p = 0.024$) in the SZ+ group, while the Rayleigh vector ($p = 0.036$) and the accumulated potency of the first 12 harmonics ($p = 0.039$), were higher in the MDD+ group. In addition, the CI was found below the value of the HC group and the range of normality for SZ+ ($p = 0.004$) and MDD+ ($p = 0.001$). In the case of IV, the degree of fragmentation was practically null in the three dual groups and significantly different from the HC group ($p = 0.001$, in all cases). Finally, BD+ patients showed a higher M5 value than the HC group ($p = 0.011$), although the value of this parameter in the three groups indicated an adequate night's rest (see Figure 1).

In the additional analyses carried out considering treatment modality as a fixed factor (see Table 5 and Figure 2), the MANCOVA analyses indicated that the dual outpatients presented the highest minimum, mesor and L10 values, and a later acrophase ($p = 0.007$) together with a delay in the central hour of the waking period with respect to those who received residential treatment. The last MANCOVA adding the diagnostic group factor, to determine whether the differences between the type of treatment differed according to the comorbid SMI, did not provide differences in any of the evaluated parameters.

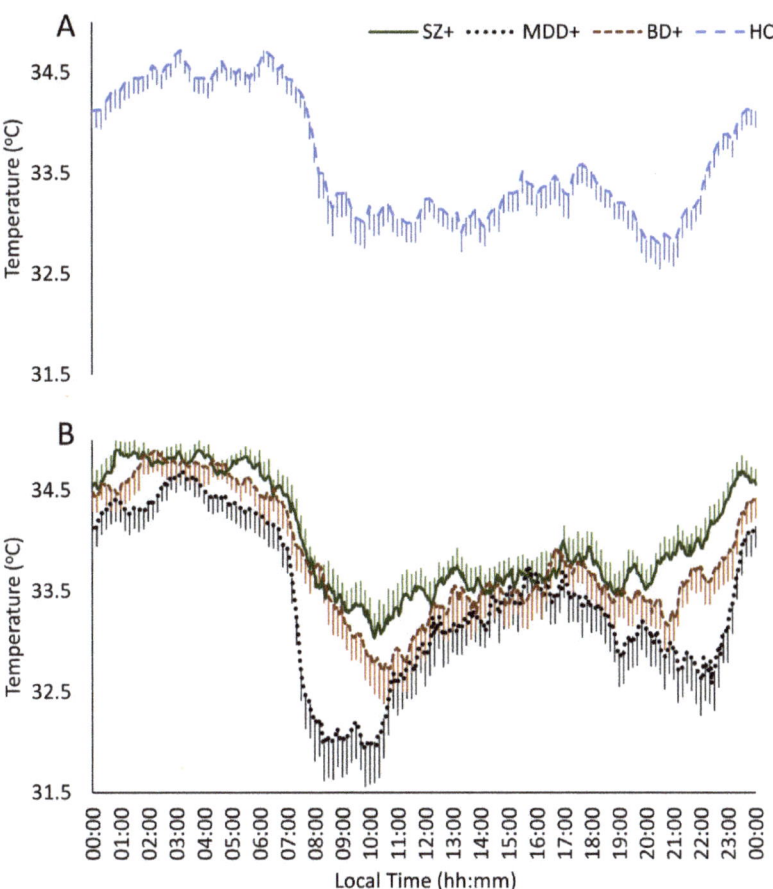

Figure 1. Distal skin temperature mean waveforms for healthy controls (**A**) and dual disorders (**B**). Waveforms data are expressed as mean ± SEM in function of local time (hours:minutes). HC: Healthy Controls (dashed blue line, $n = 40$); SZ+: Substance use disorder with comorbid schizophrenia (dashed red line, $n = 38$), MDD+: Substance use disorder with comorbid major depressive disorder (dotted black line, $n = 40$), BD+: Substance use disorder with comorbid bipolar disorder (continuous green line, $n = 36$).

Finally, the results of the correlational analysis ($p \leq 0.01$) between the DST and the clinical variables showed significant relationships with nicotine dependence. In this sense, the SZ+ group exhibited a negative relationship for the values of mesor and L10, and the Fagerström score ($r = -0.469$; $p = 0.003$ and $r = -0.438$; $p = 0.007$, respectively), that is, the higher the nicotine dependence score the lower values of both were observed. Likewise, in the MDD+ group, a negative correlation was obtained between M5 and the daily amount of cigarettes consumed ($r = -0.475$; $p = 0.004$); thus, in these patients, the higher the consumption of nicotine, the lower the temperature values in the five hours of maximum value.

Table 5. Distal skin temperature for the total sample according to treatment modality. Means, standard error and MANCOVA analyses.

	Treatment Modality		MANCOVA	
	Outpatient (n = 63)	Residential (n = 51)	$F_{(2,112)}$	ηp^2
Maximum	36.10 ± 0.06	36.01 ± 0.07	0.74	0.01
Minimum	31.56 ± 0.21	30.54 ± 0.24	9.63 **	0.08
Mesor	33.95 ± 0.11	33.52 ± 0.13	5.64 *	0.05
Amplitude	0.88 ± 0.10	1.08 ± 0.11	1.66	0.02
Acrophase [a]	01:44 ± 0.55	23:18 ± 0.62	7.59 **	0.07
Rayleigh	0.90 ± 0.02	0.91 ± 0.03	0.05	0.01
P1	0.62 ± 0.14	0.84 ± 0.16	1.03	0.01
P12	1.23 ± 0.24	1.83 ± 0.27	2.66	0.02
CI	0.39 ± 0.02	0.39 ± 0.03	0.00	0.01
IS	0.73 ± 0.02	0.72 ± 0.02	0.23	0.01
IV	0.02 ± 0.00	0.02 ± 0.00	0.60	0.01
RA_10	0.26 ± 0.02	0.32 ± 0.02	2.26	0.02
M5	35.04 ± 0.08	34.83 ± 0.09	2.75	0.02
TM5[a]	01:37 ± 0.55	01:47 ± 0.62	0.04	0.01
L10	33.22 ± 0.16	32.65 ± 0.19	4.88 *	0.04
TL10[a]	18:16 ± 0.78	15:07 ± 0.88	7.01 **	0.07

P1: first armonic power; P12: Cumulative power of the twelfth harmonic; CI: Circadianity index; IS: Interdaily stability; IV: Intradaily variability; RA_10: Relative amplitude multiplied by 10; M5: Mean value of the five consecutive hours of maximum temperature values; TM5: M5 time location; L10: Mean value of the 10 consecutive hours of minimum temperature values; TL10: L10 time location; ηp^2: Partial square index of eta (effect size). [a] Data expressed in hours and minutes (mean and standard error). * $p < 0.05$; ** $p < 0.01$.

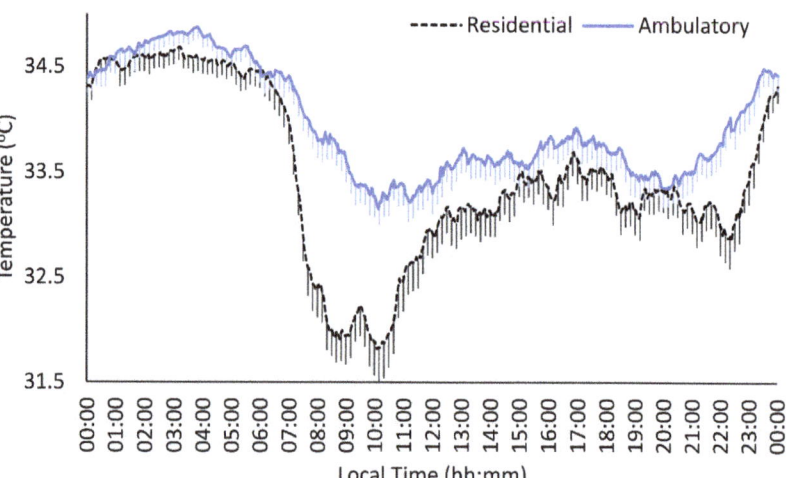

Figure 2. Distal skin temperature mean waveforms for residential treatment (dashed black line, n = 50) and ambulatory treatment (continuous blue line, n = 60). Waveforms data are expressed as mean ± SEM in function of local time (hours:minutes).

4. Discussion

This study aims to analyze differences in circadian rhythmicity in patients under treatment with SUD attending to comorbid SMI, as well as its possible relationship with epidemiological and clinical characteristics.

Regarding sociodemographic and clinical results, the three groups of dual patients showed characteristics in line with previous studies [5,60–62]. Our results indicated an important presence of factors related to a worse clinical symptomatology and prognosis, especially for patients in the SZ+ group, and are consistent with the available literature [63–65]. Moreover, for patients with SZ+ and BD+, the outpatient treatment modality was predominant, while for patients with MDD+ the residential and therapeutic community treatment was more frequent. On the other hand, the mean age of SMI onset was earlier for the SZ+ group, this observation has been associated with a worse clinical, cognitive and functional prognosis [60,66,67]. As in previous studies, our sample presented similarities in psychiatric family history, medical disease comorbidity and previous suicide attempts [68–70]. Regarding nicotine consumption, although the three groups showed a high percentage of smokers and a moderate level of dependence, the SZ+ group exhibited the highest consumption and the MDD+ the lowest one.

Moreover, the longer duration of the SUD in patients with MDD+ may be related to the older age of the group, greater latency from the onset of depression until they seek professional help or may be unsuccessful attempts at previous treatments. According to available publications, in the three groups the most commonly used substances were cocaine, alcohol and cannabis [69,71,72], with an important common pattern of polydrug use in all the groups [4,60,69,72]. While the main substance of abuse may have a specific role in clinical and circadian rhythmic variables, polydrug use as a common pattern makes difficult to address such specific analysis. On the other hand, the severity of addiction was higher in the SZ+ group (followed by MDD+) in association with the consumption of a greater number of substances [73]. All these indicators would confirm the need for continuous, comprehensive treatments that affect relapse prevention [70].

Regarding the circadian typology, and in line with a previous study [15], in the MDD+ group the morning typology was the predominant one while in the SZ+ and BD+ groups the intermediate typology was the most frequent. The highest percentage of people with morning typology was observed in patients receiving residential treatment vs. outpatient modality. This observation is consistent with previous studies [14,15,43] and points out that there could be a possible regulating effect of the circadian rhythm generated by the habits and routines imposed by a residential treatment. The restoration of an adequate circadian rhythm is an element that contributes to the clinical improvement of patients with major depression [44], and according to our results, this also could be extended to those with MDD+, SZ+ and BD+.

On the other hand, in agreement with previous data in patients with a single SMI diagnosis, such as schizophrenia and bipolar disorder [74], the total duration of daily sleep in SZ+ patients were higher than those with MDD+, placing patients with BD+ in an intermediate position. This could be explained by the delay in getting up observed in patients with SZ+, which may be related to the sedative effect of most typical/atypical antipsychotic drugs and anticholinergics they were taking [66]. Likewise, those who received outpatient treatment slept more hours a day, went to bed and got up later, and took more and longer naps. This suggests that sleep-wake rhythm time imbalances are not simply a consequence of clinical symptoms and could be influenced by treatment modality. The morningness tendency can be considered a marker of adherence to treatment and as a protective factor for relapses in both SUD and depressed patients [14,15,75]. Treatments that enhance synchronization with the environmental signals of the light-dark cycle, work on the regularity of schedules and include practice of physical exercise influence circadian recovery [19,25]. Our findings emphasize need to incorporate chronobiological adjustment strategies in dual patients under outpatient treatment modality, especially in the cases of those with SZ+ or BD+.

Regarding the circadian pattern of DST, it indicates less activation and/or greater daytime sleepiness in SZ+ patients and, to a lesser extent, also in BD+ patients. Even though there are no published data on DST in SZ+ patients, our findings are consistent with studies that have evaluated circadian functioning in patients with a diagnosis of schizophrenia only, where a lower amplitude and greater fragmentation of the activity-rest pattern were also observed [26,28,29]. In addition, we found a higher M5 value in BD+ patients compared to MDD+, that, together with a greater stability of the rhythm, points out a better night's rest [76] in BD+ patients. However, in the three groups of our sample this data was found within normality values according to population norms. The inclusion of the HC group widened the differences found in the minimum and mesor values, Rayleigh, P12, IC, IV and M5. The SZ+ group obtained a significantly higher minimum and mesor value that denotes a lower diurnal activation [76] compared to control subjects and with the MDD+ group, without differences from BD+.

It is worth mentioning the differential relationship observed between tobacco consumption and circadian rhythmicity [14] regarding the comorbid SMI. For SZ+ patients nicotine dependence was associated to the quality of wakefulness, while for patients with MDD+ nicotine dependence was linked to the sleep period (M5). Thus, tobacco consumption and its level of dependence could be considered as a modulating factor of circadian rhythmicity, which is also related to the type of SMI diagnosis. Even though this should be deepened in the future, smoking seems to impair the quality of sleep for MDD+ patients. Furthermore, the poorer quality of wakefulness shown by patients with SZ+ is minimized in those who smoke, which could be explained by the palliative effect of nicotine over the side effects of antipsychotic treatment.

On the other hand, we found more stability of the circadian rhythm (Rayleigh vector and the power of the first 12 upper harmonics) in the MDD+ group than in the HC group. A previous study [15] observed that superior stability occurred in patients in therapeutic community (residential treatment) vs. those who were in an outpatient program. Therefore, if we take into account that the majority of patients in the MDD+ group underwent treatment in therapeutic community, our results could be congruent due to the probable influence of the type of treatment on circadian rhythmicity. A result to emphasize is the lower rhythm stability index (IC) for patients with SZ+ compared to the HC group, which has been related to a more immature circadian system [58]. Furthermore, the three groups of patients showed a lower IV compared to the HC group. Furthermore, less fragmentation was also found for both the SUD and in the MDD+ groups, regardless of treatment modality [15]. Despite the absence of previous data about rhythm fragmentation in SZ+ and BD+ patients, the alteration of the IV in both cases suggests that it could be used as a psychopathological marker associated with SMIs, as it has been observed in schizophrenia [26,28] and bipolar disorder [23,39] conditions, regardless of the presence of a comorbid SUD.

Regarding treatment modality, our results suggest a better quality of both sleep and wakefulness and a more robust circadian pattern of DST in dual patients under residential treatment. The patients under outpatient treatment, however, showed less daytime activation (minimum, higher L10 value and mesor) and a more evening pattern (later acrophase) compared to patients in residential facilities. Overall, these observations reveal a low contrast in their day-to-day life [77] in consistency with previous observations made in MDD+ [15] and in depression without SUD [44]. Therefore, it is emphasized that the treatment of dual patients, regardless of their SMI comorbidity, should promote rhythmic organization, physical activity in the open air and stable feeding times to maximize a good circadian expression and a morning pattern [14,55,78].

This work has some limitations, such as the cross-sectional design with a sample composed only by men, which rules out the establishment of causal relationships and does not allow the generalization of the results to women. Likewise, the wide age range of the sample, although partially controlled with age as a covariate, might have contributed to type II error. The high pattern of polydrug use in the patients does not allow us to assess specific associations between the type of substance and circadian rhythmicity. On the other hand, the higher proportion of patients in residential treatment in the MDD+ group could have influenced some of the circadian rhythm results attributed to their diagnosis. Future studies should evaluate circadian rhythmicity at the beginning as well as during treatment in order to know the differential evolution of patients and to identify possible risk factors and predictors of therapeutic adherence.

5. Conclusions

The present work represents a first contribution to the knowledge of the differential circadian characteristics of dual diagnosis patients taking into account their comorbid SMI, as well as the relationship with sociodemographic, clinical variables and treatment modality received for the SUD. The results obtained point out the importance to consider the circadian rhythmic expression in the clinical management of dual patients, with residential treatment modality being a possible indicator of a better restoration of circadian functioning. Our findings may confirm the idea that the DST rhythm could be a biological marker of treatment adherence and a protective factor of the comorbid SMI disorder; even though future longitudinal studies are required to contrast such evidence. Progress in this line can contribute, firstly, to the detection of possible markers of vulnerability and, secondly, to establishing more appropriate therapeutic goals that incorporate chronotherapeutic strategies. All of this seems especially of interest for patients with greater circadian dysfunction such as those with SZ+, BD+ and under outpatient treatments, in whom the emphasis on maintaining changes in behavior and appropriate time habits may improve the response to treatment and prevent relapses.

Author Contributions: Conceptualization, A.A.; methodology, A.A. and J.F.N.; validation, A.A, A.B.S.-S. and J.E.M.-A.; formal analysis, A.A., A.B.S.-S. and A.M.-N.; investigation, A.B.S.-S., J.E.M.-A. and A.A.; writing—review and editing, all authors; funding acquisition, A.A. All authors have read and agreed to the published version of the manuscript.

Funding: This research was funded by Spanish Ministry of Economy, Industry and Competitiveness (PSI2015-65026-MINECO/FEDER/UE); Generalitat de Catalunya (2017SGR-748) and the Spanish Ministry of Science and Innovation (PID2020-117767GB-I00/AEI/10.13039/501100011033).

Institutional Review Board Statement: The study was conducted according to the guidelines of the Declaration of Helsinki and approved by Ethics Committee of the University of Barcelona (IRB00003099).

Informed Consent Statement: Informed consent was obtained from all subjects involved in the study.

Data Availability Statement: The data presented in this study are available on request from the corresponding author.

Acknowledgments: We thank the Mental Health division of Althaia Foundation, Gressol Man Project Foundation in Catalonia, ATRA group, Mental Health of Vall Hebron Hospital and Addiction's Division of the Maresme Health Consortium, Ethos Association, Center for Attention and Follow-up on Drug Dependencies Les Corts, Els Tres Turons Foundation, Septimània and Dianova Association for providing the sample of the study.

Conflicts of Interest: The authors declare no conflict of interest.

References

1. World Health Organization. *Lexicon of Alcohol and Drug Terms*; World Health Organization: Geneva, Switzerland, 1994.
2. Observatorio Español de las Drogas y las Adicciones. *Informe 2019 Alcohol, Tabaco y Drogas Ilegales en España*; Ministerio de sanidad, Consumo y Bienestar Social: Madrid, Spain, 2019.
3. Di Lorenzo, R.; Galliani, A.; Guicciardi, A.; Landi, G.; Ferri, P. A retrospective analysis focusing on a group of patients with dual diagnosis treated by both mental health and substance use services. *Neuropsychiatr. Dis. Treat.* **2014**, *10*, 1479–1488. [CrossRef] [PubMed]
4. Marquez-Arrico, J.E.; Río-Martínez, L.; Navarro, J.F.; Prat, G.; Adan, A. Personality profile and clinical correlates of patients with substance use disorder with and without comorbid depression under treatment. *Front. Psychiatry* **2019**, *9*, 764. [CrossRef] [PubMed]
5. Marquez-Arrico, J.E.; Adan, A. Dual diagnosis and personality traits: Current situation and future research directions. *Adicciones* **2013**, *25*, 195–202. [CrossRef] [PubMed]
6. Gulick, D.; Gamsby, J.J. Racing the clock: The role of circadian rhythmicity in addiction across the lifespan. *Pharmacol. Ther.* **2018**, *188*, 124–139. [CrossRef] [PubMed]
7. Del Capella, M.M.; Martinez-Nicolas, A.; Adan, A. Circadian rhythmic characteristics in men with substance use disorder under treatment. Influence of age of onset of substance use and duration of abstinence. *Front. Psychiatry* **2018**, *9*, 373. [CrossRef] [PubMed]

8. Perreau-Lenza, S.; Spanagela, R. Clock genes × stress × reward interactions in alcohol and substance use disorders. *Alcohol* **2015**, *49*, 351–357. [CrossRef]
9. Angarita, G.A.; Emadi, N.; Hodges, S.; Morgan, P.T. Sleep abnormalities associated with alcohol, cannabis, cocaine, and opiate use: A comprehensive review. *Addict. Sci. Clin. Pract.* **2016**, *11*, 9. [CrossRef]
10. Grau-López, L.; Grau-López, L.; Daigre, C.; Palma-Álvarez, R.F.; Rodriguez–Cintas, L.; Ros-Cucurull, E.; Roncero, C. Pharmacological treatment of insomnia symptoms in individuals with substance use disorders in Spain: A quasi-experimentals study. *Subst. Use Misuse* **2018**, *53*, 1267–1274. [CrossRef]
11. Kosobud, A.E.K.; Gillman, A.G.; Leffel, J.K.; Pecoraro, N.C.; Rebec, G.V.; Timberlake, W. Drugs of abuse can entrain circadian rhythms. *Sci. World J.* **2007**, *7*, 203–212. [CrossRef] [PubMed]
12. Kenney, S.R.; Lac, A.; Labrie, J.W.; Hummer, J.F.; Pham, A. Mental health, sleep quality, drinking motives, and alcohol-related consequences: A path-analytic model. *J. Stud. Alcohol Drugs* **2013**, *74*, 841–851. [CrossRef] [PubMed]
13. McKnight-Eily, L.R.; Eaton, D.K.; Lowry, R.; Croft, J.B.; Presley-Cantrell, L.; Perry, G.S. Relationships between hours of sleep and health-risk behaviors in US adolescent students. *Prev. Med.* **2011**, *53*, 271–273. [CrossRef] [PubMed]
14. Adan, A. A chronobiological approach to addiction. *J. Subst. Use* **2013**, *18*, 171–183. [CrossRef]
15. Antúnez, J.M.; del Capella, M.M.; Navarro, J.F.; Adan, A. Circadian rhythmicity in substance use disorder male patients with and without comorbid depression under ambulatory and therapeutic community treatment. *Chronobiol. Int.* **2016**, *33*, 1410–1421. [CrossRef] [PubMed]
16. Taylor, B.J.; Hasler, B.P. Chronotype and mental health: Recent advances. *Curr. Psychiatry Rep.* **2018**, *20*, 59. [CrossRef]
17. Logan, R.W.; Hasler, B.P.; Forbes, E.E.; Franzen, P.L.; Torregrossa, M.M.; Huang, Y.H.; Buysse, D.J.; Clark, D.B.; McClung, C.A. Impact of sleep and circadian rhythms on addiction vulnerability in adolescents. *Biol. Psychiatry* **2018**, *83*, 987–996. [CrossRef]
18. Nguyen-Louie, T.T.; Brumback, T.; Worley, M.J.; Colrain, I.M.; Matt, G.E.; Squeglia, L.M.; Tapert, S.F. Effects of sleep on substance use in adolescents: A longitudinal perspective. *Addict. Biol.* **2018**, *23*, 750–760. [CrossRef]
19. Castro, J.; Zanini, M.; da Gonçalves, B.S.B.; Coelho, F.M.S.; Bressan, R.; Bittencourt, L.; Gadelha, A.; Brietzke, E.; Tufik, S. Circadian rest-activity rhythm in individuals at risk for psychosis and bipolar disorder. *Schizophr. Res.* **2015**, *168*, 50–55. [CrossRef]
20. Chouinard, S.; Poulin, J.; Stip, E.; Godbout, R. Sleep in untreated patients with schizophrenia: A meta-analysis. *Schizophr. Bull.* **2004**, *30*, 957–967. [CrossRef]
21. De Crescenzo, F.; Economou, A.; Sharpley, A.L.; Gormez, A.; Quested, D.J. Actigraphic features of bipolar disorder: A systematic review and meta-analysis. *Sleep Med. Rev.* **2017**, *33*, 58–59. [CrossRef] [PubMed]
22. Ng, T.H.; Chung, K.F.; Ho, F.Y.Y.; Yeung, W.F.; Yung, K.P.; Lam, T.H. Sleep-wake disturbance in interepisode bipolar disorder and high-risk individuals: A systematic review and meta-analysis. *Sleep Med. Rev.* **2015**, *20*, 46–58. [CrossRef] [PubMed]
23. McGowan, N.M.; Goodwin, G.M.; Bilderbeck, A.C.; Saunders, K.E.A. Circadian rest-activity patterns in bipolar disorder and borderline personality disorder. *Transl. Psychiatry* **2019**, *9*, 195. [CrossRef] [PubMed]
24. Chen, Y.; Hong, W.; Fang, Y. Role of biological rhythm dysfunction in the development and management of bipolar disorders: A review. *Gen. Psychiatry* **2020**, *33*, e100127. [CrossRef]
25. Manoach, D.S.; Pan, J.Q.; Purcell, S.M.; Stickgold, R. Reduced sleep spindles in schizophrenia: A treatable endophenotype that links risk genes to impaired cognition? *Biol. Psychiatry* **2016**, *80*, 599–608. [CrossRef] [PubMed]
26. McKnight-Eily, L.R.; Eaton, D.K.; Lowry, R.; Croft, J.B.; Presley-Cantrell, L.; Perry, G.S. Altered circadian patterns of salivary cortisol in individuals with schizophrenia: A critical literature review. *J. Physiol. Paris* **2016**, *110*, 439–447.
27. Bromundt, V.; Köster, M.; Georgiev-Kill, A.; Opwis, K.; Wirz-Justice, A.; Stoppe, G.; Cajochen, C. Sleep-Wake cycles and cognitive functioning in schizophrenia. *Br. J. Psychiatry* **2011**, *198*, 269–276. [CrossRef] [PubMed]
28. Chung, K.F.; Poon, Y.P.Y.P.; Ng, T.K.; Kan, C.K. Correlates of sleep irregularity in schizophrenia. *Psychiatry Res.* **2018**, *270*, 705–714. [CrossRef] [PubMed]
29. Wulff, K.; Dijk, D.J.; Middleton, B.; Foster, R.G.; Joyce, E.M. Sleep and circadian rhythm disruption in schizophrenia. *Br. J. Psychiatry* **2012**, *200*, 308–316. [CrossRef] [PubMed]
30. Afonso, P.; Brissos, S.; Figueira, M.L.; Paiva, T. Schizophrenia patients with predominantly positive symptoms have more disturbed sleep-wake cycles measured by actigraphy. *Psychiatry Res.* **2011**, *189*, 62–66. [CrossRef] [PubMed]
31. Soehner, A.M.; Kaplan, K.A.; Harvey, A.G. Insomnia comorbid to severe psychiatric illness. *Sleep Med. Clin.* **2013**, *8*, 367–371. [CrossRef] [PubMed]
32. Mansour, H.A.; Wood, J.; Chowdari, K.V.; Dayal, M.; Thase, M.E.; Kupfer, D.J.; Monk, T.H.; Devlin, B.; Nimgaonkar, V.L. Circadian phase variation in bipolar I disorder. *Chronobiol. Int.* **2005**, *22*, 571–584. [CrossRef]
33. Thomas, P.; He, F.; Mazumdar, S.; Wood, J.; Bhatia, T.; Gur, R.C.; Gur, R.E.; Buysse, D.; Nimgaonkar, V.L.; Deshpande, S.N. Joint analysis of cognitive and circadian variation in schizophrenia and bipolar I disorder. *Asian J. Psychiatr.* **2018**, *38*, 96–101. [CrossRef] [PubMed]
34. Ahn, Y.M.; Chang, J.; Joo, Y.H.; Kim, S.C.; Lee, K.Y.; Kim, Y.S. Chronotype distribution in bipolar I disorder and schizophrenia in a Korean sample. *Bipolar Disord.* **2008**, *10*, 271–275. [CrossRef]
35. Melo, M.C.A.; Abreu, R.L.C.; Linhares Neto, V.B.; de Bruin, P.F.C.; de Bruin, V.M.S. Chronotype and circadian rhythm in bipolar disorder: A systematic review. *Sleep Med. Rev.* **2017**, *34*, 46–58. [CrossRef]
36. Takaesu, Y. Circadian rhythm in bipolar disorder: A review of the literature. *Psychiatry Clin. Neurosci.* **2018**, *72*, 673–682. [CrossRef] [PubMed]

37. McGowan, N.M.; Coogan, A.N. Sleep and circadian rhythm function and trait impulsivity: An actigraphy study. *Psychiatry Res.* **2018**, *268*, 251–256. [CrossRef] [PubMed]
38. Rock, P.; Goodwin, G.; Harmer, C.; Wulff, K. Daily rest-activity patterns in the bipolar phenotype: A controlled actigraphy study. *Chronobiol. Int.* **2014**, *31*, 290–296. [CrossRef] [PubMed]
39. Verkooijen, S.; van Bergen, A.H.; Knapen, S.E.; Vreeker, A.; Abramovic, L.; Pagani, L.; Jung, Y.; Riemersma-van der Lek, R.; Schoevers, R.A.; Takahashi, J.S.; et al. An actigraphy study investigating sleep in bipolar I patients, unaffected siblings and controls. *J. Affect. Disord.* **2017**, *208*, 248–254. [CrossRef] [PubMed]
40. Scott, J.; Murray, G.; Henry, C.; Morken, G.; Scott, E.; Angst, J.; Merikangas, K.R.; Hickie, I.B. Activation in bipolar disorders a systematic review. *JAMA Psychiatry* **2017**, *74*, 189–196. [CrossRef] [PubMed]
41. Moon, J.H.; Cho, C.H.; Son, G.H.; Geum, D.; Chung, S.; Kim, H.; Kang, S.G.; Park, Y.M.; Yoon, H.K.; Kim, L.; et al. Advanced circadian phase in mania and delayed circadian phase in mixed mania and depression returned to normal after treatment of bipolar disorder. *EBioMedicine* **2016**, *11*, 285–295. [CrossRef]
42. Steinan, M.K.; Morken, G.; Lagerberg, T.V.; Melle, I.; Andreassen, O.A.; Vaaler, A.E.; Scott, J. Delayed sleep phase: An important circadian subtype of sleep disturbance in bipolar disorders. *J. Affect. Disord.* **2016**, *191*, 156–163. [CrossRef] [PubMed]
43. Adan, A.; Archer, S.N.; Hidalgo, M.P.; Di Milia, L.; Natale, V.; Randler, C. Circadian typology: A comprehensive review. *Chronobiol. Int.* **2012**, *29*, 1153–1175. [CrossRef]
44. Tonon, A.C.; Carissimi, A.; Schimitt, R.L.; de Lima, L.S.; Pereira, F.D.S.; Hidalgo, M.P. How do stress, sleep quality, and chronotype associate with clinically significant depressive symptoms? A study of young male military recruits in compulsory service. *Braz. J. Psychiatry* **2020**, *42*, 54–62. [CrossRef]
45. Webb, I.C. Circadian rhythms and substance abuse: Chronobiological considerations for the treatment of addiction. *Curr. Psychiatry Rep.* **2017**, *19*, 2. [CrossRef] [PubMed]
46. American Psychiatric Association. *Diagnostic and Statistical Manual of Mental Disorders*, 5th ed.; American Psychiatric Association: Washington, DC, USA, 2013; ISBN 9780890425541.
47. First, M.B.; Spitzer, R.L.; Gibbon, M.; Williams, J.B.W. *Entrevista Clínica Estructurada Para los Trastornos del Eje I del DSM-IV, Versión Clínica*; Masson: Barcelona, Spain, 1999.
48. Kay, S.R.; Fiszbein, A.; Opler, L.A. The Positive and Negative Syndrome Scale (PANSS) for Schizophrenia. *Schizophr. Bull.* **1987**, *13*, 261–276. [CrossRef] [PubMed]
49. Peralta, V.; Cuesta, M.J. Validación de la escala de los síndromes positivo y negativo (PANSS) en una muestra de esquizofrénicos españoles. *Luso-Españolas Neurololo. Psiquiatr. Cienc. Afines.* **1994**, *22*, 171–177.
50. Young, R.C.; Biggs, J.T.; Ziegler, V.E.; Meyer, D.A. A rating scale for mania: Reliability, validity and sensitivity. *Br. J. Psychiatry* **1978**, *133*, 429–435. [CrossRef] [PubMed]
51. Hamilton, M. A rating scale for depression. *J. Neurol. Neurosurg. Psychiatry* **1960**, *23*, 56–62. [CrossRef]
52. Colom, F.; Vieta, E.; Martínez-Arán, A.; García-García, M.; Reinares, M.; Torrent, C.; Goikolea, J.; Banús, S.; Salamero, M. Versión española de una escala de evaluación de la manía: Validez y fiabilidad de la Escala de Young the Young Mania Rating Scale. *Med. Clin.* **2002**, *119*, 366–371. [CrossRef]
53. Ramos-Brieva, J.A.; Cordero-Villafafila, A. A new validation of the Hamilton Rating Scale for depression. *J. Psychiatr. Res.* **1988**, *22*, 21–28. [CrossRef]
54. Adan, A.; Caci, H.; Prat, G. Reliability of the Spanish version of the Composite Scale of Morningness. *Eur. Psychiatry* **2005**, *20*, 503–509. [CrossRef] [PubMed]
55. Martinez-Nicolas, A.; Madrid, J.A.; Rol, M.A. Day-night contrast as source of health for the human circadian system. *Chronobiol. Int.* **2014**, *31*, 382–393. [CrossRef]
56. Sosa, M.; Mondéjar, M.; Martinez-Nicolas, A.; Ortiz-Tudela, E.; Saraba, J.; Sosa, J.; Marín, R. Circadianware. Spanish Patent 08/2010/183, 3 September 2010.
57. Batinga, H.; Martinez-Nicolas, A.; Zornoza-Moreno, M.; Sánchez-Solis, M.; Larqué, E.; Mondéjar, M.T.; Moreno-Casbas, M.; García, F.J.; Campos, M.; Rol, M.A.; et al. Ontogeny and aging of the distal skin temperature rhythm in humans. *Age* **2015**, *37*, 29. [CrossRef] [PubMed]
58. Witting, W.; Kwa, I.H.; Eikelenboom, P.; Mirmiran, M.; Swaab, D.F. Alterations in the circadian rest-activity rhythm in aging and Alzheimer's disease. *Biol. Psychiatry* **1990**, *27*, 563–572. [CrossRef]
59. Richardson, J.T.E. Eta squared and partial eta squared as measures of effect size in educational research. *Educ. Res. Rev.* **2011**, *6*, 135–147. [CrossRef]
60. Benaiges, I.; Prat, G.; Adan, A. Health-related quality of life in patients with dual diagnosis: Clinical correlates. *Health Qual. Life Outcomes* **2012**, *10*, 106. [CrossRef] [PubMed]
61. Fernández-Mondragón, S.; Adan, A. Personality in male patients with substance use disorder and/or severe mental illness. *Psychiatry Res.* **2015**, *228*, 488–494. [CrossRef] [PubMed]
62. Hakulinen, C.; McGrath, J.J.; Timmerman, A.; Skipper, N.; Mortensen, P.B.; Pedersen, C.B.; Agerbo, E. The association between early-onset schizophrenia with employment, income, education, and cohabitation status: Nationwide study with 35 years of follow-up. *Soc. Psychiatry Psychiatr. Epidemiol.* **2019**, *54*, 1343–1351. [CrossRef] [PubMed]

63. Vreeker, A.; Boks, M.P.M.; Abramovic, L.; Verkooijen, S.; van Bergen, A.H.; Hillegers, M.H.J.; Spijker, A.T.; Hoencamp, E.; Regeer, E.J.; Riemersma-Van der Lek, R.F.; et al. High educational performance is a distinctive feature of bipolar disorder: A study on cognition in bipolar disorder, schizophrenia patients, relatives and controls. *Psychol. Med.* **2016**, *46*, 807–818. [CrossRef]
64. Christensen, H.N.; Diderichsen, F.; Hvidtfeldt, U.A.; Lange, T.; Andersen, P.K.; Osler, M.; Prescott, E.; Tjønneland, A.; Rod, N.H.; Andersen, I. Joint effect of alcohol consumption and educational level on alcohol-related medical events: A Danish register-based cohort study. *Epidemiology* **2017**, *28*, 872–879. [CrossRef]
65. Daigre, C.; Perea-Ortueta, M.; Berenguer, M.; Esculies, O.; Sorribes-Puertas, M.; Palma-Alvarez, R.; Martínez-Luna, N.; Ramos-Quiroga, A.; Grau-López, L. Psychiatric factors affecting recovery after a long term treatment program for substance use disorder. *Psychiatry Res.* **2019**, *276*, 283–289. [CrossRef] [PubMed]
66. Adan, A.; Arredondo, A.Y.; del Capella, M.M.; Prat, G.; Forero, D.A.; Navarro, J.F. Neurobiological underpinnings and modulating factors in schizophrenia spectrum disorders with a comorbid substance use disorder: A systematic review. *Neurosci. Biobehav. Rev.* **2017**, *75*, 361–377. [CrossRef] [PubMed]
67. Han, B.; Olfson, M.; Mojtabai, R. Depression care among depressed adults with and without comorbid substance use disorders in the United States. *Depress. Anxiety* **2017**, *34*, 291–300. [CrossRef] [PubMed]
68. Donoghue, K.; Doody, G.A.; Murray, R.M.; Jones, P.B.; Morgan, C.; Dazzan, P.; Hart, J.; Mazzoncini, R.; Maccabe, J.H. Cannabis use, gender and age of onset of schizophrenia: Data from the ÆSOP study. *Psychiatry Res.* **2014**, *215*, 528–532. [CrossRef] [PubMed]
69. Marquez-Arrico, J.E.; Adan, A. Personality in patients with substance use disorders according to the co-occurring severe mental illness: A study using the alternative five factor model. *Pers. Individ. Dif.* **2016**, *97*, 76–81. [CrossRef]
70. Szerman, N.; Peris, L. Precision psychiatry and dual disorders. *J. Dual Diagn.* **2019**, *14*, 237–246. [CrossRef] [PubMed]
71. Adan, A.; Marquez-Arrico, J.E.; Gilchrist, G. Comparison of health-related quality of life among men with different co-existing severe mental disorders in treatment for substance use. *Health Qual. Life Outcomes* **2017**, *15*, 209. [CrossRef]
72. Bassiony, M.; Seleem, D. Drug-related problems among polysubstance and monosubstance users: A cross-sectional study. *J. Subst. Use* **2020**, *25*, 392–397. [CrossRef]
73. Krawczyk, N.; Feder, K.A.; Saloner, B.; Crum, R.M.; Kealhofer, M.; Mojtabai, R. The association of psychiatric comorbidity with treatment completion among clients admitted to substance use treatment programs in a U.S. national sample. *Drug Alcohol Depend.* **2017**, *175*, 157–163. [CrossRef]
74. Meyer, N.; Faulkner, S.M.; McCutcheon, R.A.; Pillinger, T.; Dijk, D.J.; MacCabe, J.H. Sleep and circadian rhythm disturbance in remitted schizophrenia and bipolar disorder: A systematic review and meta-analysis. *Schizophr. Bull.* **2020**, *46*, 1126–1143. [CrossRef]
75. Corruble, E.; Frank, E.; Gressier, F.; Courtet, P.; Bayle, F.; Llorca, P.M.; Vaiva, G.; Gorwood, P. Morningness-eveningness and treatment response in major depressive disorder. *Chronobiol. Int.* **2014**, *31*, 283–289. [CrossRef] [PubMed]
76. Martinez-Nicolas, A.; Guaita, M.; Santamaría, J.; Montserrat, J.M.; Rol, M.Á.; Madrid, J.A. Circadian impairment of distal skin temperature rhythm in patients with sleep-disordered breathing: The effect of CPAP. *Sleep* **2017**, *40*, zsx067. [CrossRef] [PubMed]
77. Martinez-Nicolas, A.; Martinez-Madrid, M.J.; Almaida-Pagan, P.F.; Bonmati-Carrion, M.-A.; Madrid, J.A.; Rol, M.A. Assessing chronotypes by ambulatory circadian monitoring. *Front. Physiol.* **2019**, *10*, 1396. [CrossRef] [PubMed]
78. Lee, K.; Lee, H.K.; Jhung, K.; Park, J.Y. Relationship between chronotype and temperament/character among university students. *Psychiatry Res.* **2017**, *251*, 63–68. [CrossRef] [PubMed]

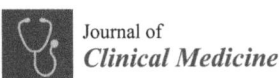

Article

Protocol for Characterization of Addiction and Dual Disorders: Effectiveness of Coadjuvant Chronotherapy in Patients with Partial Response

Ana Adan [1,2,*], José Francisco Navarro [3] and on behalf of ADDISCHRONO Group [†]

1. Department of Clinical Psychology and Psychobiology, School of Psychology, University of Barcelona, Passeig de la Vall d'Hebrón 171, 08035 Barcelona, Spain
2. Institute of Neurosciences, University of Barcelona, 08035 Barcelona, Spain
3. Department of Psychobiology, School of Psychology, University of Málaga, Campus de Teatinos s/n, 29071 Málaga, Spain; navahuma@uma.es
* Correspondence: aadan@ub.edu; Tel.: +34-93-312-5060
† Gisela Mariel Hansen, Diego A. Forero, M. Paz Hidalgo, Vincenzo Natale, Julia E. Marquez-Arrico, Alvaro Gonzalez-Sanchez, Oriol Esculies.

Abstract: This protocol aims to characterize patients with dual disorders (DD; comorbid major depression and schizophrenia) compared with patients with only a diagnosis of substance use disorder (SUD) and those with only a diagnosis of severe mental illness (SMI; major depression and schizophrenia), evaluating clinical and personality characteristics, circadian rhythmic functioning, genetic polymorphism and neuropsychological performance in order to obtain a clinical endophenotype of differential vulnerability for these diagnostic entities. Patients will be divided into three groups: DD (45 men with comorbid schizophrenia, 45 men and 30 women with major depression), SUD (n = 90, with a minimum of 30 women) and SMI males (45 with schizophrenia, 45 with major depression). All patients will be under treatment, with at least three months of SUD abstinence and/or with SMI in remission or with stabilized symptoms. Outpatients of both sexes with insufficient restoration of circadian rhythmicity with SUD (n = 30) and dual depression (n = 30) will be asked to participate in a second two-month study, being alternately assigned to the condition of the chronobiological adjuvant approach to the treatment of regular hour habits and exposure to light or to the usual treatment (control). The effect of the intervention and patient compliance will be monitored with a Kronowise KW6® ambulatory device during the first two weeks of treatment and again at weeks 4 and 8 weeks. After completing the evaluation, follow-up of the clinical evolution will be carried out at 3, 6 and 12 months. This project will allow us to analyze the functional impact of DD comorbidity and to develop the first study of chronobiological therapy in the treatment of SUD and dual depression, with results transferable to the clinical setting with cost-effective recommendations for a personalized approach.

Keywords: substance use disorder; dual disorders; major depressive disorder; schizophrenia; circadian rhythm; genetic polymorphisms; neurocognition; chronobiological therapy; exposure to natural light; clinical course

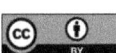

1. Introduction

Substance use disorder (SUD) affects millions of people worldwide with possible devastating personal consequences, which require a specific, intense and long-term therapeutic approach to recovery. This disorder generates a high economic cost and very significant drop-out and relapse rates. Dual disorders (DD), defined as the coexistence of an SUD and a severe mental illness (SMI) not secondary to the first, have become increasingly prevalent in recent years [1]. Among the comorbidities of SUD, diagnoses of major depression and schizophrenia are the most frequent. In addition, about 50% of schizophrenic patients and 32% of patients with affective disorders also have an SUD, excluding nicotine and caffeine [2,3].

In both SUD and DD, the male sex is most prevalent in the clinical setting (around 80%), with cocaine or alcohol being the substances that produce the most frequent dependence in Spain and other European countries, followed by cannabis [4,5], although most patients develop a pattern of polyconsumption. Currently, DD has an enormous clinical impact due to the difficulty in diagnosis and therapeutic management, as well as its high healthcare cost. Thus, it has been demonstrated that DD patients are more likely to exhibit an increase in symptoms, more relapses, hospitalizations, medical illnesses and suicidal risk, as well as greater victimization, social isolation and premature death [6,7]. Patients with DD also tend to show poor adherence, worse treatment response and lower quality of life [8,9] as compared to those with a single pathological condition.

1.1. Circadian Rhythmicity

The alteration of the circadian rhythmic system (amplitude reduction, phase delay, lower interdaily stability, worse sleep quality and wakefulness) has been considered a possible marker for SUDs [10], major depression [11,12] and schizophrenia [13,14]. In young people with affective disorders in early stages, alterations are related to social and occupational functioning [15], whereas in adolescents at risk of developing psychosis, they are related to the severity of psychotic symptoms and the deterioration of social functioning at one year of follow-up [14]. In the middle and advanced phases, circadian involvement may meet chronodisruption criteria and is correlated with symptomatic severity, more remission difficulty, worse prognosis and worse quality of life in patients [16]. However, research has focused on the presence of sleep disorders in SUD (with 70% of patients who come to treatment), major depression and schizophrenia [17] and, to a lesser extent, in the rhythms of circadian markers, such as body temperature.

Numerous review studies have proposed, from the observations of circadian dysregulation in SUD patients prior to treatment and during detoxification, that it would be useful to incorporate chronobiological strategies both in the therapeutic approach [17,18] and in prevention [19], similar to how these strategies have been applied in patients with seasonal or non-seasonal depression. A lower contrast between day and night (reduced amplitude) and a greater fragmentation of the rhythm and fragility of the sleep–wake cycle have been considered poor indicators of circadian rhythmicity, which may reflect an immaturity of the circadian system [20]. Our group has demonstrated that patients in treatment with only SUD [21] and, to a greater extent, with dual depression [22] exhibit a lower percentage of rhythm, interdaily stability and amplitude due to less adequate diurnal values related to onset age of consumption, severity of addiction, withdrawal time and type of treatment (residential/outpatient). These observations suggest a slower restoration of the homeostatic process (S), and the need for sleep during wakefulness compared to the circadian process (C) of the revised Borbély model [23].

Despite the increasing interest and the possible clinical utility attributed to chronobiology for the understanding and management of SUD and DD, studies with humans, although offering very promising data, are very limited. The development of ambulatory devices for the evaluation of a set of objective parameters of the functioning of the circadian system, such as the Kronowise KW6® (Kronohealth, Murcia, Spain) (distal body temperature, activity, intensity and type of environmental light), offers enormous possibilities to advance knowledge of variables key to clinical practice. Body temperature is considered a good estimator of circadian endogenous rhythmic expression, whereas exposure to light is valued as an indicator of synchronization with the solar cycle and of activity expressing the circadian behavioral habits of individuals. Its use in this investigation may result in obtaining a clinical marker of response to treatment and risk of relapse, with very affordable technology and costs and with good acceptance by patients.

1.2. Genetic Polymorphisms and Clock Genes

Molecular genetics plays an important role in the identification of new risk factors and pathophysiological mechanisms for the vast majority of neuropsychiatric disorders, which are useful for the development of new approaches for both diagnosis and treatment. Single nucleotide polymorphisms (SNPs) represent the most frequently studied type of genetic variation in human molecular genomics. Currently, the human SNP database includes more than 30 million of SNPs (http://www.ncbi.nlm.nih.gov/SNP; accessed on 21 March 2022). A fraction of SNPs has direct functional effects and is the basis for a large number of interindividual differences, as well as being involved in the predisposition to diseases and endophenotypes related to the individual response to drugs, among many others [24].

Among the circadian or clock genes, the Period genes (*PER2* and *PER3*) stand out for their implications, encoding proteins that are increased during the night hours and decreased during daytime. These inform the NSQ cells and peripheral organs as to what time it is approximately. There is a complex interaction between the clock genes and the functioning of the organism, with a bidirectional relationship between circadian rhythmic expression and various mental disorders. Thus, certain characteristics of circadian rhythmicity (phase delay and reduced amplitude, among others) influence the risk of developing an SUD, and this, in turn, is a factor that impairs proper circadian rhythmicity by modifying the gene expression of clock genes [17]. Genetic studies support the thesis that circadian genes are directly involved in the regulation of the dopaminergic reward circuit and that in vulnerable individuals, alterations of the circadian system could contribute to modifying the value of the reward and the motivation for substance use. In this sense, neuroimaging studies show altered neuronal responses towards the reward in evening subjects [19].

In humans, the *PER2* gene has the greatest influence on NSQ and is only expressed in the CNS. Polymorphisms in this gene have been associated with compulsive stress-mediated alcohol consumption, in addition to being involved in the expression of period and phase. Research with animal models of addiction has shown that a reduced expression of Per2 is related to a decreased production of the MAOA enzyme, as well as to increases in dopamine and improvements in depressive symptomatology [12,25], whereas D2R activity contributes to reducing the expression and rhythm of Per2 in the reinforcement system (striatum) [18]. Thus, serotonin at adequate levels regulates the circadian expression of Per2 (low during the day and elevated at night) [25]. The *PER3* gene, the most robust of the rhythmic genes, has been related to the circadian typology phase in response to morning light exposure and to differences in cognitive impact (executive functions and memory) [26]. *PER3* polymorphisms and levels of their gene expression have also been associated with addiction, schizophrenia and major depression, as well as response to SSRI-type antidepressants [12,26].

PER2 (rs934945) has been found, in Latin American participants, to be associated with morning alertness and activity planning, whereas *PER3* (rs2640909) is associated with morningness–eveningness (phase) [27]. Therefore, we intend to further analyze this aspect in the present investigation. We are not aware of any study exploring the presence of these polymorphisms in patients with SUD or DD. Our interest in this work, being aware of the small number of participants regarding the current genetic research in consortium and with global databases, is to try to establish their possible relationships with the other variables under study.

In relation to other genetic polymorphisms, there are numerous studies in patients diagnosed with SUD, major depression or schizophrenia, whereas in DD, knowledge is very limited, with heterogeneous data. Based on the diagnoses and variables considered in the present study, we focused our interest on the exploration of the *BDNF* (brain-derived neurotrophic factor; rs6265), *APOE* rs429358, rs7412 (E2, E3 and E4) and *MAOA* (uVNTR) genes, considering their implications for cognitive performance and circadian rhythmic expression, as well as the possible relationship with the response to the proposed chronobiological intervention.

BDNF rs6265 (Val66Met) is one of the main candidate genes in major depression [28] and in schizophrenia [29], and it has been implicated in cognitive deficits exhibited by the patients. Likewise, the existence of *BDNF* polymorphisms has been confirmed in DD patients with schizophrenia [30] and with altered cognitive performance. The data on *APOE*, which acts as a regulator of several mechanisms of cerebral plasticity, are controversial in schizophrenia, with both positive and negative conclusions but with some involvement as a protective factor in Asian populations [31]. In healthy individuals, a polymorphism in the promoter region of the *MAOA* gene has been related to the quality of wakefulness [32], whereas polymorphisms in *MAOA* have been associated with major depression and with suicidal behavior in men [33].

1.3. Cognitive Performance

Neuropsychological impairment associated with SUD, both psychotic and depressive, is a field of study with numerous published papers [34] (for review). Different cognitive deficits have also been identified in SUD, associated with problems of behavioral inhibition, decision making, sustained attention and strategy planning [35,36]. In all cases, there is evidence that deficits do not always recover after the remission of the disorder and that cognitive rehabilitation and psychosocial interventions in the therapeutic approach are key factors for recovery.

The data collected in patients with DD are scarce and heterogeneous, although—to a greater or lesser extent—deficits in attention, memory and executive functions are consistently observed, in agreement with neurochemical and neurofunctional affectations. These deficits have been described both in relation to schizophrenia [37,38], with deficits in flexibility and inhibition in executive functions, and affective disorders/major depression, in which the magnitude of the deficits is comparable to that observed in SUD [39]. Various studies carried out by our group suggest that a complete neuropsychological evaluation is necessary, although compatible with the pressure of clinical practice, and that the affectation is modulated by factors such as age, the age at onset of SUD, the main type of dependence drug and premorbid Intellectual Quotient (IQ) in both SUD [40] and dual schizophrenia [41–43]. That is, in dual schizophrenia, there is a complex model in which young patients have less vulnerability than those with only schizophrenia due to the presence of neurocognitive deficits, regardless of the domain studied, although these deficits become evident around age 50, associated with the risk of neurodegeneration and the main type of drug consumed. In relation to decision making, this is less appropriate in patients with dual schizophrenia regarding SUD, and the existence of suicide attempts seems to be a determining factor [44].

Until now, the combined measurement of neurocognition, circadian rhythmicity and molecular genetics in the diagnostic entities that we propose to study has never been addressed. This research could allow us to elucidate the presence of endogenous and exogenous explanatory factors and, if possible, with a predictive capacity of clinical interest.

1.4. Personality Characteristics

There is a large amount of evidence that indicates that certain personality characteristics, evaluated with multiple questionnaires that underlie different theoretical models, would be risk factors for the development of addictive behaviors and psychopathological disorders, also related to cognitive performance, clinical course and adherence to treatment. The existence of a vulnerability endophenotype is currently pointed out to develop an association between SUD and high Neuroticism-Anxiety and Impulsivity-Sensation-Seeking. If the disorder is developed, greater severity of addiction, craving and relapse are related to high scores of both personality traits [7]. In addition, treatment dropout occurs to a greater extent in patients with low scores in the Reward Dependency and Persistence traits [45].

Despite the heterogeneity of designs of previous studies with DD, we can point out that in male patients, there is a specific personality pattern, where SUD men tend to present with high Neuroticism-Anxiety and Impulsivity-Sensation-Seeking characteristics, and SMI men tend to show high Avoidance and low Persistence, regardless of whether SMI involves schizophrenia or major depression [46]. In dual depression, low Activity scores (ZKPQ) are specifically observed, being more evident with an early age at onset of SUD [7]. Low Activity is a feature present in the evening typology [47], and although it must be further analyzed, it could configure the personality endophenotype of dual depression and be related to polymorphisms of the *PER2* clock genes and *PER3*. On the other hand, in dual schizophrenia, low scores in Sociability are specifically observed [48], although this finding should be replicated in future studies with a greater number of patients and control of variables.

The implementation of therapeutic interventions aimed at the management of extreme personality traits has been more effective in individuals at high-risk of developing SUD than in classical cognitive or motivational therapies [49]. Similarly, in SUD patients, personality traits are beginning to be considered as a clinical marker, suggesting their usefulness in personalized treatments [50]. Our research aims to expand existing knowledge to DD, also linking it with clinical aspects of circadian rhythmicity and neurocognition to configure relevant and useful information in the therapeutic approach during the early remission phase. We consider the psychobiological-based personality questionnaires the most sensitive for this purpose, so we have been using the revised Cloninger Temperament and Character Inventory (TCI-R) and the Zuckerman-Kuhlman Personality Questionnaire (ZKPQ) based on the model of personality of the five alternative factors.

1.5. Chronobiological Therapeutic Approach to SUD and DD

The establishment of habits with regular sleep–wake schedules, meals and daily activities is very beneficial to maintain health and essential to recover it. In addition, these should be synchronized to the light–dark cycle with a morning pattern phase in which the contrast between light of day and night darkness is enhanced. It has been observed that the stability of habits is a protective factor for the development of mood disorders and to prevent relapses if they occur [12,51]. This therapeutic approach is based on fundamentals of chronobiology, although its implementation has been called "social rhythm therapy", and it has been applied with good results in patients with bipolar disorder (see [51] for a review). The guidelines recommending stable habits and synchronization to the solar cycle are usually successfully incorporated into the withdrawal treatment of SUD, especially in the residential regime, regardless of the therapeutic approach [19,22]. However, investigation of the therapeutic effects of the establishment of habits in humans is scarce; information on compliance by outpatients and longitudinal efficacy data have not been collected in any case.

Because light is the main synchronizer of the human circadian clock, exposure to light has been proposed as a significant element to be incorporated into "social rhythm therapy" [51], whether natural or artificial light and preferably in the early hours of the morning [52]. Light has serotoninergic and melatoninergic agonist effects, which underlie the therapeutic actions explored so far.

Exposure to bright artificial light, ideally white full-spectrum light, is necessary when exposure to natural (solar) light is insufficient or not available, and it is the most frequent option in studies that have addressed the efficacy of light therapy. This has shown efficacy in reducing depressive symptoms in both seasonal and non-seasonal depression [53], as well as in insomnia and circadian sleep disorders (see [54] for a meta-analysis) at an intensity of between 2500 and 10,000 lux without differing greatly in the results for depression treatment [55]. Although exposure to light in the treatment of non-seasonal depression is effective in monotherapy regardless of sex, showing a faster response than that of antidepressants, some studies indicate greater symptomatic improvement in combination with antidepressant drugs (i.e., fluoxetine) [56,57]. The most common exposure periods are between 7 and 14 days, although it is suggested as ideal to maintain the treatment for between two and five weeks for non-seasonal depression [55]. A recent meta-analysis [58] concluded that bright white light, starting at 1000 lux, also improves daytime alertness and cognitive performance.

The study of exposure to natural light has provided data of interest, especially in the field of depression. Wirz-Justice et al. [52] observed that patients with seasonal depression responded to an hour of walking exposed to the light in winter (Switzerland) after only one week and also responded better than to exposure to artificial light of 2800 lux. The hospitalization time in patients with non-seasonal depression decreases if spaces are better illuminated, which has been observed in Mediterranean latitudes regardless of the season of the year [59], as well as further north in Holland [60]. In adults of not very advanced age, it promotes and adjusts the secretion phase of nocturnal melatonin [61], which in turn can correct abnormal functional patterns in the dopaminergic reinforcement system [62]. The intensity of natural light reaches therapeutic values without a problem, since it is estimated to be 3000 lux on a cloudy day, 10,000 lux on a normal day (approximate intensity of 45 min after sunrise) and 50,000 lux on a sunny day [61] (https://www.scribd.com/document/359698224/LightLevels-outdoor-indoor-es, accessed on 21 March 2022).

The rhythmic restoration difficulties observed in SUD patients [21] and dual depressive patients [22,63] under treatment, especially due to a worse quality of the daytime period, can benefit from incorporating adjunctive treatment of hourly habits and light exposure. This promotes the improvement of daytime activation, with its consequent benefits in the cognitive and affective state, and can reduce depressive symptomatology and the dysphoria of the withdrawal process in the case of dual patients. Natural light in our latitude (Barcelona, 41°38N) is suitable for this intervention, even in the shortest photoperiod months of the year [64].

Our project aims to obtain a clinical endophenotype of the differential vulnerability of DD, focusing on the two most common SMIs comorbid to SUD (major depression and schizophrenia) in clinical practice. For this purpose, a selection of measurements (circadian rhythm, genetic polymorphisms, neurocognition and personality traits) was included that may result in adherence and clinical course markers (with an emphasis on relapses) (Study 1). We also evaluated the efficacy of incorporating regular habits and exposure to natural light as an adjunctive therapy to the clinical management of patients with SUD and dual depression who show partial response to treatment compared to patients with similar characteristics who received the usual treatment (Study 2). Both studies represent a novel approach that may result in a significant advance in this field of knowledge.

2. Hypothesis and Objectives

2.1. Initial Hypothesis

1. Patients with DD will show worse social, clinical and quality of life characteristics, the SMI group being in an intermediate position and the SUD group showing the best profile in the majority of variables. Sex will influence this characterization, with worse clinical profiles in women.
2. Alterations of the circadian rhythmicity of peripheral temperature (lower amplitude and stability, phase delay, low percentage of rhythm, lower index of circadian function), with a predominance of endogenous deterioration, will be more present in patients with DD and SMI than in SUD patients, being related to the severity of the addiction, concomitant symptomatology, current age of patients and age at onset of the disorder.
3. Polymorphisms in the proposed candidate genes will contribute to prediction of clinical (MAOA), circadian (PER2 and PER3) and functioning profiles in neuropsychological tests (BDNF, MAOA) in patients.
4. Cognitive performance in neuropsychological tasks (attention, short and long-term verbal memory, working memory, cognitive flexibility and executive functions) will affect both SUD and DD patients compared to normative data. These will be modulated by sex and other variables, such as age, age at onset of the disorder, suicide attempts, tobacco use, main dependence substance, comorbid mental disorder, etc. The cognitive skills of patients with DD will be better than those of patients who only suffer from SMI (intradisorder comparisons).

5. The personality pattern of the SUD and DD patients will be characterized by the endophenotype of high Impulsivity-Sensation Seeking and Anxiety-Neuroticism, a pattern that will be configured with the additional feature of low Activity in dual depression and low Sociability in dual schizophrenia. This will differ between genders, with high Impulsivity-Sensation Seeking in men and high Anxiety-Neuroticism in women.
6. The deterioration of circadian rhythmic activity and cognitive performance will be related to a lower adherence to treatment and a higher rate of relapse, evaluated during a year of follow-up. In both cases, comorbidity will worsen the success of the treatment, with a greater impact on dual schizophrenia than on dual depression.
7. Chronobiological intervention in SUD and dual depression will improve rhythmic expression (increase in amplitude and interdaily stability of peripheral temperature). Benefits will be obtained in diurnal activation, mood and quality of life related to health and adherence to treatment in the early remission phase for both sexes. This will be observed in both diagnostic groups, with greater magnitude in the dual depression group and with respect to the control groups that follow the usual treatment in spite of criteria compliance. The positive data of the intervention will indicate the greater involvement and difficulty of restoring the S process than the C process (Borbély model) and will be associated with the presence of PER2 polymorphisms (rs934945) and worse cognitive performance prior to the intervention.

2.2. General Objectives

1) To study in patients with DD (major depression and comorbid schizophrenia) compared to SUD-only patients and SMI-only (major depression and schizophrenia) patients, as well as their clinical characteristics, circadian rhythmic functioning, presence of genetic polymorphisms, neuropsychological performance and personality characteristics in order to obtain a possible clinically cost-effective endophenotype of differential vulnerability for the diagnostic entities considered.
2) To establish clinical markers of treatment adherence, prognosis of evolution and risk of relapse (one year follow-up) that can be considered in the therapeutic approach.
3) To evaluate the benefit of incorporating regularly scheduled habits and exposure to natural light in the treatment of SUD and dual patients who exhibit difficulties regaining circadian rhythmicity after three months of treatment.

2.3. Specific Objectives

For study 1:

1. To describe the presence of genetic polymorphisms and the characteristics of circadian rhythmicity, neurocognitive performance and personality traits in patients with DD (comorbid schizophrenia and major depression) compared to patients diagnosed with SMI only and with SUD only. The registration of the endogenous and environmental components underlying circadian rhythmicity, the selection of polymorphisms of circadian genes and related to cognition, as well as the exhaustive consideration of cognitive performance and personality characteristics facilitates a novel and robust approach.
2. To describe the differential aspects in circadian rhythmicity, genetic polymorphisms, neurocognitive performance, personality traits and health-related quality of life in patients with DD according to comorbid SMI (major depressive disorder and schizophrenia).
3. To determine the presence of the variables most affected or with greater specific weight among those evaluated according to the characteristics of the SUD (age at onset, severity, etc.) and the comorbid diagnosis (major depressive disorder and schizophrenia). The influence of sex will be explored in the case of SUD and dual depression.
4. To explore relationships between clinical variables and the presence of rhythmic and/or cognitive deterioration, as well as genetic polymorphisms and extreme personality traits in the DD, SUD and SMI groups. These will be studied in SUD and dual depression conditions according to sex. This information will lead us to consider

possible indicators/markers of vulnerability to be considered in clinical evaluation or treatment for an individualized approach.

5. To elucidate among the set of studied variables possible single or combined indicators of treatment adherence, as well as prognosis of evolution and relapses in SUD and DD to be used in future treatment and/or prevention for these patients.

For study 2:

1. To evaluate the benefits of adjuvant chronobiological therapy (regular habits in the schedule and exposure to natural light) for two months in abstinent patients with SUD and dual depression who show rhythmic restoration difficulties at three months of treatment.
2. To explore possible predictive variables of response to the efficacy of chronobiological therapy (genetic polymorphisms, cognitive performance, personality characteristics) in SUD and dual depressive patients of both sexes.
3. To compare the differential effects of chronobiological therapy with respect to usual treatment according to diagnosis (SUD and dual depression) and sex in terms of time and magnitude of the response in circadian rhythmicity (peripheral temperature and activity), clinical symptomatology and health-related quality of life.
4. To study the evolution of the chronobiological intervention of the SUD and dual depressive patients of both sexes with a one-year follow-up, also comparing the evolution of patients with the same diagnosis and similar clinical characteristics under usual treatment.

3. Materials and Methods

3.1. Participants

For study 1, patients between aged 20 and 50 who presented only SUD, DD (dual depression or dual schizophrenia) and only SMI (major depressive disorder and schizophrenia) according to the Diagnostic and Statistical Manual of Mental Disorders (DSM-5) criteria [65]. A minimum of 90 patients will be included in each group, half of them diagnosed with major depressive disorder and schizophrenia in the DD and SMI groups. In the SUD group a minimum of 30 women will be included, whereas in the dual depression group a minimum of 20 women will be added to the sample of 45 men. Likewise, associated with the inclusion criteria of the second study, 45 DD patients with dual depression is the minimum, but we should probably include about 10 to 15 more. In all cases, the inclusion of nicotine and caffeine consumers will be allowed. Participation in the study will be voluntary and unpaid, after signing of informed consent by the patient or his legal tutors. See Figure 1.

For study 2, outpatients with a diagnosis of SUD and dual depression with a partial restoration of circadian rhythmicity will be selected. At least 30 patients will be included in each group, and ideally, 50% will be women. This will be determined based on the inclusion criteria of peripheral temperature values of SUD patients obtained by Capella et al. [21], which can be considered normative due to the high number of patients studied. Candidates will be those with an L10 (average 10 h with a minimum value) greater than 33 °C, an amplitude of less than 0.80 and an interdaily stability of rhythm of less than 0.5 (range 0–1). In addition, the daily distribution of activity and its exposure to light will be assessed not due to selection criteria but to individually emphasize the implementation of scheduled habits. The exclusion criteria will be: (a) presence of ocular pathologies (retinopathies, cataracts, etc.); (b) skin problems and/or eye sensitivity and photophobia; (c) obesity and metabolic syndrome; (d) practice of daily or weekly intense physical exercise; and (e) treatment with drugs known to modify circadian rhythmicity or produce sedative effects (i.e., agomelatine, antipsychotics, mood stabilizers and hypnotics). Patients will be alternately assigned to the condition of chronobiological approach adjuvant to the treatment of regular hour habits and exposure to light or to the usual treatment (control) with only the evaluations.

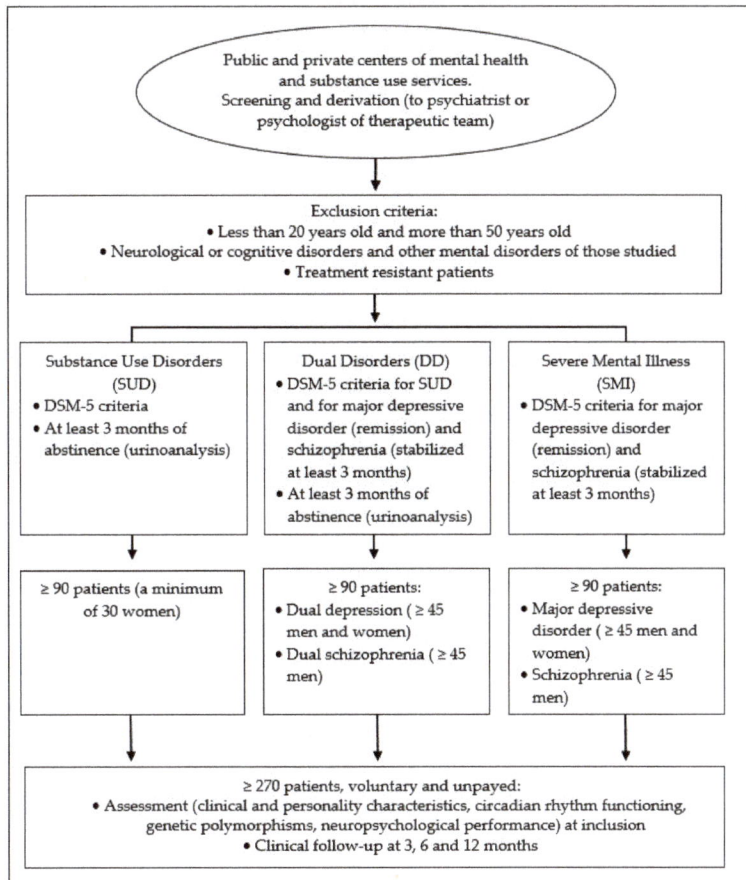

Figure 1. Inclusion and exclusion criteria of the groups of patients participating in Study 1.

Sample size. Starting with the population of patients from the referring centers, with adherence to treatment during the inclusion period, the sample should be 239 patients (with a 95% confidence level and a 5% margin of error), compared to the 270 proposed in study 1. This would be an adequate sample size for the subsequent contrasts to be analyzed. For study 2, there are no data on patients with rhythmic alteration in SUD or dual depression, but the sample of our study exceeds that of all previous work on treatment with natural light in other more prevalent pathologies.

3.2. Instruments

Clinical evaluation. Sociodemographic data, family and personal psychiatric history, presence and characteristics of current diagnoses will be collected, along with age at onset, pharmacological treatments, tobacco consumption (if so, the Fagerström dependence questionnaire will be applied), caffeine consumption, assistance framework and treatment program, withdrawal time, relapses and previous suicide attempts, number of hospital admissions and duration and presence/absence of psychosocial problems. The health-related quality of life assessment will also be incorporated (SF-36 questionnaire) [66].

To rule out that the comorbid mental disorder in DD is secondary, the Spanish version of the Psychiatric Research Interview for Substance and Mental Disorders for DSM-5 (PRISM-5) [67] will be used. The severity of the SUD will be assessed using the Drug Abuse

Screening Test (DAST-20) [68], the intensity of the depressive symptomatology using the Hamilton depression scale (HDRS) [69], the psychotic symptomatology with the PANSS scale [70] and suicidal risk using the Plutchik scale [71], all of them the Spanish version.

The evolution will be followed at 3, 6 and 12 months of inclusion in the study (application in pdf with closed fields that can be filled in on the computer), preferably through the contact professional of the center of origin or by the team's researchers in a hetero-assessed manner, with the patient and consulting their medical history.

Circadian rhythmicity pattern. A Kronowise KW6® ambulatory device (Kronohealth SL, University of Murcia, Spain) will be used to objectively record circadian rhythmicity. This integrates the measurement of peripheral/distal skin temperature, activity level by means of a 3-axis accelerometer and body position, as well as four light channels (average and peak of visible light, blue or circadian light that mimics the spectrum of melanopsin of retinal ganglion cells and infrared radiation). This integrated register allows for collection of variables that influence circadian rhythmicity (body position, physical activity, exposure to light, sleep and food schedules, etc.) in an objective and validated way [20,72]. An easy-to-use programming and reading-analysis software (Circadianware™, Kronohealth, Murcia, Spain) has been developed and provides a complete circadian report. The device consists of a clock system placed around the non-dominant wrist, with a micro-USB connection for programming, data download and battery charging. Patients in study 1 should wear the device for 2 days, and those in study 2 will be monitored continuously during the first two weeks and at weeks 4 and 8, except in moments of personal hygiene, during which they can be removed (indicated in the "event" option of the Kronowise KW6®). In addition to the usual sleep schedule, on the days of registration, bedtime and waking up times will be considered by the event marker available in the device. The use of ambulatory instruments in mental health represents a significant progress both in assessment and, as recently evidenced, in therapeutic management [73,74].

Self-assessed information on circadian typology will also be collected using the Composite Morningness Scale (CSM) [75], mood rhythmicity pattern (MrhI) [76] and seasonal variations (SPAQ) [77], in all cases with validated instruments in the Spanish population. For study 2, patients will fill in eight unipolar visual analogue scales [78] daily after natural light exposition and during the two months of the intervention in order to assess subjective activation and mood status.

Genetic determinations. A 2 mL sample of saliva (Salivette Oragene-DNA (OG-500)) will be taken after 30 min of not having had any liquid or solid intake, including chewing gums or smoking. The saliva samples will be stored at room temperature in a light-preserved place until processed. For the extraction of genomic DNA, an aliquot of saliva will be used, following the manufacturer's protocol (Oragene). A Qubit fluorometer (Invitrogen, Carlsbad, CA) will be used to determine DNA concentrations. The DNA samples will be adjusted to a final concentration of 10 ng/ul in TE-4 (10 mM Tris-HCl, 0.1 mM EDTA, pH 7.5) and stored at 4 °C until use. Molecular genetics analyses will be performed using previously validated real-time PCR-based methodologies, using Taqman probes for the PER2 polymorphisms (rs934945), PER3 (rs2640909), BDNF rs6265 (Val66Met), APOE rs429358 and rs7412 (E2, E3 and E4). The VNTR in MAOA will be genotyped by analyzing the amplified PCR fragments and run on agarose gel electrophoresis.

Neuropsychological evaluation. The battery of standardized neuropsychological tests is based on the evaluation of functions that may be affected in our sample. A measurement is avoided based on aspects such as reaction time or fine motor skills, since these may be influenced by the effects of the various psychopharmacological treatments used by patients, especially those with DD. The functions assessed and the tests applied are the following:

(a) Cubes (manipulative IQ) and Vocabulary (verbal IQ) from the WAIS-III [79].
(b) Attention. Block of direct digits from the WAIS-III Digit test [79].
(c) Short and long-term verbal declarative memory will be evaluated by the Rey's Verbal Auditory Learning Test (RAVLT).

(d) Executive functions. Trail Making Test (Part A and B) and block of reverse digits from the WAIS-III Digits test for working memory; the Tower of Hanoi in its computerized version of 4 disks for planning and problem resolution; and the Wisconsin Card Sorting Task (WCST, Computerized Wisconsin Card Sort Task Version 4, 2003, Estevez-Gonzalez, Barcelona, Spain) for cognitive flexibility, concept creation, problem solving, inhibition and learning.

Finally, information will be collected with the Prefrontal Symptom Inventory (ISP) [80], consisting of 46 items that evaluate three factors: executive control problems (motivational, control and attention problems), social behavior problems and emotional control problems. This inventory has been validated in an adult clinical population with SUD, and convergence data with neuropsychological measures are also available [81].

Personality characteristics. Two personality questionnaires will be used that have been sensitive to numerous psychopathological disorders, including SUDs, and with positive data also in DD. Both are available in validated Spanish versions with population norms:

(a) Revised Temperament and Character Inventory (TCI-R) [82], based on the 7-factor personality model, consisting of 240 items with a response format on a 5-point Likert scale (1: strongly disagree and 5: totally agree). This considers 4 dimensions of Temperament of greater constitutional weight (Sensation Seeking, Persistence, Reward Dependency and Avoidance of Danger) and 3 of Character determined by more acquired personality aspects (Cooperation, Determination and Transcendence).

(b) Zuckerman-Kuhlman Personality Questionnaire (ZKPQ) [83], based on the Five-Factor Alternative Model and composed of a total of 99 dichotomous items (true–false). The Spanish version will be used, for which there are normative data [84]. The ZKPQ measures the dimensions of Neuroticism-Anxiety (N-Anx), Aggression-Hostility (Agg-Host), Activity (Act), Sociability (Sy) and Impulsivity-Sensation Seeking (ImSS).

3.3. General Procedure

Study 1. Candidates to participate in the study will be added gradually, as they are derived by the psychiatrist or psychologist in the therapeutic team from the clinical centers, who will have briefly explained what the study consists of. The study objective will be explained to all patients at the first visit (inclusion), along with the measurements to be carried out and number of sessions involving their participation. Those who accept will sign an informed consent (tutors in the case of incapacitation) and will be evaluated in the patient's usual care center, preferably in morning sessions (9:00 a.m.–2:00 p.m.).

The collection of epidemiological and clinical information, as well as the application of the instruments, will be carried out by means of an individualized data collection booklet that will be completed either by the experimenter (hetero-application) or by the patient (self-application), depending on the case. Those tests that have a computerized version will be presented and answered on a computer. These are mostly performance tests that the subjects must answer individually. For the completion of the information, 3 individual sessions with the patient will be required, with a variable duration depending on the time it takes to respond but that will not exceed 2.5 h. The breakdown of sessions is presented in Figure 2.

A report of the results will be prepared for the clinical centers, and the return to the patient will be carried out by us or by a professional of the therapeutic team, according to the center's decision.

Study 2. Outpatients of both sexes with a diagnosis of SUD and dual depression who have provided a circadian registry of peripheral temperature with a partial restoration of circadian rhythmicity will be proposed to participate in a chronobiological intervention complementary to the usual treatment. Those patients of both groups who agree to participate (given the link with the centers, a very high affirmative response is expected) will be assigned alternately to the treatment condition (habits and exposure to light) or to the control condition, with only routine treatment and ambulatory evaluations of rhythmic and subjective measures, as well as scheduled visits. The instructions of habits and exposure to natural light that will be stipulated for patients are presented in Box 1.

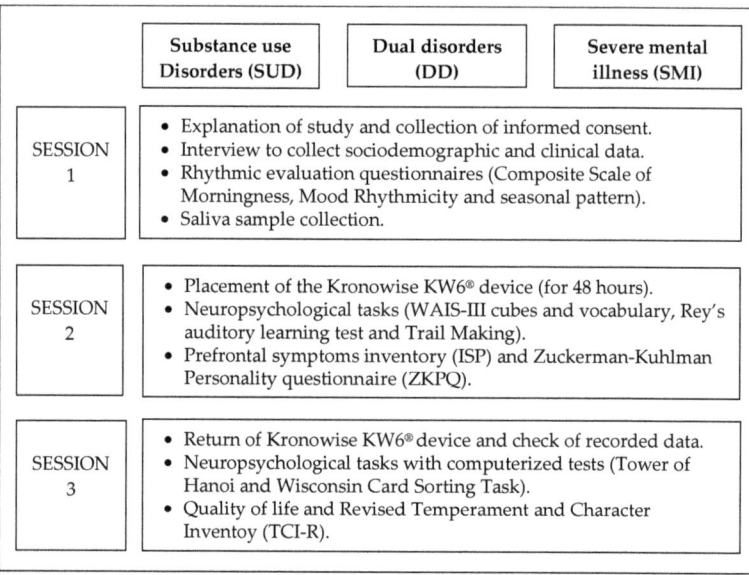

Figure 2. Breakdown of measurements for the sessions in study 1.

Box 1. Instructions of habits and exposure to natural light stipulated for patients assigned to treatment condition in study 2. The text will be printed on a plasticized card that will be delivered on the day of inclusion to the patient so that they have it on hand and can check whenever they want.

Hourly habits:
- Get up before 08:00 a.m. and go to bed no later than 11:00 p.m.
- Sleep schedules will be regular, without changes on weekends or holidays.
- Have breakfast after getting up, lunch before 2:00 p.m. and dinner at about 9:00 p.m. After eating, you can rest, but please avoid falling asleep.
- Avoid bright blue light (electronic devices) one hour before going to sleep.

Daily exposure to natural light:
Go out every day between 9:00 and 11:00 a.m. for a one-hour walk. You can take short rest breaks, but it is better to keep moving and walking while exposed to daylight. Do not wear sunglasses or glasses that darken in contact with light. If weather conditions make it impossible to go outside, place yourself at the time of the walk next to a window with outside light for an hour while doing some activity (for example reading).

The intervention will last two months with the following visits and planned evaluations:
- Visit 1 (inclusion). Explanation of the study differentiated according to the assigned condition and collection of informed consent. Placement of the Kronowise KW6® device that will be worn continuously until the next visit, emphasizing that the patient should register daily the time of getting up, having meals and going to bed. Specification of the rules to be followed in relation to hourly habits and exposure to natural light and delivery of the reminder card for treatment condition. Delivery and collection of the subjective assessment in 8 visual analogue scales (4 of activation and 4 of affective state) to be filled out by the patient each day until the next visit.

- Visit 2 (at 2 weeks of inclusion). Assessment of compliance with the chronobiological approach by the patient and possible adverse effects referred to us (open evaluation). Collection of the Kronowise KW6® device and the visual analogue scales of these first 15 days and delivery of those that will be filled in the next 15 days. Application of the HAM-17 scale in patients with dual depression.
- Visit 3 (at 4 weeks of inclusion). Assessment of compliance with the chronobiological approach by the patient and possible adverse effects referred to us (open evaluation). Collection of visual analogue scale and delivery of those that must be completed until the next visit. Placement of the Kronowise KW6® device that will be worn continuously for a week (it will be delivered on a routine visit to the center after the registration week). Application of the SF-36 to all patients and the HAM-17 scale in dual depression patients.
- Visit 4 (at 8 weeks of inclusion). Assessment of compliance with the chronobiological approach by the patient and possible adverse effects referred to us (open evaluation). Collection of the visual analogue scales and placement of the Kronowise KW6® device that will be worn continuously for a week. Application of the SF-36 to all patients and the HAM-17 scale in dual depression patients.
- Visit 5 (at 9 weeks of inclusion). Assessment of compliance with the chronobiological approach by the patient. Collection of visual analogue scales and Kronowise KW6® device. Recommendation to continue with the approach if the patient is satisfied and his sociolaboral activity allows it.

For the follow-ups at 3 (12 weeks), 6 and 12 months of inclusion, the same information will be collected from the patients in study 1 with a personal visit whenever possible.

Patients who agree to participate will sign a second informed consent that includes, for the intervention condition, the commitment to adhere to the recommendations of daily habits and daily exposure to natural light and to wear the Kronowise KW6® device during the established periods, with specification of the control about their activity both night and day. Patients assigned to the control group will sign another simplified informed consent. Thanks to continuous ambulatory registry, adherence to both the schedules and the daily session of exposure to natural light will be controlled, along with the quantification of the intensity and type of light exposed and duration/intensity of physical exercise throughout the record. This prevents us from requiring the patient to register daily, even for shorter time periods of essential information, such as that collected with sleep diaries.

3.4. Statistical Analysis

The time series obtained from the Kronowise KW6® records, using the Circadianware™ software, will be subjected to a classic rhythmometric analysis with the cosinor method (maximum, minimum, mesor, amplitude, acrophase and % of the rhythm), as well as to an analysis non-parametric (interdaily stability, intraday variability, relative amplitude, etc.). The circadian function index (CFI) is calculated with the average of IS, IV and RA, ranging from 0 (absence of rhythm) to 1 (robust circadian rhythm).

The SNPStats program [85] will be used to calculate allelic and genotypic frequencies, as well as Hardy–Weinberg equilibrium analysis (with an χ^2 test) to explore the association of SNP genotypes, with quantitative measures of the evaluated variables. A corrected linear regression model will be used for age and sex (when applicable). An approach based on the false discovery rate (FDR, q value) will be applied for the correction of multiple statistical tests, using the QVALUE program. The exploration of gene–gene and environment–gene interactions will be carried out with the MDR program and the multilocus genetic profile (MGP) method.

All independent and dependent variables collected in the study will be incorporated through a double entry system in a computer file after conversion of the data involving hours to the centesimal system. In the dependent variables for which population scales are available (i.e., percentiles), these will be considered or Z or T scores will be calculated as appropriate. Descriptive statistics and a complete correlational analysis will be calculated for the different variables considered. Subsequently, different covariance analyses (ANCOVA/MANCOVA) will be carried out for the rhythmic pattern, neuropsychological performance and personality factors, as dependent variables, introducing group (DD, SUD, SMI) as an independent variable and the age as covariate in all cases. The same analyses will be carried out for the SUD and dual depressive patients, incorporating sex as a factor. If the conditions for the analyses are not met, equivalent non-parametric tests will be used. The need to apply Bonferroni correction for multiple comparisons will also be assessed. The consideration of other independent variables to be included as covariates will be determined from the descriptive and correlational analyses (residential/outpatient treatment, age at onset of the disorder, months of abstinence, etc.). All analyses will also be performed comparing only the DD and SMI groups according to the type of mental disorder. For study 2, repeated measures analyses will be carried out with the different temporal measurements and with intervention (treatment and control), diagnosis (SUD and dual depression) and sex as factors, as well as contrasts between groups at each time considered. In all cases, the eta squared partial statistic (η_p^2) will be estimated to measure the effect sizes. Linear or logistic regression models will be carried out, if applicable, that include as predictive variables those present in the clinical history in relation to the measurements made in both studies and, of these, in relation to the information of the follow-ups. The analyses will be carried out with the SPSS/PC+ statistical package (SPSS Inc., Chicago, IL, USA), and the statistical tests will be considered bilaterally, with a type I error established at 5%.

3.5. Management and Collection of Research Data

The protocols for the two studies are in accordance with Spanish legislation (Biomedical Research Law, BOE 4 July 2007, Research on data collection in humans). Our research adheres to the ethical standards of the Declaration of Helsinki [86] and of research in chronobiology [87]. Furthermore, the procedures will be carried out in accordance with international recommendations in the field of ethics of human genetic studies [88]. Participation in the studies does not imply risks for patients, as there are no invasive registries or interventions with known risky side effects.

Data collected from the research group for the Project will be digitized and stored on the University's Microsoft OneDrive for Business. The Microsoft Agreement includes Terms and Conditions that are compliant with EU Data Protection Law and the National Bioethics Committee rules and regulations. Only researchers working for the Project will have access to the data, using their username and passwords to access the files.

4. Discussion

The results of this project can contribute significantly to the knowledge about patients with SUD and DD both at a basic or theoretical level and for intervention and relapse prevention. All the results obtained from the two studies, but especially the relationships between the different variables evaluated (clinical characteristics, genetic polymorphisms, circadian rhythmicity, neurocognitive functioning and personality traits), will represent, in most cases, the first data obtained in the field both at national and international level. The adjuvant chronobiological therapy intervention will be the first study to be carried out with this type of patients and with an objective outpatient evaluation that provides us with information on patient compliance and changes in circadian rhythmicity. The consideration of sex in SUD and dual depression is a pending task due to the non-proportional prevalence of cases in the clinic, which we will carry out in a novel way both at the level of characterization and intervention.

Currently, both SUD and DD are disorders of high prevalence in drug dependence and mental health care worldwide, with difficulties in therapeutic management and with high relapse rates. The search for biomarkers or endophenotypes likely to improve adherence and response to treatment is a relevant pending issue. Furthermore, exploring the option of improving the approach by means of chronobiological strategies will be a pioneering contribution that can be transferred to the clinical setting, as well as being disseminated at a social and media level.

Likewise, our research can provide recommendations in relation to considering aspects that benefit the evaluation and diagnosis protocols and/or the convenience of incorporating some strategies in the therapeutic management of patients (i.e., cognitive rehabilitation), including the sex dimension. We also hope to delimit some cost-effective markers of adherence, prognosis and risk of relapse, as well as the existence of rhythmic characteristics in combination with modifiable genetic polymorphisms in case they are found to be altered. With all this, the present research will result in a contribution in line with the general objectives proposed by the WHO for mental illnesses [89] and specifically in the clinical management of patients with addiction and DD [90]. Finally, the proposed intervention, if it proves to be useful, will be the first work carried out worldwide with a potential clinical sample (SUD and dual depression) that could unquestionably benefit from it.

From a social-impact point of view, since the Nobel medicine/physiology award of 2017 (Jeffrey C. Hall, Michael Rosbash and Michael W. Young) for research on the molecular mechanisms that control circadian rhythms, media interest in chronobiology has notably increased. DD is a health issue to which the media are beginning to be sensitive, especially promoted by the debate on the legal situation of cannabis and the coexistence of psychotic disorders among its consumers. The media have also recently echoed the impact that the coronavirus pandemic has generated on consumption patterns and increases in SUD. The dissemination of the results of study 1 will make visible the high presence of psychiatric comorbidity in SUD, as well as its personal and social impact, together with recommendations based on useful markers in clinical management. The data from the chronobiological intervention, if positive results are obtained, will undoubtedly be likely to be disseminated not only in our country but internationally.

Author Contributions: Conceptualization, A.A.; methodology, A.A. and J.F.N.; funding acquisition, A.A.; writing—review and editing, all authors. All authors have read and agreed to the published version of the manuscript.

Funding: This research was funded by the grant PID2020-117767GB-I00 of the Spanish Ministry of Science and Innovation (MCIN/AEI/10.13039/501100011033), the Generalitat of Catalunya (2017SGR-748) and by Consejería de Economía, Innovación, Ciencia y Empleo, Junta de Andalucía, Spain (Group CTS-195).

Institutional Review Board Statement: The study will be conducted according to the guidelines of the Declaration of Helsinki and was approved by Ethics Committee of the University of Barcelona (IRB00003099).

Informed Consent Statement: Informed consent will be obtained from all subjects involved in the two studies.

Conflicts of Interest: The authors declare no conflict of interest.

References

1. Adan, A.; Torrens, M. Special Issue: Diagnosis and management of addiction and other mental disorders (dual disorders). *J. Clin. Med.* **2021**, *10*, 1307. [CrossRef] [PubMed]
2. Hunt, S.E.; Large, M.M.; Cleary, M.; Lai, H.M.X.; Saunders, J.B. Prevalence of comorbid substance use in schizophrenia spectrum disorders in community and clinical settings, 1990–2017: Systematic review and meta-analysis. *Drug Alcohol Depend.* **2018**, *191*, 234–258. [CrossRef] [PubMed]
3. Xiong Lai, H.M.; Cleary, M.; Sitharthan, T.; Hunt, S.E. Prevalence of comorbid substance use, anxiety and mood disorders in epidemiological surveys, 1990–2014: Systematic review and meta-analysis. *Drug Alcohol Dep.* **2015**, *154*, 1–13.
4. Arias, F.; Szerman, N.; Vega, P.; Meias, B.; Basurte, I.; Morant, C.; Ochoa, E.; Poyo, F.; Babín, F. Madrid study on the prevalence and characteristics of outpatients with dual pathology in community mental health and substance misuse services. *Adicciones* **2013**, *25*, 118–127. [CrossRef] [PubMed]
5. European Monitoring Centre for Drug and Drug Addiction. *Comorbidity of Substance Use and Mental Disorders in Europe, EMCDDA Insights*; Publications Office of the European Union: Luxemburg, 2019.
6. Olivares, J.M.; Sermon, J.; Hemels, M.; Schreiner, A. Definitions and drivers of relapse in patients with schizophrenia: A systematic literature review. *Ann. Gen. Psychiatry* **2013**, *12*, 32. [CrossRef] [PubMed]

7. Marquez-Arrico, J.E.; Río-Martínez, L.; Navarro, J.F.; Prat, G.; Adan, A. Personality profile and clinical correlates of patients with substance use disorder with and without comorbid depression under treatment. *Front. Psychiatry* **2019**, *9*, 764. [CrossRef]
8. Marquez-Arrico, J.E.; Navarro, J.F.; Adan, A. Health-Related Quality of Life in male patients under treatment for substance use disorders with and without major depressive disorder: Influence in clinical course at one-year Follow-up. *J. Clin. Med.* **2020**, *9*, 3110. [CrossRef] [PubMed]
9. Torrens, M.; Mestre-Pintó, J.I.; Montanari, L.; Vicente, J.; Domingo-Salvany, A. Patología dual: Una perspectiva europea. *Adicciones* **2017**, *29*, 3–5. [CrossRef] [PubMed]
10. Rosenwasser, A.M. Circadian clock genes: Non-circadian roles in sleep, addiction, and psychiatric disorders? *Neurosci. Biobehav. Rev.* **2010**, *34*, 1249–1255. [CrossRef] [PubMed]
11. Carpenter, J.S.; Robillard, R.; Hermens, D.F.; Naismith, S.L.; Gordon, C.; Scott, E.M.; Hickie, I.B. Sleep-wake profiles and circadian rhythms of core temperature and melatonin in young people with affective disorders. *J. Psychiatry Res.* **2017**, *94*, 131–138. [CrossRef] [PubMed]
12. Zaki, N.F.W.; Spence, D.W.; BaHammam, A.S.; Pandi-Perumal, S.R.; Cardinali, D.P.; Brown, G.M. Chronobiological theories of mood disorders. *Eur. Arch. Psychiatry Clin. Neurosci.* **2018**, *268*, 107–118. [CrossRef] [PubMed]
13. Lewy, A.J.; Lefler, B.J.; Emens, J.S.; Bauer, V.K. The circadian basis of winter depression. *Proc. Natl. Acad. Sci. USA* **2006**, *103*, 7414–7419. [CrossRef]
14. Lunsford-Avery, J.R.; da Silva, B.; Brietzke, E.; Bressan, R.A.; Gadelha, A.; Auerbach, R.P.; Mittal, V.A. Adolescents at clinical-high risk for Psychosis: Circadian rhythm disturbances predict worsened prognosis at 1-year follow-up. *Schizophr. Res.* **2017**, *189*, 37–42. [CrossRef] [PubMed]
15. Carpenter, J.S.; Abelmann, A.C.; Hatton, S.E.; Robillard, R.; Hermens, D.F.; Bennet, M.R.; Logopoulos, J.; Hickie, I.B. Pineal volume and evening melatonin in young people with affective disorders. *Brain Imaging Behav.* **2017**, *11*, 1741–1750. [CrossRef] [PubMed]
16. Webb, I.C. Circadian rhythms and substance abuse: Chronobiological considerations for the treatment of addiction. *Curr. Psychiatry Rep.* **2017**, *19*, 12. [CrossRef] [PubMed]
17. Robillard, R.; Hermens, D.F.; Naismith, S.L.; White, D.; Rogers, N.L.; Ip, T.K.Y.; Mullin, S.J.; Alvares, G.A.; Guastella, A.J.; Smith, K.L.; et al. Ambulatory sleep-wake patterns and variability in young people with emerging mental disorders. *J. Psychiatry Neurosci.* **2015**, *40*, 28–37. [CrossRef]
18. DePoy, L.M.; McClung, C.A.; Logan, R.W. Neural mechanisms of circadian regulation of neural and drug reward. *Neural Plast.* **2017**, *2017*, 5720842. [CrossRef] [PubMed]
19. Logan, R.W.; Hasler, B.P.; Forbes, E.E.; Franzen, P.L.; Torregrossa, M.M.; Huang, Y.H.; Buysse, D.J.; Clark, D.B.; McClung, C.A. Impact of sleep and circadian rhythms on addiction vulnerability in adolescents. *Biol. Psychiatry* **2018**, *83*, 987–996. [CrossRef]
20. Martínez-Nicolás, A.; Madrid, J.A.; García, F.J.; Campos, M.; Moreno-Casbas, M.T.; Almaida-Pagán, P.F.; Lucas-Sánchez, A.; Rol, M.A. Circadian monitoring as an aging predictor. *Sci. Rep.* **2018**, *8*, 15027. [CrossRef]
21. Capella, M.M.; Martinez-Nicolas, A.; Adan, A. Circadian rhythmic characteristics in men with substance use disorder under treatment. Influence of age of onset and duration of abstinence. *Front. Psychiatry* **2018**, *9*, 373. [CrossRef]
22. Antúnez, J.M.; Capella, M.M.; Navarro, J.F.; Adan, A. Circadian rhythmicity in substance use disorder male patients with and without comorbid depression under ambulatory and therapeutic community treatment. *Chronobiol. Int.* **2016**, *33*, 1410–1421. [CrossRef] [PubMed]
23. Borbély, A.A.; Daan, S.; Wirs-Justice, A.; Deboer, T. The two-process model of sleep regulation: A reappraisal. *J. Sleep Res.* **2016**, *25*, 131–143. [CrossRef] [PubMed]
24. Mitropoulos, K.; Al Jaibeji, H.; Forero, D.A.; Laissue, P.; Wonkam, A.; Lopez-Correa, C.; Mohamed, Z.; Chantratita, W.; Lee, M.T.; Llerena, A.; et al. Success stories in genomic medicine from resource-limited countries. *Hum. Genom.* **2015**, *18*, 11. [CrossRef] [PubMed]
25. Kim, M.; de la Peña, J.B.; Cheong, J.H.; Kim, H.J. Neurobiological functions of the period circadian clock 2 gene (*Per2*). *Biomol. Ther.* **2018**, *26*, 358–367. [CrossRef]
26. Archer, S.N.; Schmidt, C.; Vandewalle, G.; Dijk, D.-J. Phenotyping of PER3 variants reveals widespread effects on circadian preference, sleep regulation, and health. *Sleep Med. Rev.* **2018**, *40*, 109–126. [CrossRef]
27. Ojeda, D.A.; Perea, C.S.; Niño, C.L.; Gutiérrez, R.M.; López-León, S.; Arboleda, H.; Camargo, A.; Adan, A.; Forero, D.A. A novel association of two non-synonymous polymorphisms in Per2 and Per3 genes with specific diurnal preference subscales. *Neurosci. Lett.* **2013**, *553*, 52–56. [CrossRef]
28. Losenkov, I.S.; Mulder, N.J.; Levchul, L.A.; Vyalova, N.M.; Looenen, A.J.M.; Bosker, F.J.; Simutkin, G.G.; Boiko, A.S.; Bokhan, N.A.; Wilffert, B.; et al. Association between BDNF gene variant Rs6265 and the severity of depression in antidepressant treatment-free depressed patients. *Front. Psychiatry* **2020**, *11*, 38. [CrossRef]
29. Nieto, R.R.; Carrasco, A.; Corral, S.; Castillo, R.; Gaspar, P.A.; Bustamante, M.L.; Silva, H. BDNF as a biomarker of cognition in schizophrenia/psychosis: An updated review. *Front. Psychiatry* **2021**, *12*, 662407. [CrossRef]
30. Cheah, S.-Y.; Lawford, B.R.; Young, R.M.; Connor, J.P.; Morris, C.P.; Voisey, J. BDNF SNPs are implicated in comorbid alcohol dependence in schizophrenia but not in alcohol-dependent patients without schizophrenia. *Alcohol Alcohol.* **2014**, *49*, 491–497. [CrossRef]

31. González-Castro, T.E.; Tovilla-Zárate, C.A.; Hernández-Díaz, Y.; Fresán, A.; Juarez-Rojop, I.E.; Ble-Castillo, J.; López-Narváez, L.; Genis, A.; Hernández-Alvarado, M.M. No association between ApoE and schizophrenia: Evidence of systematic review and updated meta-analysis. *Schizophr. Res.* **2015**, *169*, 355–368. [CrossRef]
32. Ojeda, D.A.; Niño, C.L.; López-León, S.; Camargo, A.; Adan, A.; Forero, D.A. A functional polymorphism in the promoter region of MAOA gene is associated with sleepiness in healthy subjects. *J. Neurol. Sci.* **2014**, *337*, 176–179. [CrossRef] [PubMed]
33. Ursic, K.; Zupanc, T.; Paska, A.V. Analysis of promotor polymorphism in monoamine oxidase A (MAOA) gene in completed suicide on Slovenian population. *Neurosci. Lett.* **2018**, *673*, 111–115. [CrossRef] [PubMed]
34. Martinez-Arán, A.; Vieta, E. Cognition as a target in schizophrenia, bipolar disorder and depression. *Eur. Neuropsychopharmacol.* **2015**, *25*, 151–157. [CrossRef] [PubMed]
35. Volkow, N.D.; Koob, G.; McLellan, A.T. Neurobiological advances from the brain disease model of addiction. *N. Engl. J. Med.* **2016**, *374*, 363–371. [CrossRef]
36. Schmidt, T.P.; Pennington, D.L.; Cardoos, S.L.; Durazzo, T.C.; Meyerhoff, D.J. Neurocognition and inhibitory control in polysubstance use disorders: Comparison with alcohol use disorders and changes in abstinence. *J. Clin. Exp. Neuropsychol.* **2017**, *39*, 22–34. [CrossRef]
37. Wobrock, T.; Falkai, P.; Schneider-Axmann, T.; Hasan, A.; Derks, E.M.; Boter, H.; Rybakovski, J.K.; Libiger, J.; Dollfus, S.; López-Ibor, J.J.; et al. Comorbid substance abuse in first-episode schizophrenia: Effects on cognition and psychopathology in the EUFEST study. *Schizophr. Res.* **2013**, *147*, 132–139. [CrossRef]
38. Duijkers, J.; Vissers, C.; Egger, J. Unraveling executive funtioning in dual diagnosis. *Front. Psychol.* **2016**, *7*, 974. [CrossRef]
39. Hunt, S.A.; Kay-Lambkin, F.J.; Baker, A.L.; Michie, P.T. Systematic review of neurocognition in people with co-occurring alcohol misuse and depression. *J. Affect. Disord.* **2015**, *179*, 51–64. [CrossRef]
40. Capella, M.M.; Benaiges, I.; Adan, A. Neuropsychological performance in polyconsumer men under treatment. Influence of age of onset of substance use. *Sci. Rep.* **2015**, *5*, 12038. [CrossRef]
41. Benaiges, I.; Serra-Grabulosa, J.M.; Adan, A. Neuropsychological functioning and age-related changes in schizophrenia and/or cocaine dependence. *Prog. Neuropsychopharm. Biol. Psychiatry* **2013**, *40*, 298–305. [CrossRef]
42. Benaiges, I.; Serra-Grabulosa, J.M.; Prat, G.; Adan, A. Executive functioning in individuals with schizophrenia and/or cocaine dependence. *Hum. Psychopharmacol. Clin. Exp.* **2013**, *28*, 29–39. [CrossRef]
43. Adan, A.; Arredondo, A.Y.; Capella, M.M.; Prat, G.; Forero, D.; Navarro, J.F. Neurobiological underpinnings and modulating factors in psychotic disorders with a comorbid substance use disorder: A systematic review. *Neurosci. Biobehav. Rev.* **2017**, *75*, 361–377. [CrossRef] [PubMed]
44. Adan, A.; Capella, M.M.; Prat, G.; Forero, D.A.; López-Vera, S.; Navarro, J.F. Executive functioning in males with schizophrenia and substance use disorders. Influence of lifetime suicide attempts. *PLoS ONE* **2017**, *12*, e0169943. [CrossRef]
45. Marquez-Arrico, J.E.; López-Vera, S.; Prat, G.; Adan, A. Temperament and character dimensions in male patients with substance use disorders: Differences relating to psychiatric comorbidity. *Psychiatry Res.* **2016**, *237*, 1–8. [CrossRef] [PubMed]
46. Fernández-Mondragon, S.; Adan, A. Personality in male patients with substance use disorder and/or severe mental illness. *Psychiatry Res.* **2015**, *228*, 488–494. [CrossRef] [PubMed]
47. Adan, A.; Archer, S.N.; Hidalgo, M.P.; Di Milia, L.; Natale, V.; Randler, C. Circadian typology: A comprehensive review. *Chronobiol. Int.* **2012**, *29*, 1153–1175. [CrossRef]
48. Marquez-Arrico, J.E.; Adan, A. Personality in patients with substance use disorders according to the co-occurring severe mental illness: A study using the Alternative Five Factor Model. *Pers. Individ. Differ.* **2016**, *97*, 76–81. [CrossRef]
49. Conrod, P.J. Personality-targeted interventions for substance use and misuse. *Curr. Addict. Rep.* **2016**, *3*, 426–436. [CrossRef]
50. Szerman, N.; Peris, L. Precision psychiatry and dual disorders. *J. Dual Diagn.* **2019**, *14*, 237–246. [CrossRef] [PubMed]
51. Haynes, P.L.; Gengler, D.; Kelly, M. Social rhythm therapies for mood disorders: An update. *Curr. Psychiatry Rep.* **2016**, *18*, 75. [CrossRef]
52. Wirz-Justice, A.; Graw, P.; Kräuchi, K.; Sarrafzadeh, A.; English, J.; Arend, J.; Sand, L. "Natural" light treatment of seasonal affective disorder. *J. Affect. Disord.* **1996**, *37*, 109–120. [CrossRef]
53. Kripke, D.F. A breakthrouggh treatment for major depression. *J. Clin. Psychiatry* **2015**, *76*, e661. [CrossRef] [PubMed]
54. van Maanen, A.; Meijer, A.M.; van der Heijen, K.B.; Oort, F.J. The effects of light therapy on sleep problems: A systematic review and meta-analysis. *Sleep Med. Rev.* **2016**, *29*, 52–62. [CrossRef] [PubMed]
55. Al-Karawi, D.; Jubair, L. Bright light therapy for nonseasonal depression: Meta-analysis of clinical trials. *J. Affect. Disord.* **2016**, *198*, 64–71. [CrossRef]
56. Lam, R.W.; Levitt, A.J.; Levitan, R.D.; Michalak, E.E.; Cheung, A.H.; Morehouse, R.; Ramasubbu, R.; Yatham, L.N.; Tam, E.M. Efficacy of bright light treatment, fluoxetine, and the combination in patients with nonseasonal major depressive disorder: A randomized clinical trial. *JAMA Psychiatry* **2016**, *73*, 56–63. [CrossRef]
57. Levitan, R.D.; Levitt, A.J.; Michalak, E.E.; Morehouse, R.; Ramasubbu, R.; Yatman, L.N.; Tam, E.M.; Lam, R.W. Apetitive symptoms differentially predict treatment response to fluoxetine, light, and placebo in nonseasonal major depression. *J. Clin. Psychiatry* **2018**, *79*, 17m11856. [CrossRef]
58. Xu, Q.; Lang, C.P. Revisiting the alerting effects of light: A systematic review. *Sleep Med. Rev.* **2018**, *41*, 39–49. [CrossRef]
59. Cañellas, F.; Mestre, L.; Belber, M.; Fronters, G.; Rey, M.A.; Rial, R. Increased daylight availability reduces length of hospitalisation in depressive patients. *Eur. Arch. Psychiatry Clin. Neurosci.* **2016**, *266*, 277–280. [CrossRef]

60. Gbyl, K.; Østergaard Madsen, H.; Dunker Svendsen, S.; Petersen, P.M.; Hageman, I.; Volf, C.; Martiny, K. Depressed patients hospitalized in southeast-facing rooms are discharged earlier than patients in northwest-facing rooms. *Neuropsychobiology* **2016**, *74*, 193–201. [CrossRef]
61. Tekieh, T.; Lockley, S.W.; Robinson, P.A.; McCloskey, S.; Zobaer, M.S.; Postnova, S. Modeling melanopsin mediated effects of light on circadian phase, melatonin suppression, and subjective sleepiness. *J. Pineal Res.* **2020**, *69*, e12681. [CrossRef]
62. Siporin, S. Lighting the darkness of addiction: Can phototherapy enhance contingence-management-based treatment of substance-related and addictive disorders? *J. Addict. Nurs.* **2014**, *25*, 197–203. [CrossRef]
63. Serrano-Serrano, A.; Márquez-Arrico, J.E.; Navarro, J.F.; Martinez-Nicolas, A.; Adan, A. Circadian characteristics in patients under treatment for substance use disorders and severe mental illness (schizophrenia, major depression and bipolar disorder). *J. Clin. Med.* **2021**, *10*, 4388. [CrossRef] [PubMed]
64. Martinez-Nicolas, A.; Martinez-Madrid, M.J.; Almaida-Pagan, P.F.; Bonmati-Carrion, M.A.; Madrid, J.A.; Rol, M.A. Assessing chronotypes by ambulatory circadian monitoring. *Front. Physiol.* **2019**, *10*, 1396. [CrossRef]
65. American Psychiatric Association. *Diagnostic and Statistical Manual of Mental Disorders*, 5th ed.; American Psychiatric Publishing: Washington, DC, USA, 2013; ISBN 9780890425541.
66. Ware, J.E.; Sherbourne, C.D. The MOS 36-item short-form health survey (SF-36). *Med. Care* **1992**, *30*, 473–483. [CrossRef]
67. Hasin, D.S.; Trautman, K.D.; Miele, G.M.; Samet, S.; Smith, M.; Endicott, J. *Psychiatric Research Interview for Substance and Mental Disorders for DSM-5 (PRISM-5)*; Department of Psychiatry, Columbia University: New York, NY, USA, 2021.
68. Gálvez, B.P.; Fernández, L.G. Validación española del Drug Abuse Screening Test (DAST-20 y DAST-10). *Health Addict.* **2010**, *10*, 35–50.
69. Hamilton, M. A rating scale for depression. *J. Neurol. Neurosurg. Psychiatry* **1960**, *23*, 56–62. [CrossRef]
70. Peralta, V.; Cuesta, M.J. Validación de la escala de los síndromes positivo y negativo (PANSS) en una muestra de esquizofrénicos españoles. *Actas Luso-Españolas Neurol. Psiquiatr. Cienc. Afines* **1994**, *22*, 171–177.
71. Plutchik, R.; van Praag, H.M.; Conte, H.R.; Picard, S. Correlates of suicide and violence risk 1: The suicide risk measure. *Compr. Psychiatry* **1989**, *30*, 296–302. [CrossRef]
72. Bonmati-Carrion, M.A.; Middleton, B.; Revell, V.; Skene, D.J.; Rol, M.A.; Madrid, J.A. Circadian phase assessment by ambulatory monitoring in humans: Correlation with dim light melatonin onset. *Chronobiol. Int.* **2014**, *31*, 37–51. [CrossRef] [PubMed]
73. Afid, I.J.; Farkhan, M.; Kurdi, O.; Maula, M.I.; Ammarullah, M.I.; Setiyana, B.; Jamari, J.; Winarni, T.I. Effect of short-term deep-pressure portable seat on behavioral and biological stress in children with autism spectrum disorders: A pilot study. *Bioengineering* **2022**, *9*, 48.
74. Maula, M.I.; Aji, A.L.; Aliyafi, M.B.; Afid, I.J.; Ammurallah, M.I.; Winarni, T.I.; Jamari, J. The subjective comfort test of autism hug machine portable seat. *J. Intellect. Disabil. Diagn. Treat.* **2021**, *9*, 182–188. [CrossRef]
75. Adan, A.; Caci, H.; Prat, G. Reliability of the Spanish version of the Composite Scale of Morningness. *Eur. Psychiatry* **2005**, *20*, 503–509. [CrossRef] [PubMed]
76. Carissimi, A.; Oliveira, M.; Frey, B.N.; Navarro, J.F.; Hidalgo, M.P.; Adan, A. Validation and psychometric properties of the Spanish Mood Rhythm Instrument. *Biol. Rhythm Res.* **2022**, in press. [CrossRef]
77. Adan, A.; Natale, V.; Fabbri, M. Propiedades psicométricas de la versión castellana del cuestionario de evaluación de patrón estacional (Seasonal Pattern Assessment Questionnaire, SPAQ). *Rev. Latinoam. Psicol.* **2006**, *38*, 59–69.
78. Monk, T.H. A visual analogue scale technique to measure global vigor and affect. *Psychiatry Res.* **1989**, *27*, 89–99. [CrossRef]
79. Wechsler, D. WAIS-III. In *Escala de Inteligencia Para Adultos de Wechsler*, 3rd ed.; TEA Ediciones: Madrid, Spain, 2001.
80. Ruiz-Sánchez de León, J.M.; Pedrero-Pérez, E.J.; Lozoya-Delgado, P.; Llanero-Luque, M.; Rojo-Mota, G.; Puerta-García, C. Inventario de síntomas frontales para la evaluación clínica de las adicciones en la vida diaria: Proceso de creación y propiedades psicométricas. *Rev. Neurol.* **2012**, *54*, 649–663.
81. Pedrero-Pérez, E.J.; Ruiz-Sánchez de León, J.M.; Rojo-Mota, G.; Morales-Alonso, S.; Pedrero-Aguilar, J.; Lorenzo-Luque, I.; González-Sánchez, A. Inventario de síntomas prefrontales (ISP): Validez ecológica y convergencia con medidas neuropsicológicas. *Rev. Neurol.* **2016**, *63*, 241–251. [CrossRef]
82. Cloninger, C.R. *The Temperament and Character Inventory-Revised*; Center for Psychobiology of the Personality, Washington University: St. Louis, MO, USA, 1999.
83. Zuckerman, M.; Kuhlman, D.M.; Joireman, J.; Teta, P.; Kraft, M.A. comparison of three structural models for personality: The Big Three, the Big Five, and the Alternative Five. *J. Personality Soc. Psychol.* **1993**, *65*, 757–768. [CrossRef]
84. Gomá-Freixenet, M.; Valero, S. Spanish normative data of the Zuckerman-Kuhlman Personality Questionnaire in a general population sample. *Psicothema* **2008**, *20*, 324–330.
85. Sole, X.; Guino, E.; Valls, J.; Iniesta, R.; Moreno, V. SNPStats: A web tool for the analysis of association studies. *Bioinformatics* **2006**, *22*, 1928–1929. [CrossRef]
86. World Medical Association WMA declaration of Helsinki: Ethical principles for medical research involving human subjects. *JAMA* **2013**, *310*, 2191–2194. [CrossRef] [PubMed]
87. Portaluppi, F.; Smolensky, M.H.; Touitou, Y. Ethics and methods for biological rhythm research on animals and human beings. *Chronobiol. Int.* **2010**, *27*, 1911–1929. [CrossRef]
88. Beskow, L.M.; Burke, W.; Merz, J.F.; Barr, P.A.; Terry, S.; Penchaszadeh, V.B.; Gostin, L.O.; Gwinn, M.; Khoury, M.J. Informed consent for population-based research involving genetics. *JAMA* **2001**, *286*, 2315–2321. [CrossRef] [PubMed]

89. World Health Organization. *Comprehensive Mental Health Action Plan 2013–2030*; World Health Organization: Geneva, Swizerland, 2021; Available online: https://www.who.int/publications/i/item/9789240031029 (accessed on 21 March 2022).
90. Volkow, N.D.; Torrens, M.; Poznyak, V.; Sáenz, E.; Busse, A.; Kashino, W.; Krupchanka, D.; Kestel, D.; Campello, G.; Gerra, G. Managing dual disorders: A statement by the Informal Scientific Network, UN Commission on Narcotic Drugs. *World Psychiatry* **2020**, *19*, 396–397. [CrossRef] [PubMed]

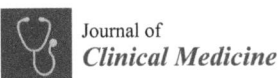

Article

Exploring the Association between Gambling-Related Offenses, Substance Use, Psychiatric Comorbidities, and Treatment Outcome

Cristina Vintró-Alcaraz [1,2,3,†], Gemma Mestre-Bach [4,†], Roser Granero [2,3,5], Elena Caravaca [1], Mónica Gómez-Peña [1,3], Laura Moragas [1,3], Isabel Baenas [1,2,3], Amparo del Pino-Gutiérrez [1,2,3,6], Susana Valero-Solís [1,3], Milagros Lara-Huallipe [1,3], Bernat Mora-Maltas [1,3], Eduardo Valenciano-Mendoza [1,3], Elías Guillen-Guzmán [3,7], Ester Codina [1,3], José M. Menchón [1,8,9], Fernando Fernández-Aranda [1,2,3,9,*] and Susana Jiménez-Murcia [1,2,3,9,*]

1. Department of Psychiatry, Bellvitge University Hospital-Bellvitge Biomedical Research Institute (IDIBELL), 08907 Barcelona, Spain
2. Centro de Investigación Biomédica en Red Fisiopatología Obesidad y Nutrición (CIBERObn), Instituto de Salud Carlos III, 28029 Madrid, Spain
3. Psychoneurobiology of Eating and Addictive Behaviors Group, Neurosciences Programme, Bellvitge Biomedical Research Institute (IDIBELL), 08908 Barcelona, Spain
4. Facultad de Ciencias de la Salud, Universidad Internacional de La Rioja, 26006 La Rioja, Spain
5. Departament de Psicobiologia i Metodologia de les Ciències de la Salut, Universitat Autònoma de Barcelona, 08193 Barcelona, Spain
6. Department of Public Health, Mental Health and Mother-Infant Nursing, School of Nursing, University of Barcelona, 08907 Barcelona, Spain
7. Department of Child and Adolescent Psychiatry and Psychology, Institute of Neurosciences, Hospital Clinic Barcelona, 08036 Barcelona, Spain
8. Centro de Investigación Biomédica en Red Salud Mental (CIBERSAM), Instituto de Salud Carlos III, 08907 Barcelona, Spain
9. Department of Clinical Sciences, School of Medicine and Health Sciences, University of Barcelona, 08907 Barcelona, Spain
* Correspondence: ffernandez@bellvitgehospital.cat (F.F.-A.); sjimenez@bellvitgehospital.cat (S.J.-M.)
† These authors contributed equally to this work.

Abstract: Several studies have explored the association between gambling disorder (GD) and gambling-related crimes. However, it is still unclear how the commission of these offenses influences treatment outcomes. In this longitudinal study we sought: (1) to explore sociodemographic and clinical differences (e.g., psychiatric comorbidities) between individuals with GD who had committed gambling-related illegal acts (differentiating into those who had had legal consequences ($n = 31$) and those who had not ($n = 55$)), and patients with GD who had not committed crimes ($n = 85$); and (2) to compare the treatment outcome of these three groups, considering dropouts and relapses. Several sociodemographic and clinical variables were assessed, including the presence of substance use, and comorbid mental disorders. Patients received 16 sessions of cognitive-behavioral therapy. Patients who reported an absence of gambling-related illegal behavior were older, and showed the lowest GD severity, the most functional psychopathological state, the lowest impulsivity levels, and a more adaptive personality profile. Patients who had committed offenses with legal consequences presented the highest risk of dropout and relapses, higher number of psychological symptoms, higher likelihood of any other mental disorders, and greater prevalence of tobacco and illegal drugs use. Our findings uphold that patients who have committed gambling-related offenses show a more complex clinical profile that may interfere with their adherence to treatment.

Keywords: gambling disorder; gambling-related offenses; dropout; relapse; psychopathology; personality; substance use; psychiatric comorbidity; impulsivity

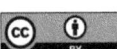

Citation: Vintró-Alcaraz, C.; Mestre-Bach, G.; Granero, R.; Caravaca, E.; Gómez-Peña, M.; Moragas, L.; Baenas, I.; del Pino-Gutiérrez, A.; Valero-Solís, S.; Lara-Huallipe, M.; et al. Exploring the Association between Gambling-Related Offenses, Substance Use, Psychiatric Comorbidities, and Treatment Outcome. *J. Clin. Med.* 2022, *11*, 4669. https://doi.org/10.3390/jcm11164669

Academic Editors: Ana Adan and Marta Torrens

Received: 5 July 2022
Accepted: 3 August 2022
Published: 10 August 2022

Publisher's Note: MDPI stays neutral with regard to jurisdictional claims in published maps and institutional affiliations.

Copyright: © 2022 by the authors. Licensee MDPI, Basel, Switzerland. This article is an open access article distributed under the terms and conditions of the Creative Commons Attribution (CC BY) license (https://creativecommons.org/licenses/by/4.0/).

1. Introduction

Gambling disorder (GD) is a psychiatric disorder characterized by recurrent and persistent problematic gambling behavior often associated with certain personality traits, cognitive distortions, and co-occurring psychopathology [1,2]. Moreover, GD, similar to other addictions, is characterized by cognitive deficits and alterations in underlying neurobiological mechanisms mainly related to impulsivity, compulsivity, reward/punishment processing, and decision-making [3,4]. GD is leading to clinically significant distress and usually also leads to relevant financial problems [5], which in some cases has been increased in the context of the COVID-19 pandemic [6].

Financial problems arising from GD can lead to the commission of illegal acts, although there is no consensus about the specific causality of this association [7]. Gambling-related crimes are usually committed for two specific purposes: (1) to obtain money to finance the gambling behavior and/or (2) to recoup financial shortfalls resulting from the gambling behavior [8]. Usually, non-violent, income-producing, and property-related offenses are carried out, such as fraud, robbery, forgery, and theft [9,10].

The commission of gambling-related offenses was contemplated as a diagnostic criterion in previous versions of the Diagnostic and Statistical Manual of Mental Disorders (DSM), although in the latest version, the DSM-5 [1], this criterion was eliminated since many authors considered it to be a criterion associated with the severity of the GD, rather than a diagnostic criterion itself [11,12]. Although it is not currently considered a diagnostic criterion, it remains a relevant clinical criterion [13], and numerous research studies have been conducted to explore reasons for which not all individuals engage in gambling-related offenses. Distinct clinical and sociodemographic differences have been identified between individuals with GD who commit illegal acts and those who do not. Some authors have found that committing gambling-related crimes was associated, at the sociodemographic level, with younger age, lower income, and being unemployed [14,15]. At the clinical level, crimes have been linked with greater psychopathology and impulsivity levels, higher GD severity (associated, in turn, with an increased risk of criminal recidivism), earlier GD onset, greater gambling-related debts, and longer duration of the disorder [14,16–20]. In addition, it has been suggested that gambling-related offenses may be a mediating factor between personality traits (such as novelty seeking, for instance) and GD severity [21].

Therefore, those individuals with GD who commit gambling-related illegal behaviors show a clinical profile characterized by a greater severity, which could interfere with GD treatment outcomes. In addition, it has been suggested that substance use and psychiatric comorbidities (e.g., depression, anxiety, and attention-deficit/hyperactivity disorder) may mediate the association between illegal acts and GD [15,22,23].

Ledgerwood et al. [24] observed that those patients with GD who had committed crimes maintained a higher GD severity throughout the cognitive-behavioral treatment (CBT), compared to those who had not committed crimes. However, the treatment outcome of these specific patients has scarcely been explored. Likewise, the commission of offenses, and the specific role of substance use and psychiatric comorbidities have not been explored in depth and there is a paucity of studies that distinguish between those crimes that have entailed legal consequences and those cases where gamblers escaped detection or charge [8]. To address these relevant empirical limitations, the present longitudinal study had two central objectives: (1) to explore sociodemographic and clinical differences between individuals with GD who had committed gambling-related illegal acts (differentiating into those that had had legal consequences and those that had not, and also exploring substance use and psychiatric comorbidities), and patients with GD who had not committed crimes; and (2) to compare the treatment outcome of these three groups, considering dropouts and relapses. We hypothesized that, of the three groups, patients with GD who had committed gambling-related crimes with legal consequences would present a more impaired clinical profile and, consequently, a worse response to treatment.

2. Materials and Methods

2.1. Participants and Procedure

The sample consisted of 117 consecutive treatment-seeking patients with GD. They were recruited between April 2017 and May 2018 at the Behavioral Addictions Unit within the Department of Psychiatry, at a Spanish University Hospital. They were referred through general practitioners or via other health professionals, such as mental health institutions.

Two face-to-face clinical interviews were conducted by experienced psychologists and psychiatrists before a diagnosis was given. The inclusion criteria were: (1) adult participants (18 years old or more); (b) both genders; (c) sufficient proficiency in Spanish to understand the assessment; and (d) patients who sought treatment for GD as their primary mental health concern and who met DSM criteria for GD. Exclusion criteria included the presence of (1) intellectual disability; (2) an organic mental disorder; (3) a neurodegenerative condition; or (4) an active psychotic disorder. Additional sociodemographic and clinical information was taken through self-report instruments and a specific face-to-face interview was done individually to explore gambling-related illegal acts before initiating outpatient treatment. Participants were classified into three different groups according to their criminal behavior: patients with no history of gambling-related illegal acts (n = 85; Illegal−), patients with a history of gambling-related illegal acts without legal repercussions (n = 55; Illegal + Cons−), and patients who had committed gambling-related illegal acts that had legal consequences (n = 31; Illegal + Cons+). This classification has already been used in previous studies [25]. Only those patients who reported illegal acts on both DSM-IV-TR criterion 8 [26] and the clinical interview were included in the illegal acts groups.

2.2. Treatment

The CBT group treatment program received by the participants of the present study consisted of 16 weekly outpatient sessions at our public University Hospital, lasting 90 min each session. The treatment program has already been described elsewhere [27] and it has reported short and medium-term effectiveness [28,29]. The groups were conducted by an experienced clinical psychologist and a licensed co-therapist. The goal of this intervention was to educate patients on how to implement CBT strategies to minimize gambling behavior and eventually obtain full abstinence. The topics addressed in the different sessions included: psychoeducation about GD (its course, diagnostic criteria, risk factors, etc.), cognitive restructuring focused on cognitive distortions (e.g., the illusion of control and magical thinking), stimulus control (money management, self-exclusion programs, avoidance of potential triggers, etc.), emotion-regulation skills training, response prevention, and other relapse prevention techniques.

Throughout the 16 sessions, attendance, control of spending, as well as the occurrence of relapses and dropouts were recorded weekly by the clinical psychologist. In this study, a relapse was understood as the occurrence of a full gambling episode once CBT had begun. This conceptualization is common in many studies assessing patients with GD [28,30]. Failure to attend 3 consecutive sessions was considered a dropout.

2.3. Measures

DSM-5M-5 [1]

Patients were diagnosed with pathological gambling if they met DSM-IV-TR criteria [26]. We used DSM-IV-TR criteria because the 8th criterion explores the presence of gambling-related illegal acts. Noteworthy, with the release of the DSM-5 [1], the term "pathological gambling" was replaced with "GD". All patient diagnoses were post-hoc reassessed and recodified to avoid the confounding effect of increased GD severity in patients with a criminal history. In this regard, only patients who met DSM-5 criteria for GD were included in the present study. The internal consistency in our study sample was α = 0.818.

South Oaks Gambling Screen (SOGS) [31]

The SOGS is a 20-item diagnostic questionnaire that ascertains GD severity. It discriminates between probable pathological, problem, and non-problem gamblers. Both reliability and validity of the Spanish validation of this tool are high [32], and the test–retest reliability ($R = 0.98$, $p < 0.01$) and internal consistency (Cronbach's $\alpha = 0.94$) are excellent. In our study sample, this questionnaire achieved adequate internal consistency ($\alpha = 0.734$).

Symptom Checklist-Revised (SCL-90-R) [33]

This questionnaire assesses a broad range of psychological problems and psychopathological symptoms. It contains 90 items measuring nine primary symptom dimensions and it also yields a global score (Global Severity Index (GSI)), which is a widely used index of psychopathological distress. The Spanish validation obtained good psychometrical properties, with a mean internal consistency of 0.75 (Cronbach's alpha) [34]. The internal consistency estimated in the study sample for the global scale was excellent ($\alpha = 0.98$: $\alpha = 0.891$ for somatization, $\alpha = 0.896$ for obsession-compulsion, $\alpha = 0.877$ for interpersonal sensitivity, $\alpha = 0.917$ for depression, $\alpha = 0.895$ for anxiety, $\alpha = 0.873$ for hostility, $\alpha = 0.832$ for phobic anxiety, $\alpha = 0.798$ for paranoid ideation, and $\alpha = 0.855$ for psychoticism).

Impulsive Behavior Scale (UPPS-P) [35]

This questionnaire assesses 5 dimensions of impulsive behavior through self-report on 59 items: lack of premeditation, lack of perseverance, sensation-seeking, negative urgency, and positive urgency. The Spanish adaptation showed good reliability (Cronbach's α between 0.79 and 0.93) and external validity [36]. In our sample, internal consistency was $\alpha = 0.923$: $\alpha = 0.854$ for negative urgency, $\alpha = 0.917$ for positive urgency, $\alpha = 0.818$ for lack of premeditation, $\alpha = 0.754$ for lack of perseverance, and $\alpha = 0.866$ for sensation-seeking.

Temperament and Character Inventory-Revised (TCI-R) [37]

It is a 240-item self-reported questionnaire that measures seven personality dimensions: four temperament (novelty seeking, harm avoidance, reward dependence, and persistence) and three character dimensions (self-directedness, cooperativeness, and self-transcendence). We used the Spanish version which showed adequate internal consistency (Cronbach's alpha α mean value of 0.87) [38]. In the present study, internal consistency was between adequate ($\alpha = 0.701$ for reward dependence, $\alpha = 0.726$ for novelty-seeking, $\alpha = 0.745$ for harm avoidance, and $\alpha = 0.772$ for cooperativeness) to good ($\alpha = 0.819$ for self-transcendence, $\alpha = 0.846$ for self-directedness, and $\alpha = 0.862$ for persistence).

Other sociodemographic and clinical variables

Additional sociodemographic and clinical variables related to gambling, as well as substance use, and psychiatric comorbidities were assessed by means of a semi-structured face-to-face clinical interview described elsewhere [27]. Socioeconomic status was obtained using the Hollingshead Factor Index, based on the educational attainment and occupational prestige domains [39]. Gambling-related crimes were explored through a face-to-face interview designed for this study by two forensic experts in the field.

2.4. Statistical Analysis

Stata17 for Windows was used for statistical analysis [40]. Analysis of variance (ANOVA) was used for the comparison of quantitative variables between the groups, and chi-square tests (χ^2) for the comparison of categorical variables. For these comparisons, the effect sizes were estimated with the standardized Cohen's-d for mean differences and Cramer's-phi (φ) for proportion differences. In addition, Finner's correction was used to control the potential increase in the Type-I error due to the use of multiple null-hypothesis tests (Finner-method is an alternative procedure to the classic Bonferroni-method) [41].

Kaplan-Meier product-limit estimator was used to obtain the cumulate survival curve for the rate to dropout and relapse, and Long Rank (Mantel-Cox procedure) compared the resulting functions between the groups [42].

2.5. Ethics

The present study was carried out in accordance with the latest version of the Declaration of Helsinki. The Research Ethics Committee of Bellvitge University Hospital approved the study, and signed informed consent was obtained from all participants.

3. Results

3.1. Description of the Sample

Most participants in the study were men (93.0%), with primary (51.5%) or secondary (45.0%) education levels, single (48.0%) or married (37.4%), employed (60.2%), and pertained to mean-low or low socioeconomic levels (91.8%). No statistical differences between groups were found for the sociodemographic variables (see Table 1).

Table 1. Comparison between the groups for sociodemographic variables.

		Total (n = 171)		Illegal− (n = 85)		Illegal + Cons− (n = 55)		Illegal + Cons+ (n = 31)		p
		n	%	n	%	n	%	n	%	
Gender	Women	12	7.0%	7	8.2%	4	7.3%	1	3.2%	0.643
	Men	159	93.0%	78	91.8%	51	92.7%	30	96.8%	
Education	Primary	88	51.5%	42	49.4%	31	56.4%	15	48.4%	0.740
	Secondary	77	45.0%	41	48.2%	22	40.0%	14	45.2%	
	University	6	3.5%	2	2.4%	2	3.6%	2	6.5%	
Civil status	Single	82	48.0%	33	38.8%	31	56.4%	18	58.1%	0.163
	Married	64	37.4%	39	45.9%	17	30.9%	8	25.8%	
	Divorced	25	14.6%	13	15.3%	7	12.7%	5	16.1%	
Social Index	Mean-high	1	0.6%	1	1.2%	0	0.0%	0	0.0%	0.965
	Mean	13	7.6%	6	7.1%	4	7.3%	3	9.7%	
	Mean-low	66	38.6%	32	37.6%	23	41.8%	11	35.5%	
	Low	91	53.2%	46	54.1%	28	50.9%	17	54.8%	
Employment	Unemployed	68	39.8%	32	37.6%	22	40.0%	14	45.2%	0.764
	Employed	103	60.2%	53	62.4%	33	60.0%	17	54.8%	
Age (years-old); mean-SD		41.38	13.40	45.86	14.00	36.31	10.90	38.10	11.82	**<0.001 ***

Note. Illegal−: without illegal behavior. Illegal + Cons−: with illegal behavior and without legal consequences. Illegal + Cons+: with illegal behavior and with legal consequences. SD: standard deviation. * Bold: significant comparison.

3.2. Comparison of the Clinical Profile between the Groups

Table 2 contains the results of the ANOVA comparing the clinical profiles. Patients who reported an absence of gambling-related illegal behavior achieved the oldest mean age, the latest age of onset of gambling-related problems, the lowest GD severity levels (DSM-5 criteria, the SOGS total, and the cumulated debts related to the gambling activity), the most functional psychopathological state (lowest means in the SCL-90-R scales), the lowest impulsivity levels, and a personality profile with the lowest novelty seeking and the highest self-directedness and cooperativeness levels. For patients who reported illegal acts, the presence of legal consequences was associated to higher mean scores in somatization, anxiety, phobic anxiety, and novelty seeking.

Table 3 includes the comparison between the groups for the presence of psychiatric comorbidities and substance use. Compared with the other conditions, the group characterized by the presence of illegal acts without legal consequences achieved higher likelihood of any comorbid mental disorder. The prevalence of other mental disorders different to depression, anxiety, and bipolar disorders was lower within the patients without illegal behaviors. The absence of illegal acts was also related to lower likelihood of substance use, specifically tobacco and illegal drugs.

Table 2. Comparison between the groups for clinical profiles.

	Illegal− (n = 85)		Illegal + Cons− (n = 55)		Illegal + Cons+ (n = 31)		Illegal + Co− vs. Illegal−		Illegal + Co+ vs. Illegal−		Illegal + Co+ vs. Illegal + Co−	
	Mean	SD	Mean	SD	Mean	SD	p	|d|	p	|d|	p	|d|
Age (years-old)	45.86	14.00	36.31	10.90	38.10	11.82	<0.001 *	0.76 †	0.004 *	0.60 †	0.531	0.16
Onset GD (years-old)	31.35	12.62	25.42	8.87	25.18	8.18	0.003 *	0.54 †	0.008 *	0.58 †	0.922	0.03
Duration GD (years)	6.05	7.32	5.87	6.09	7.74	6.64	0.883	0.03	0.238	0.24	0.224	0.29
DSM-5 criteria	6.47	2.06	7.53	1.78	7.74	1.73	0.002 *	0.55 †	0.002 *	0.67 †	0.619	0.12
SOGS-total	9.69	2.99	11.53	3.21	12.55	3.36	0.001 *	0.59 †	<0.001 *	0.90 †	0.149	0.31
Debts (euros)	5757	9943	9914	14,639	9219	14,195	0.050 *	0.33	0.049 *	0.28	0.744	0.05
SCL-90R Somatization	0.88	0.78	0.93	0.80	1.47	0.90	0.694	0.07	0.001 *	0.70 †	0.003 *	0.63 †
SCL-90R Obsessive-comp.	1.05	0.86	1.37	0.88	1.53	0.89	0.037 *	0.36	0.009 *	0.55 †	0.395	0.19
SCL-90R Sensitivity	0.93	0.89	1.13	0.80	1.49	0.83	0.176	0.24	0.002 *	0.65 †	0.060	0.45
SCL-90R Depression	1.37	0.98	1.69	0.87	2.01	0.92	0.052	0.34	0.001 *	0.68 †	0.123	0.36
SCL-90R Anxiety	0.93	0.82	1.09	0.70	1.50	0.94	0.246	0.21	0.001 *	0.65 †	0.025 *	0.50 †
SCL-90R Hostility	0.77	0.87	1.18	1.00	1.14	0.83	0.011 *	0.43	0.056	0.43	0.860	0.04
SCL-90R Phobic anxiety	0.46	0.62	0.51	0.71	0.88	0.89	0.646	0.08	0.005 *	0.55 †	0.023 *	0.45
SCL-90R Paranoia	0.78	0.80	1.12	0.82	1.33	0.88	0.020 *	0.41	0.002 *	0.65 †	0.245	0.25
SCL-90R Psychotic	0.81	0.76	1.05	0.74	1.30	0.91	0.070	0.33	0.003 *	0.59 †	0.155	0.30
SCL-90R GSI	0.96	0.74	1.19	0.68	1.51	0.78	0.073	0.32	<0.001 *	0.72 †	0.052	0.44
SCL-90R PST	42.08	23.48	50.51	20.60	57.77	18.84	0.027 *	0.38	0.001 *	0.74 †	0.140	0.37
SCL-90R PSDI	1.82	0.64	2.00	0.54	2.25	0.70	0.101	0.30	0.001 *	0.64 †	0.077	0.40
UPPS-P Premeditation	23.35	5.23	24.42	6.33	26.26	5.96	0.285	0.18	0.017 *	0.52 †	0.155	0.30
UPPS-P Perseverance	21.84	4.93	23.13	5.30	23.97	4.19	0.132	0.25	0.041 *	0.47	0.449	0.18
UPPS-P Sensation	25.79	7.64	29.93	8.36	29.94	7.73	0.003 *	0.52 †	0.013 *	0.54 †	0.996	0.00
UPPS-P Positive urgency	28.96	7.79	32.60	10.67	34.39	9.69	0.023 *	0.39	0.005 *	0.62 †	0.386	0.18
UPPS-P Negative urgency	30.06	6.55	32.76	8.00	34.97	5.61	0.025 *	0.37	0.001 *	0.81 †	0.157	0.32
UPPS-P Total	129.4	21.40	142.8	24.15	149.6	21.03	0.001 *	0.59 †	<0.001 *	0.96 †	0.175	0.30
TCI-R Novelty seeking	106.1	11.96	110.5	13.41	118.0	14.19	0.052	0.34	<0.001 *	0.91 †	0.009 *	0.55 †
TCI-R Harm avoidance	101.7	18.91	100.0	17.36	104.3	13.20	0.577	0.09	0.487	0.16	0.281	0.28
TCI-R Reward dependence	99.1	13.47	96.1	14.76	95.0	10.46	0.196	0.21	0.150	0.34	0.727	0.08
TCI-R Persistence	103.7	19.38	106.1	17.27	111.0	16.83	0.463	0.13	0.061	0.40	0.233	0.29
TCI-R Self-directedness	134.2	20.26	123.9	22.10	116.4	20.34	0.005 *	0.52 †	<0.0001 *	0.88 †	0.109	0.36
TCI-R Cooperativeness	132.4	16.46	129.7	16.68	124.1	14.83	0.335	0.16	0.017 *	0.53 †	0.132	0.35
TCI-R Self-transcendence	60.2	13.69	63.4	13.88	66.3	13.27	0.185	0.23	0.037 *	0.45	0.348	0.21

Note. Illegal−: without illegal behavior. Illegal + Cons−: with illegal behavior and without legal consequences. Illegal + Cons+: with illegal behavior and with legal consequences. SD: standard deviation. GD: gambling disorder. SOGS: South Oaks Gambling Screen. SCL-90-R: Symptom Checklist-Revised. UPPS-P: Urgency, Premeditation, Perseverance, Sensation Seeking, Positive Urgency. TCI-R: Temperament and Character Inventory-Revised. * Bold: significant comparison. † Effect size within the range mild-moderate to high-large (|d| > 0.50).

Table 3. Comparison between the groups for comorbid mental disorders and substances.

	Illegal− (n = 85)		Illegal + Cons− (n = 55)		Illegal + Cons+ (n = 31)		Illegal + Co− vs. Illegal−		Illegal + Co+ vs. Illegal−		Illegal + Co+ vs. Illegal + Co−	
	n	%	n	%	n	%	p	|φ|	p	|φ|	p	|φ|
Any mental disorder	16	18.8%	18	32.7%	6	19.4%	0.061	0.158 †	0.948	0.006	0.184	0.143 †
Depression	5	5.9%	4	7.3%	1	3.2%	0.743	0.028	0.568	0.053	0.441	0.083
Anxiety	4	4.7%	4	7.3%	1	3.2%	0.553	−0.050	0.289	0.098	0.450	0.081
Bipolar	3	3.5%	1	1.8%	0	0.0%	0.523	0.054	0.728	0.032	0.441	0.083
Other	3	3.5%	9	16.4%	3	9.7%	0.008 *	0.224 †	0.186	0.123 †	0.390	0.093
Any substance	46	54.1%	38	69.1%	19	61.3%	0.077	0.149 †	0.491	0.064	0.463	0.079
Tobacco	41	48.2%	35	63.6%	16	51.6%	0.074	0.151 †	0.747	0.030	0.276	0.118 †
Alcohol	11	12.9%	6	10.9%	5	16.1%	0.719	0.030	0.659	0.041	0.486	0.075
Illegal drugs	1	1.2%	8	14.5%	5	16.1%	0.002 *	0.266 †	0.001 *	0.299 †	0.844	0.021

Note. Illegal−: without illegal behavior. Illegal + Cons−: with illegal behavior and without legal consequences. Illegal + Cons+: with illegal behavior and with legal consequences. |φ|: Phi-statistic. * Bold: significant comparison. † Effect size within the range mild-moderate to high-large (|φ| > 0.10).

3.3. Comparison of the Therapy Outcomes between the Groups

Table 4 shows the risk of dropout and relapses and the comparison between the groups. For both outcomes, the highest likelihood was associated to the presence of illegal behavior with legal consequences (64.5% of dropout and 32.3% of relapses). Regarding the cumulative survival functions, the patients who reported both illegal behaviors with legal consequences also achieved the highest rate of dropout and relapse during the treatment (Figure 1).

Table 4. Comparison between the groups for CBT outcomes.

		Illegal− (n = 85)		Illegal + Cons− (n = 55)		Illegal + Cons+ (n = 31)		Illegal + Co− vs. Illegal−		Illegal + Co+ vs. Illegal−		Illegal + Co+ vs. Illegal + Co−	
		n	%	n	%	n	%	p	|φ|	p	|φ|	p	|φ|
Dropout	Present	43	50.6%	23	41.8%	20	64.5%	0.310	0.086	0.183	0.124 †	**0.043 ***	0.218 †
	Absent	42	49.4%	32	58.2%	11	35.5%						
Relapses	Present	19	22.4%	17	30.9%	10	32.3%	0.258	0.096	0.276	0.101 †	0.897	0.014
	Absent	66	77.6%	38	69.1%	21	67.7%						

Note. Illegal−: without illegal behavior. Illegal + Cons−: with illegal behavior and without legal consequences. Illegal + Cons+: with illegal behavior and with legal consequences. CBT: cognitive-behavioral treatment. |φ|: Phi-statistic. * Bold: significant comparison. † Effect size within the range mild-moderate to high-large (|φ| > 0.10).

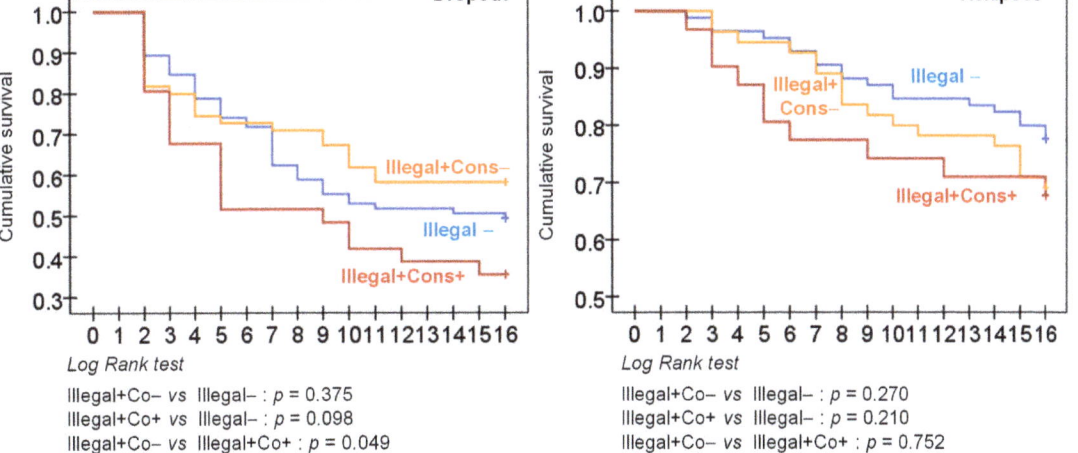

Figure 1. Survival functions for the rate of dropout and relapses. Note. Illegal−: without illegal behavior. Illegal + Cons−: with illegal behavior and without legal consequences. Illegal + Cons+: with illegal behavior and with legal consequences.

4. Discussion

The present study aimed to explore sociodemographic and clinical differences between individuals with GD who had committed gambling-related illegal acts (differentiating into those who had had legal consequences and those who had not), and patients with GD who had not committed crimes. Moreover, we aimed to compare the treatment outcome of these three groups, considering dropouts and relapses.

Regarding sociodemographic factors, the proportion of patients included in the present study was mostly male. This clinical reality supports previous studies, which have highlighted a male-female ratio of individuals with GD of 2.8:1.0 [43]. GD remains, therefore, a disorder more prevalent in men, although it is progressively increasing in women [44,45].

In addition, no differences were found between groups in terms of years of schooling, given that most patients had primary or secondary levels of education and a low or medium-low socioeconomic level. These findings are consistent with previous studies, which also found no differences between patients who had committed illegal acts and those who had not [16,20]. However, they are inconsistent with other research that has highlighted an inverse relationship between education and the risk of committing crimes [46], as well as between social stratification and delinquency [47].

Patients who had committed illegal acts (with or without legal consequences) were younger than those who had not. These findings support the age-of-crime curve, which proposes a bell-shaped pattern in the association between age and crime [48,49]. In adolescence and young adulthood, there would therefore be a greater probability of committing crimes that would subsequently decrease with age. Age was the only sociodemographic factor in which significant differences were found between groups, as occurred in previous studies [24].

Regarding clinical features, patients who had not committed gambling-related illegal acts showed lower GD severity than those who had (with or without legal consequences). Previous studies also reported higher levels of GD severity in those patients who had committed gambling-related crimes [19,25,50,51]. These findings would lend support to the fact that illegal acts are a clear indicator of GD severity, rather than a diagnostic criterion per se [11,12], and that it is unlikely that an individual would commit illegal acts in the absence of other diagnostic criteria for GD [52]. It should be noted, however, that contrary to our hypotheses, no differences in GD severity were observed between the group that had committed illegal acts with legal consequences and the group that had committed them without legal consequences. We had hypothesized a different clinical profile between both groups estimating that those crimes with legal consequences might be more severe than those without legal repercussions. However, it is possible that not having legal consequences does not imply less severity of the crime, but simply that the crime was not detected.

Those patients who had committed gambling-related illegal acts also reported greater levels of impulsivity compared to those who had not. However, no significant differences in impulsivity were detected between individuals who had committed gambling-related illegal acts with or without legal consequences. In this line, previous studies suggested that among the different dimensions of impulsivity contemplated by the UPPS-P model, positive urgency (understood as acting rashly when facing intense positive emotions) and lack of premeditation (defined as the tendency to act without taking into account the possible consequences of the behavior) were predictors of the presence of illegal acts in individuals with GD, and could therefore be considered a risk factor [16].

Furthermore, individuals who had committed illegal acts (and more specifically the group without legal consequences) showed a higher probability of presenting psychiatric comorbidity. These findings are consistent with previous studies, which suggested that comorbid mental disorders may be relevant mediating factors in the association between gambling behavior and crime [22,23]. Moreover, the absence of gambling-related illegal acts was also associated with a lower likelihood of substance use, specifically tobacco and illegal drugs. Previous studies in this line have suggested that the co-occurrence of GD and substance use may enhance a disinhibition effect in the individual, and this may increase the likelihood of committing illegal acts related to gambling [15]. The patients who had not committed gambling-related crimes showed a more adaptive personality profile, with lower novelty seeking and higher self-directedness and cooperativeness levels, compared to those who had committed crimes. These results coincide with previous studies [16], suggesting that especially self-directedness, characterized by greater self-control and skills for achieving goals [37], could to some extent be preventing the commission of illegal acts. In addition, these patients showed lower levels of psychopathology compared to the groups that had committed crimes, as observed in previous studies [20].

Finally, to the best of our knowledge, to date, no study has studied in depth the association between the commission of gambling-related crimes and response to treatment, specifically, dropout and relapse rates. Both dropout and relapse are considered essential to assess GD treatment outcome, along with other variables such as gambling behavior measures (e.g., monthly net expenditure and gambling frequency) and measures of GD-related problems (e.g., social, legal, and financial difficulties) [53]. In the present study, consistent with our hypothesis, the illegal acts with legal consequences group presented a higher risk of both dropout and relapse compared to the other two groups. Therefore, although no significant differences were observed in terms of sociodemographic and clinical factors regarding the presence/absence of legal consequences, it is a relevant factor to consider when analyzing treatment outcomes.

It should be noted that the groups that had committed illegal acts presented a more impaired clinical profile, with greater severity of the disorder and psychopathology, more maladaptive personality traits, and higher levels of impulsivity. All these factors could be interfering with dropout and relapse rates, as previous studies suggest [54,55]. In the specific case of gambling-related offenses, Ledgerwood et al. [24] observed that GD severity was maintained throughout CBT in the group of patients who had committed illegal acts, compared to those who had not. Therefore, the authors suggested that the profile of gamblers with associated offenses might require treatments of longer duration and intensity in order to achieve an effective reduction of GD symptomatology. Gambling-related illegal acts and their legal consequences would therefore be factors to contemplate when analyzing the treatment adherence of this type of patient, as well as when designing treatment programs focused on this specific clinical population.

Limitations and Future Studies

The present study presents several limitations. First, although an attempt was made to reduce the probability of bias by assessing the commission of gambling-related crimes using two independent clinical interviews (one with DSM criteria and the other specific to illegal acts), both focus on self-reporting, so that failure to disclose these crimes by patients may occur, as previous studies have highlighted [8]. Similarly, psychiatric comorbidity and substance use were self-reported by patients at the initial clinical interview, prior to the beginning of therapy. Therefore, it should be noted that the diagnoses reported may be biased. Second, although the present study reports the presence/absence of legal consequences (a previously unexplored factor), it does not include relevant data associated with criminal behavior, such as the typology of the crime or recidivism. Third, this study included only treatment-seeking individuals, so this may be a more problem-conscious gambler profile. Future studies could also include non-treatment seeking gamblers to contrast the clinical profiles. Fourth, the different clinical factors included (personality, psychopathology and impulsivity) have been evaluated through self-report questionnaires, with their consequent limitations. Finally, although gender is an important factor to take into account in the recovery processes [56], the present study has not explored gender differences.

5. Conclusions

Patients who reported an absence of gambling-related illegal behavior were older, and showed the lowest GD severity, the most functional psychopathological state, the lowest impulsivity levels, and a more adaptive personality profile. Patients who had committed offenses with legal consequences presented the highest risk of dropout and relapses, higher number of psychological symptoms, higher likelihood of any other mental disorders, and greater prevalence of tobacco and illegal drugs use. Our findings uphold that patients who have committed gambling-related offenses show a more complex clinical profile that may interfere with their adherence to treatment. Therefore, specific treatment plans are required for this type of patient.

Author Contributions: C.V.-A.: conceptualization, writing—original draft; G.M.-B.: conceptualization, writing—original draft; R.G.: formal analysis, methodology; E.C. (Elena Caravaca): investigation; M.G.-P.: investigation; L.M.: investigation; I.B.: investigation; A.d.P.-G.: investigation; S.V.-S.: investigation; M.L.-H.: investigation; B.M.-M.: investigation; E.V.-M.: investigation; E.G.-G.: investigation; E.C. (Ester Codina): investigation; J.M.M.: funding acquisition; F.F.-A.: writing—review and editing, funding acquisition; S.J.-M.: writing—review and editing, project administration, funding acquisition. All authors have read and agreed to the published version of the manuscript.

Funding: CERCA Programme/Generalitat de Catalunya gave institutional support. This work was additionally supported by a grant from the Ministerio de Ciencia, Innovación y Universidades (grant RTI2018-101837-B-100). The research was funded by the Delegación del Gobierno para el Plan Nacional sobre Drogas (2019I47 and 2021I031), Instituto de Salud Carlos III (ISCIII) (PI17/01167 and PI207132) and co-funded by FEDER funds/European Regional Development Fund (ERDF), a way to build Europe. CIBEROBN and CIBERSAM are both initiatives of ISCIII. CVA is supported by a predoctoral grant awarded by the Ministerio de Educación, Cultura y Deporte (FPU16/01453). GMB was supported by a postdoctoral grant by FUNCIVA. IB was partially supported by a Post-Residency Grant from Research Committee of the University Hospital of Bellvitge (HUB; Barcelona, Spain) 2020–2021. RG is supported by The Catalan Institution for Research and Advanced Studies (ICREA-2021 Academia Program). The funders had no role in the study design, data collection and analysis, decision to publish or preparation of the manuscript.

Institutional Review Board Statement: The study was conducted in accordance with the Declaration of Helsinki, and approved by the Ethics Committee of the Hospital Universitari de Bellvitge PR307/06 (8 February 2007).

Informed Consent Statement: Informed consent was obtained from all subjects involved in the study.

Data Availability Statement: The datasets analyzed during the current study are not publicly available due to patient confidentiality and other ethical reasons but are available from the corresponding author on reasonable request.

Conflicts of Interest: F.F.-A. received consultancy honoraria from Novo Nordisk and editorial honoraria as EIC from Wiley. The rest of the authors declare no conflict of interest. The funders had no role in the design of the study; in the collection, analyses, or interpretation of data; in the writing of the manuscript, or in the decision to publish the results.

References

1. APA. *Diagnostic and Statistical Manual of Mental Disorders*, 5th ed.; American Psychiatric Association: Washington, DC, USA, 2013.
2. Potenza, M.N.; Balodis, I.M.; Derevensky, J.; Grant, J.E.; Petry, N.M.; Verdejo-Garcia, A.; Yip, S.W. Gambling Disorder. *Nat. Rev. Dis. Prim.* **2019**, *5*, 51. [CrossRef] [PubMed]
3. Fauth-Bühler, M.; Mann, K.; Potenza, M.N. Pathological Gambling: A Review of the Neurobiological Evidence Relevant for Its Classification as an Addictive Disorder. *Addict. Biol.* **2017**, *22*, 885–897. [CrossRef] [PubMed]
4. Micla, R.; Cubała, W.J.; Mazurkiewicz, D.W.; Jakuszkowiak-Wojten, K. The Neurobiology of Addiction. A Vulnerability/Resilience Perspective. *Eur. J. Psychiatry* **2018**, *32*, 139–148. [CrossRef]
5. Takeuchi, H.; Tsurumi, K.; Murao, T.; Mizuta, H.; Kawada, R.; Murai, T.; Takahashi, H. Framing Effects on Financial and Health Problems in Gambling Disorder. *Addict. Behav.* **2020**, *110*, 106502. [CrossRef]
6. Miela, R.J.; Cubała, W.J.; Jakuszkowiak-Wojten, K.; Mazurkiewicz, D.W. Gambling Behaviours and Treatment Uptake among Vulnerable Populations during COVID-19 Crisis. *J. Gambl. Issues* **2021**, *48*, 233–252. [CrossRef]
7. Dennison, C.R.; Finkeldey, J.G.; Rocheleau, G.C. Confounding Bias in the Relationship Between Problem Gambling and Crime. *J Gambl. Stud.* **2021**, *37*, 427–444. [CrossRef]
8. Adolphe, A.; Khatib, L.; van Golde, C.; Gainsbury, S.M.; Blaszczynski, A. Crime and Gambling Disorders: A Systematic Review. *J. Gambl. Stud.* **2018**, *35*, 395–414. [CrossRef]
9. Laursen, B.; Plauborg, R.; Ekholm, O.; Larsen, C.V.L.; Juel, K. Problem Gambling Associated with Violent and Criminal Behaviour: A Danish Population-Based Survey and Register Study. *J. Gambl. Stud.* **2016**, *32*, 25–34. [CrossRef]
10. Folino, J.O.; Abait, P.E. Pathological Gambling and Criminality. *Curr. Opin. Psychiatry* **2009**, *22*, 477–481. [CrossRef]
11. Granero, R.; Penelo, E.; Stinchfield, R.; Fernández-Aranda, F.; Aymamí, N.; Gómez-Peña, M.; Fagundo, A.B.; Sauchelli, S.; Islam, M.A.; Menchón, J.M.; et al. Contribution of Illegal Acts to Pathological Gambling Diagnosis: DSM-5 Implications. *J. Addict. Dis.* **2014**, *33*, 41–52. [CrossRef]
12. Petry, N.M.; Blanco, C.; Stinchfield, R.; Volberg, R. An Empirical Evaluation of Proposed Changes for Gambling Diagnosis in the DSM-5. *Addiction* **2013**, *108*, 575–581. [CrossRef] [PubMed]
13. Turner, N.E.; Stinchfield, R.; McCready, J.; McAvoy, S.; Ferentzy, P. Endorsement of Criminal Behavior Amongst Offenders: Implications for DSM-5 Gambling Disorder. *J. Gambl. Stud.* **2016**, *32*, 35–45. [CrossRef] [PubMed]
14. Mestre-Bach, G.; Granero, R.; Vintró-Alcaraz, C.; Juvé-Segura, G.; Marimon-Escudero, M.; Rivas-Pérez, S.; Valenciano-Mendoza, E.; Mora-Maltas, B.; del Pino-Gutierrez, A.; Gómez-Peña, M.; et al. Youth and Gambling Disorder: What about Criminal Behavior? *Addict. Behav.* **2021**, *113*, 106684. [CrossRef] [PubMed]
15. Gorsane, M.A.; Reynaud, M.; Vénisse, J.L.; Legauffre, C.; Valleur, M.; Magalon, D.; Fatséas, M.; Chéreau-Boudet, I.; Guilleux, A.; Challet-Bouju, G.; et al. Gambling Disorder-Related Illegal Acts: Regression Model of Associated Factors. *J. Behav. Addict.* **2017**, *6*, 64–73. [CrossRef]
16. Mestre-Bach, G.; Steward, T.; Granero, R.; Fernández-Aranda, F.; Talón-Navarro, M.T.; Cuquerella, À.; Baño, M.; Moragas, L.; del Pino-Gutiérrez, A.; Aymamí, N.; et al. Gambling and Impulsivity Traits: A Recipe for Criminal Behavior? *Front. Psychiatry* **2018**, *9*, 6. [CrossRef]
17. April, L.M.; Weinstock, J. The Relationship Between Gambling Severity and Risk of Criminal Recidivism. *J. Forensic Sci.* **2018**, *63*, 1201–1206. [CrossRef]
18. Ellis, J.D.; Lister, J.J.; Struble, C.A.; Cairncross, M.; Carr, M.M.; Ledgerwood, D.M. Client and Clinician-Rated Characteristics of Problem Gamblers with and without History of Gambling-Related Illegal Behaviors. *Addict. Behav.* **2018**, *84*, 1–6. [CrossRef]

19. Potenza, M.N.; Steinberg, M.A.; McLaughlin, S.D.; Wu, R.; Rounsaville, B.J.; O'Malley, S.S. Illegal Behaviors in Problem Gambling: Analysis of Data from a Gambling Helpline. *J. Am. Acad. Psychiatry Law* **2000**, *28*, 389–403.
20. Mestre-Bach, G.; Steward, T.; Granero, R.; Fernández-Aranda, F.; Talón-Navarro, M.T.; Cuquerella, À.; del Pino-Gutiérrez, A.; Aymamí, N.; Gómez-Peña, M.; Mallorquí-Bagué, N.; et al. Sociodemographic and Psychopathological Predictors of Criminal Behavior in Women with Gambling Disorder. *Addict. Behav.* **2018**, *80*, 124–129. [CrossRef]
21. Jiménez-Murcia, S.; Granero, R.; Fernandez-Aranda, F.; Sauvaget, A.; Fransson, A.; Hakansson, A.; Mestre-Bach, G.; Steward, T.; Stinchfield, R.; Moragas, L.; et al. A Comparison of DSM-IV-TR and DSM-5 Diagnostic Criteria for Gambling Disorder in a Large Clinical Sample. *Front. Psychol.* **2019**, *10*, 931. [CrossRef]
22. Preston, D.L.; McAvoy, S.; Saunders, C.; Gillam, L.; Saied, A.; Turner, N.E. Problem Gambling and Mental Health Comorbidity in Canadian Federal Ofenders. *Crim. Justice Behav.* **2012**, *39*, 1373–1388. [CrossRef]
23. Meyer, G.; Stadler, M.A. Criminal Behavior Associated with Pathological Gambling. *J. Gambl. Stud.* **1999**, *15*, 29–43. [CrossRef] [PubMed]
24. Ledgerwood, D.M.; Weinstock, J.; Morasco, B.J.; Petry, N.M. Clinical Features and Treatment Prognosis of Pathological Gamblers with and without Recent Gambling-Related Illegal Behavior. *J. Am. Acad. Psychiatry Law* **2007**, *35*, 294–301. [PubMed]
25. Vintró-Alcaraz, C.; Mestre-Bach, G.; Granero, R.; Cuquerella, À.; Talón-Navarro, M.T.; Valenciano-Mendoza, E.; Mora-Maltas, B.; del Pino-Gutiérrez, A.; Gómez-Peña, M.; Moragas, L.; et al. Identifying Associated Factors for Illegal Acts among Patients with Gambling Disorder and ADHD. *J. Gambl. Stud.* **2021**, *2021*, 1–15. [CrossRef] [PubMed]
26. Apa. *Diagnostic and Statistical Manual of Mental Disorders, Text Revision (DSM-IV-TR)*, 4th ed.; American Psychiatric Association: Washington, DC, USA, 2000; Volume 1, ISBN 0-89042-334-2.
27. Jiménez-Murcia, S.; Aymamí-Sanromà, M.N.; Gómez-Peña, M.; Álvarez-Moya, E.M.; Vallejo, J. *Protocols de Tractament Cognitivo-conductual Pel Joc Patològic i d'altres Addiccions No Tòxiques. [Cognitive-Behavioral Treatment Protocols for Pathological Gambling and Other Nonsubstance Addictions]*; Hospital Universitari de Bellvitge: Barcelona, Spain, 2006.
28. Jiménez-Murcia, S.; Tremblay, J.; Stinchfield, R.; Granero, R.; Fernández-Aranda, F.; Mestre-Bach, G.; Steward, T.; del Pino-Gutiérrez, A.; Baño, M.; Moragas, L.; et al. The Involvement of a Concerned Significant Other in Gambling Disorder Treatment Outcome. *J. Gambl. Stud.* **2016**, *33*, 937–953. [CrossRef]
29. Mestre-Bach, G.; Steward, T.; Granero, R.; Fernández-Aranda, F.; del Pino-Gutiérrez, A.; Mallorquí-Bagué, N.; Mena-Moreno, T.; Vintró-Alcaraz, C.; Moragas, L.; Aymamí, N.; et al. The Predictive Capacity of DSM-5 Symptom Severity and Impulsivity on Response to Cognitive-Behavioral Therapy for Gambling Disorder: A 2-Year Longitudinal Study. *Eur. Psychiatry* **2019**, *55*, 67–73. [CrossRef]
30. Müller, K.W.; Wölfling, K.; Dickenhorst, U.; Beutel, M.E.; Medenwaldt, J.; Koch, A. Recovery, Relapse, or Else? Treatment Outcomes in Gambling Disorder from a Multicenter Follow-up Study. *Eur. Psychiatry* **2017**, *43*, 28–34. [CrossRef]
31. Lesieur, H.R.; Blume, S.B. The South Oaks Gambling Screen (SOGS): A New Instrument for the Identification of Pathological Gamblers. *Am. J. Psychiatry* **1987**, *144*, 1184–1188. [CrossRef]
32. Echeburúa, E.; Báez, C.; Fernández, J.; Páez, D. Cuestionario de Juego Patológico de South Oaks (SOGS): Validación Española. *Análisis y Modif. Conduct.* **1994**, *74*, 769–791.
33. Derogatis, L.R. *SCL-90-R: Symptom Checklist-90-R. Administration, Scoring and Procedures Manuall—II for the Revised Version*; Clinical Psychometric Research: Towson, MD, USA, 1994.
34. Derogatis, L.R. *SCL-90-R: Cuestionario de 90 Síntomas-Manual*; TEA Editorial: Madrid, Spain, 2002.
35. Whiteside, S.P.; Lynam, D.R.; Miller, J.D.; Reynolds, S.K. Validation of the UPPS Impulsive Behavior Scale: A Four Factor Model of Impulsivity. *ProQuest Diss. Theses* **2001**, *574*, 90. [CrossRef]
36. Verdejo-García, A.; Lozano, Ó.; Moya, M.; Alcázar, M.Á.; Pérez-García, M. Psychometric Properties of a Spanish Version of the UPPS–P Impulsive Behavior Scale: Reliability, Validity and Association With Trait and Cognitive Impulsivity. *J. Pers. Assess.* **2010**, *92*, 70–77. [CrossRef] [PubMed]
37. Cloninger, C. *The Temperament and Character Inventory-Revised*; Washington University: St Louis, MS, USA, 1999.
38. Gutiérrez-Zotes, J.A.; Bayón, C.; Montserrat, C.; Valero, J.; Labad, A.; Cloninger, C.R. Temperament and Character Inventory-Revised (TCI-R). Standardization and Normative Data in a General Population Sample. *Actas Españolas Psiquiatr.* **2004**, *32*, 8–15.
39. Hollingshead, A.B. Four Factor Index of Social Status. *Yale Journal of Sociology.* **2011**, *8*, 21–51.
40. Stata-Corp. *Stata Statistical Software: Release 17*; Stata Press Publication, StataCorp LLC.: College Station, TX, USA, 2021.
41. Finner, H.; Roters, M. On the False Discovery Rate and Expected Type I Errors. *Biometrical J.* **2001**, *43*, 985–1005. [CrossRef]
42. Singer, J.B.; Willett, J.B. *Applied Longitudinal Data Analysis: Modeling Change and Event Occurrence*; Oxford University Press: New York, NY, USA, 2003.
43. Blanco, C.; Hasin, D.S.; Petry, N.; Stinson, F.S.; Grant, B.F. Sex Differences in Subclinical and DSM-IV Pathological Gambling: Results from the National Epidemiologic Survey on Alcohol and Related Conditions. *Psychol. Med.* **2006**, *36*, 943–953. [CrossRef] [PubMed]
44. McCarthy, S.; Thomas, S.L.; Bellringer, M.E.; Cassidy, R. Women and Gambling-Related Harm: A Narrative Literature Review and Implications for Research, Policy, and Practice 11 Medical and Health Sciences 1117 Public Health and Health Services 16 Studies in Human Society 1605 Policy and Administration. *Harm Reduct. J.* **2019**, *16*, 1–11. [CrossRef]

45. Hare, S. *Study of Gambling and Health in Victoria: Findings from the Victorian Prevalence Study 2014*; Victorian Responsible Gambling Foundation: Victoria, Australia, 2015.
46. Swisher, R.R.; Dennison, C.R. Educational Pathways and Change in Crime Between Adolescence and Early Adulthood. *J. Res. Crime Delinq.* **2016**, *53*, 840–871. [CrossRef]
47. Hernández de Frutos, T. Social Stratification and Delinquency. Forty Years of Sociological Discrepancy. *Rev. Int. Sociol.* **2006**, *45*, 199–232. [CrossRef]
48. Farrington, D. Age and Crime. In *Crime Justice*; University of Chicago Press: Chicago, IL, USA, 1986.
49. Piquero, A.; Farrington, D.; Blumstein, A. *Key Issues in Criminal Career Research: New Analyses of the Cambridge Study in Delinquent Development*; Cambridge University Press: New York, NY, USA, 2007.
50. Kuoppamäki, S.M.; Kääriäinen, J.; Lind, K. Examining Gambling-Related Crime Reports in the National Finnish Police Register. *J. Gambl. Stud.* **2013**, *30*, 967–983. [CrossRef]
51. Turner, N.E.; Preston, D.L.; Saunders, C.; McAvoy, S.; Jain, U. The Relationship of Problem Gambling to Criminal Behavior in a Sample of Canadian Male Federal Offenders. *J. Gambl. Stud.* **2009**, *25*, 153–169. [CrossRef]
52. Stinchfield, R. Reliability, Validity, and Classification Accuracy of the South Oaks Gambling Screen (SOGS). *Am. J. Psychiatry* **2003**, *27*, 1–19. [CrossRef]
53. Walker, M.; Toneatto, T.; Potenza, M.N.; Petry, N.; Ladouceur, R.; Hodgins, D.C.; El-Guebaly, N.; Echeburua, E.; Blaszczynski, A. A Framework for Reporting Outcomes in Problem Gambling Treatment Research: The Banff, Alberta Consensus. *Addiction* **2006**, *101*, 504–511. [CrossRef] [PubMed]
54. Maniaci, G.; La Cascia, C.; Picone, F.; Lipari, A.; Cannizzaro, C.; La Barbera, D. Predictors of Early Dropout in Treatment for Gambling Disorder: The Role of Personality Disorders and Clinical Syndromes. *Psychiatry Res.* **2017**, *257*, 540–545. [CrossRef]
55. Ronzitti, S.; Soldini, E.; Smith, N.; Clerici, M.; Bowden-Jones, H. Gambling Disorder: Exploring Pre-Treatment and In-Treatment Dropout Predictors. A UK Study. *J. Gambl. Stud.* **2017**, *33*, 1277–1292. [CrossRef] [PubMed]
56. Neale, J.; Nettleton, S.; Pickering, L. Gender Sameness and Difference in Recovery from Heroin Dependence: A Qualitative Exploration. *Int. J. Drug Policy* **2014**, *25*, 3–12. [CrossRef] [PubMed]

MDPI
St. Alban-Anlage 66
4052 Basel
Switzerland
Tel. +41 61 683 77 34
Fax +41 61 302 89 18
www.mdpi.com

Journal of Clinical Medicine Editorial Office
E-mail: jcm@mdpi.com
www.mdpi.com/journal/jcm

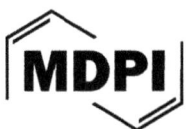

www.ingramcontent.com/pod-product-compliance
Lightning Source LLC
LaVergne TN
LVHW070625100526
838202LV00012B/726